Basic
Medical Sciences
for MRCP Part 1

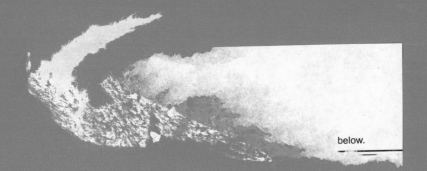

below.

Commissioning Editor: Ellen Green
Project Development Manager: Janice Urquhart
Project Manager: Nancy Arnott
Designer: Erik Bigland
Illustration Manager: Bruce Hogarth
Illustrator: David Gardner

Basic
Medical Sciences
for MRCP Part 1

Philippa J. Easterbrook MB BChir BSc(Hons) MRCP DTM&H MPH

Head of Department, Professor of HIV Medicine and Consultant
Physician in Infectious Diseases, Guy's, King's and St Thomas' School
of Medicine, King's College Hospital, London;
Formerly Senior Lecturer in Infectious Diseases, Imperial College School
of Medicine, Chelsea and Westminster Hospital, London

THIRD EDITION

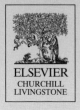

ELSEVIER
CHURCHILL
LIVINGSTONE

EDINBURGH LONDON NEW YORK OXFORD PHILADELPHIA ST LOUIS
SYDNEY TORONTO 2005

First published 1994
Second edition 1999
Third edition 2005

ISBN 0 443 07326 0
International edition ISBN 0 443 07327 9

British Library Cataloguing in Publication Data
A catalogue record for this book is available from the British Library

Library of Congress Cataloging in Publication Data
A catalog record for this book is available from the Library of Congress

Note
Medical knowledge is constantly changing. Standard safety precautions must be followed, but as new research and clinical experience broaden our knowledge, changes in treatment and drug therapy may become necessary or appropriate. Readers are advised to check the most current product information provided by the manufacturer of each drug to be administered to verify the recommended dose, the method and duration of administration, and contraindications. It is the responsibility of the practitioner, relying on experience and knowledge of the patient, to determine dosages and the best treatment for each individual patient. Neither the Publisher nor the author assumes any liability for any injury and/or damage to persons or property arising from this publication.

The Publisher

Working together to grow
libraries in developing countries

www.elsevier.com | www.bookaid.org | www.sabre.org

ELSEVIER   BOOK AID International   Sabre Foundation

your source for books,
journals and multimedia
in the health sciences
www.elsevierhealth.com

The
publisher's
policy is to use
paper manufactured
from sustainable forests

Printed in China

Preface

Both MRCP (UK) parts 1 and 2 examinations require a sound knowledge and understanding of the basic sciences. This concise but comprehensive revision guide summarizes the core basic sciences relevant to the MRCP examination in eight chapters: Genetics and molecular medicine, Microbiology, Immunology, Anatomy, Physiology, Biochemistry, Cell biology and clinical chemistry, Statistics and epidemiology, and Clinical pharmacology. It is intended primarily for MRCP part 1 and 2 candidates, although those studying for other postgraduate examinations, such as the US Medical Licensing Examination (MLE) and PLAB, may also find it useful. Information is presented in the form of lists, tables, flow diagrams and simple illustrations, and each chapter is prefaced by a summary of the key topics covered to provide a useful framework for revision of the important concepts and facts. No book of this length covering such a wide area could hope to be comprehensive, and I have therefore concentrated on recurring examination themes, topical issues, and recent developments reported in the scientific and medical literature. When a particular topic is unfamiliar or a point needs further clarification, one of the many excellent basic science textbooks should be consulted. A number of practice Best of Five MCQs in the basic sciences for MRCP are also available.

In this third edition, all chapters have been extensively updated with new material to reflect recent developments, particularly in molecular medicine, immunology and microbiology. We have also improved the layout. Topics of particular relevance are highlighted in shaded boxes; and a second colour has been used to enhance the clarity of tables and figures.

Acknowledgements
I am grateful to many former colleagues in Oxford, Baltimore and London who provided valuable criticism on earlier editions. Thanks also to the team at Elsevier in Edinburgh for their project management and to David Gardner for his skilled art work.

I would appreciate any corrections, clarifications or suggestions for future editions.

London   PJE

The MRCP (UK) Part 1 Examination
The purpose of the MRCP Part 1 exam is to test the candidates' broad knowledge and understanding of basic clinical science; their awareness of important new advances in disease mechanisms; and their ability to apply their knowledge and problem-solving skills to clinical situations.

The MRCP Part 1 exam consists of two papers, each lasting three hours. Each paper comprises 100 MCQs in a 'Best of Five' format, where a candidate must choose one best answer from five possible answers. Each MCQ has a question stem, which may contain clinical information, followed by five branches. Candidates are required to select the one branch that represents the best answer to the question. There is no negative marking, and one mark is awarded for each correct answer. No marks are given for an incorrect answer, or for answers in excess of the one required. Normal ranges for all laboratory measurements are quoted in the exam paper.

The general composition of the paper by topic and speciality is as follows:

Basic and clinical science questions comprise at least 25% of the paper with **25 questions**

Cell, molecular and membrane biology	2
Clinical anatomy	3
Clinical biochemistry and metabolism	4
Clinical physiology	4
Genetics	3
Immunology	4
Statistics, epidemiology and evidence-based medicine	5

Clinical pharmacology, therapeutics and toxicology account for **15 questions**

Clinical specialities account for **60 questions**, but many of these questions also test knowledge of underlying scientific principles.

Cardiology	15
Gastroenterology and hepatology	15
Clinical haematology and oncology	15
Infectious and sexually transmitted diseases	15
Endocrinology	15
Nephrology	8
Neurology	15
Respiratory medicine	15
Rheumatology	15
Psychiatry	15
Dermatology	8
Ophthalmology	4

Questions in each speciality are randomized across both papers. Further details on the exam are available from www.mrcpuk.org/mrcppt.

Contents

1 GENETICS AND MOLECULAR MEDICINE   1

2 MICROBIOLOGY   39

3 IMMUNOLOGY   87

4 ANATOMY   133

5 PHYSIOLOGY   179

6 BIOCHEMISTRY, CELL BIOLOGY AND CLINICAL CHEMISTRY   239

7 STATISTICS AND EPIDEMIOLOGY   305

8 CLINICAL PHARMACOLOGY   337

INDEX   415

1

GENETICS AND MOLECULAR MEDICINE

GLOSSARY 2

NUCLEIC ACIDS 6
Nucleic acid structure 6
  DNA 7
  RNA 7
Protein synthesis 8
  Genetic code 9
  Control of protein synthesis 10
  Cell cycle 11

RECOMBINANT DNA TECHNOLOGY
  11
  Applications 11
Basic techniques of gene analysis 11
  DNA probe hybridization 11
  Gene mapping 12
  Gene cloning 13
  Gene sequencing 14
  Polymerase chain reaction 16
Gene therapy 18

CHROMOSOMAL ABNORMALITIES 18
Autosomal disorders 19
  Trisomies 19
  Deletions 20
  Philadelphia chromosome 20
Sex chromosome disorders 20

SINGLE-GENE ABNORMALITIES 22
Autosomal dominant inheritance 22
Autosomal recessive inheritance 23

Sex-linked dominant inheritance 24
Sex-linked recessive inheritance 25
Mitochondrial genetic disorders 26
Dynamic/unstable mutations: triplet or
    trinucleotide repeat diseases 27
Molecular basis of single-gene disorders
  27

**PRENATAL AND POSTNATAL
    DIAGNOSIS** 28
Prenatal: indications 28
Postnatal diagnosis 29

**MULTIFACTORIAL OR POLYGENIC
    INHERITANCE** 29
Population genetics 31

ONCOGENESIS 32
  Regulation of gene expression 32
  The somatic evolution of cancer 32
  Oncogenes 33
  Tumour suppressor genes and inherited
    family cancer syndromes 34
  Mismatch repair genes 35
  Apoptosis 35

IMMUNOGENETICS 36
The major histocompatibility complex
  36
  Classification of diseases associated
    with HLA 37

GENETICS AND MOLECULAR MEDICINE

GLOSSARY

Alleles	Alternative forms of a gene found at the same locus on a particular chromosome.
Amplification	(i) Treatment designed to increase the proportion of plasmid DNA relative to that of bacterial DNA. (ii) Replication of a gene library in bulk. (See polymerase chain reaction, p. 16.)
Aneuploidy	A chromosome profile with fewer or greater than the normal diploid number: e.g. 45 (Turner's syndrome) or 47 (Down's syndrome) chromosomes.
Antisense technology	Use of synthetic nucleotide sequences, complementary to specific DNA or RNA sequences, to block expression of a gene.
Autosome	Any chromosome other than the sex chromosomes: i.e. 22 pairs in humans.
Barr body	All X chromosomes in excess of one per cell are inactivated so that only one is active (Lyon hypothesis), which is visible in interphase as a dark-staining Barr body: i.e. no Barr body in male or XO female.
cDNA	A single-stranded DNA complementary to an RNA, synthesized from it by the enzyme reverse transcriptase in vitro; often used as a probe in chromosome mapping.
Chimera	An individual composed of two populations of cells from different genotypes: e.g. blood group chimerism.
Chromatids	Equal halves of a chromosome following replication.
Chromosome mapping	The assigning of a gene or other DNA sequence to a particular position on a specific chromosome.
Clone	A cell line derived by mitosis from a single diploid cell.
Cloning	The isolation of a particular gene or DNA sequence. In recombinant technology, genes or DNA sequences are cloned by inserting them into a bacterium or other microorganism, which is then selected and propagated.
Concordant twins	Members of a pair of twins exhibiting the same trait. (See also Discordant twins.)
Conserved sequence	A DNA sequence that has remained virtually unchanged throughout evolution. This is usually taken to imply that the sequence has an important function.
Deletion	A chromosomal aberration in which part of the chromosome is lost.
Diploid	The chromosome number of a somatic cell: i.e. 46 in humans.
Discordant twins	Only one twin has the trait. (See also Concordant twins.)
Dizygotic twins	Twins produced by two separately fertilized ova: i.e. no more genetically similar than brothers and sisters. (See also monozygotic twins.)

DNA fingerprinting	A pattern of DNA sequences, e.g. tandem repeat sequences, unique to an individual. This DNA profile can be detected in cells (e.g. blood or semen) and can be used in criminal cases and paternity suits.
Exon	Portion of the DNA that codes for the final mRNA and is then translated into protein.
Expressivity	Variation in the level of expression of a particular gene.
Gamete	Haploid sperm or egg cell.
Gene	A region of DNA that encodes a protein.
Gene therapy	See page 18.
Genome	The complete set of genes of an organism and the intervening DNA sequences. The Human Genome Project was an international research programme aimed at mapping all the genes in the human genome.
Genotype	The genetic constitution of an individual, usually at a particular locus.
Haploid	The chromosome number of a normal gamete: i.e. 23 in humans.
Haplotype	The particular combination of alleles in a defined region of a chromosome. Originally used to define the HLA type of an individual, it is now routinely used to describe any combination of alleles, such as those used in prenatal diagnosis by genetic linkage.
Heteroploidy	Abnormal appearance of the karyotype due to alteration in (i) the number of chromosomes or (ii) their shape and form.
Homologous chromosomes	The two matching members of a pair of chromosomes.
Hybridization	The joining of the complementary sequences of DNA (or DNA and RNA) by base pairing.
Index case	See Proband.
In situ hybridization	Use of a labelled probe to detect any complementary DNA or RNA sequence in a tissue section, cultured cell or cloned bacterial cell.
Intron	Intervening sequence on DNA that does not appear in the final RNA transcript.
Karyotype	The presentation of a cellular chromosome profile. Normal human karyotype is 44 autosomes and two sex chromosomes – XX female, XY male.
Library	A collection of DNA clones representing either all expressed genes i.e. a cDNA library, or a whole genome i.e. a genomic library.
Linkage disequilibrium	The association of two linked alleles more frequently than would be expected by chance.
Linkage map	A map of the relative positions of gene loci on a chromosome, deduced from the frequency with which they are inherited together.

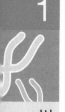

Locus	Site of a gene on a chromosome.
Meiosis	Sex cell division or reduction division. Formation of gametes with half the number of chromosomes (haploid) as the parent cell (diploid): i.e. 23.
Mitosis	Somatic cell division: each daughter cell has the same complement of chromosomes as the parent: i.e. 46.
Monozygotic twins	Twins produced from a single fertilized ovum. (See also Dizygotic twins.)
Mosaic	An individual with abnormal genotypic or phenotypic variation from cell to cell within the same tissue.
Non-disjunction	The failure of two members of a chromosome to separate during cell division, so that both pass to the same daughter cell.
Northern blotting	See page 13.
Oncogenes	Genes of either viral or mammalian origin that cause transformation of cells in culture. In normal cells, they are 'switched-off' or downregulated. They have copies in both viruses (v-onc) and mammalian cells (c-onc or protooncogenes) and have products that are essential to normal cell function or development. These include proteins (guanine-nucleotide binding proteins), cell surface receptors (epidermal growth factor receptor), and cellular growth factors (platelet-derived growth factor).
Penetrance	The proportion of individuals with a given genotype (usually a disease-causing mutation) manifesting a phenotype (usually a disease).
Phage	Virus that multiplies in bacteria.
Phenotype	The characteristics of an organism which result from an interaction between gene (the genotype) and environment.
Physical mapping	A linear map of the location of genes on a chromosome, as determined by the physical detection of overlaps between cloned DNA fragments rather than by linkage analysis.
Plasmid	An autonomously replicating DNA element, separate from the chromosome. These units, which only occur in bacteria, can be used as vectors of small fragments of foreign DNA.
Pleiotropy	The production of multiple effects by a single gene.
Polymerase chain reaction	See page 16.
Polymorphism	The occurrence in one population of two or more genetically determined forms (alleles), all of which are too frequent to be ascribed to mutation: e.g. blood group systems, the HLA system and various forms of G6PDH deficiency.

Polyploidy	Homologous chromosome numbers in more than two complete sets: i.e. three sets: triploid or 69 chromosomes; four sets: tetraploid or 92 chromosomes.
Primer (oligonucleotide primer)	A short DNA sequence used to initiate the synthesis of DNA, as in a polymerase chain reaction.
Proband or propositus	The family member who first presents with a given trait.
Probe	A specific DNA sequence, radioactively or fluorescently labelled, used with hybridization techniques to detect complementary sequences in a sample of genetic material.
Protooncogene	See page 33.
Reporter gene	A gene whose product can be used as a genetic 'label'. For example, a gene for neomycin resistance incorporated into a plasmid before transfection allows the detection of successfully transfected cells.
Restriction endonuclease	An enzyme that cleaves DNA at a specific site.
Restriction fragment length polymorphism (RFLP)	See page 13.
Reverse transcription	DNA synthesis from RNA templates, catalysed by the enzyme reverse transcriptase. It is used to synthesize DNA for probes and occurs naturally in retroviruses.
Southern blotting	See page 13.
Splicing	The removal of introns from messenger RNA and the joining together of adjacent exons.
Tandem repeat sequences	Multiple copies of a short DNA sequence lying in a series along a chromosome; used in physical mapping, linkage mapping and also in DNA fingerprinting because each person's pattern of tandem repeats is likely to be unique.
Tetraploid	See Polyploidy.
Transfection	The transfer of new genetic material into cells.
Translocation	The transfer of genetic material from one chromosome to another non-homologous chromosome.
Transposition	Movement from one site in the genome to another.
Transposon	A segment of DNA that can move from one position in the genome to another.
Triploid	See Polyploidy.
Trisomy	The presence of an extra chromosome, rather than the usual diploid set: i.e. 47 in humans.
Tumour suppressor gene (antioncogene)	See page 34.

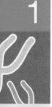

Vector	A DNA molecule, usually derived from a virus or bacterial plasmid, which acts as a vehicle to introduce foreign DNA into host cells for cloning, and then to recover it.
Zygote	Fertilized egg.

NUCLEIC ACIDS

NUCLEIC ACID STRUCTURE

All nucleic acids are polynucleotides. A nucleotide consists of three components (Fig. 1.1):
1. A base
2. A pentose sugar
3. 1–3 phosphate groups.

There are two kinds of nucleic acids (Table 1.1):
- **Deoxyribonucleic acid (DNA)**
- **Ribonucleic acid (RNA).**

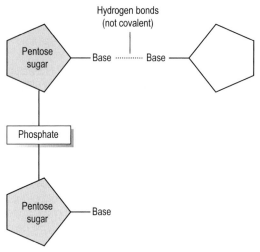

Fig. 1.1 Nucleotide structure.

Table 1.1 Structure of nucleic acids

Nucleic acid	Sugar	Bases		Monomeric unit*
		Purines†	Pyrimidines	
DNA	2′ Deoxyribose	Adenine (A) Guanine (G)	Thymidine (T) Cytosine (C)	Deoxyribonucleotides, e.g. adenylic acid (AMP), thymidylic acid (TMP)
RNA	Ribose	Adenine (A) Guanine (G)	Uracil (U) Cytosine (C)	Ribonucleotides, e.g. adenylic acid (AMP), uridylic acid (UMP)

*If the sugar is not phosphorylated, the structure is called a nucleoside.
†Xanthine and hypoxanthine are also purines.

Table 1.2 Proportions of different types of nuclear DNA	
Type of DNA	*Percentage of total DNA*
1. Single copy	70
2. Repetitive DNA	30
(a) Tandem repeats	(10)
Microsatellites	
Minisatellites	
Macrosatellites	
(b) Interspersed repeats	(20)
Short interspersed repeats (SINES)	
Long interspersed repeats (LINES)	

DNA (Tables 1.1 and 1.2)

- Double-stranded, double helix. Found primarily in the chromosomes of the cell nucleus.
- Two polynucleotide chains are antiparallel (i.e. one chain runs in a 5′ to 3′ direction; the other runs 3′ to 5′) and held together by hydrogen bonds between the bases:

> – adenine pairs only with thymidine (2 hydrogen bonds)
> – guanine pairs only with cytosine (3 hydrogen bonds).

- In each *diploid cell* double-stranded DNA is distributed between 23 pairs of chromosomes, comprising about 3.5×10^9 base pairs.
- Approximately 90% of the cell's DNA exists as a nucleoprotein called chromatin. Chromatin is comprised of DNA and both histone and non-histone proteins.

Mitochondrial DNA (mtDNA) (see also p. 26)

- Mitochondria contain their own DNA which differs from that of the rest of the cell.
- Codes for: 22 tRNAs
  2 mt rRNAs
  3 proteins, which are all subunits of the oxidative phosphorylation pathway.

Satellite DNA

- Highly repetitive DNA which comprises approximately 25% of the genome. Some sequences have no known function.
- Subsets of satellites can be classified according to their sequence motifs, length and size into:
  1. Satellite DNA (5–200 base pairs)
  2. Minisatellite DNA: Hypervariable family (10–60 base pairs), and Telomeric family (6 base pairs).
  3. Microsatellite DNA (1–4 base pairs).

RNA (Table 1.1)

- Single-stranded; 90% is present in the cell cytoplasm and 10% in the nucleolus.
- Three forms:
  1. **Messenger RNA (mRNA)** is the template for polypeptide synthesis. It has a cap at the 5′ end, and a poly A tail at the 3′ end (Fig. 1.2).
  2. **Transfer RNA (tRNA)** brings activated amino acids into position along the mRNA template. It forms a cloverleaf structure that contains many unusual nucleotides.

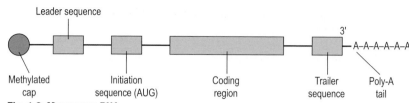

Fig. 1.2 **Messenger RNA.**

3. **Ribosomal RNA (rRNA)** is a component of ribosomes which functions as a non-specific site of polypeptide synthesis. In eukaryotic cells there are four rRNA molecules of 18, 28, 5 and 5.8s.

PROTEIN SYNTHESIS (Fig. 1.3)

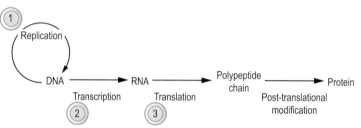

Fig. 1.3 **Protein synthesis.**

1. DNA replication (Fig. 1.4)
- Replication is semiconservative, i.e. each daughter molecule receives one strand from the parent DNA molecule.
- Unwinding proteins, *DNA-directed RNA polymerase, DNA polymerase and ligase are also required*.
- DNA polymerases synthesize the new strand in a 5′ to 3′ direction. They are the enzymes responsible for DNA chain synthesis. Four have been identified: α, β, γ and δ.
- Discontinuous replication, i.e. one or both DNA strands may be synthesized in pieces known as Okazaki fragments, which are then linked together to yield a continuous DNA chain.

2. Transcription
- Synthesis of complete RNA molecules from DNA.
- Takes place in the nucleus. One of the two DNA strands acts as a template for the formation of an mRNA molecule with a complementary base sequence.

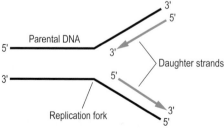

Fig. 1.4 **DNA replication.**

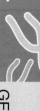

- Transcription yields three types of RNA: mRNA, tRNA and rRNA.
- Fully conservative replication.
- Synthesis in 5′ → 3′ direction.
- Controlled by the interaction between specific DNA sequence motifs (*cis* elements) and DNA-binding proteins (transactivating factors).
- **DNA-dependent RNA polymerase** is required to recognize and bind to sequences called promoters (located upstream of transcription start site) to initiate transcription. RNA polymerase must also cooperate with other proteins (transcription factors) which control transcription, together with specific enhancers or repressors, to form an initiation complex (see Note below).
- **Processing:** the RNA must be further modified to make it functionally active, e.g. non-coding introns (i.e. 'junk' sequences) cut out, intervening exons (i.e. coding sequences) spliced or joined together, and in some cases polyadenylation before delivery of mRNA to the cytoplasm. The process of gene splicing occurs in the nucleus by means of an RNA–protein complex called the splicesome. These consist of a core structure made up of 3 subunits called small nuclear ribonuclear proteins (sn-RNPs pronounced 'snarps') and non-sn-RNP splicing factors. Antibodies against these ribonucleoproteins are found in patients with SLE.

> **Note:** Unlike DNA polymerase, RNA polymerase can initiate the synthesis of new strands: There are 3 types of chromosomally encoded RNA polymerase (I, II and III), which recognize different types of RNA molecule. The RNA of an RNA virus is replicated by an RNA-dependent RNA polymerase. Oncogenic RNA viruses synthesize DNA from RNA, and insert the DNA into the chromosomes of animal cells. This reverse transcription is mediated by an RNA-directed DNA polymerase (*reverse transcriptase*).

3. Translation
- Protein synthesis according to the amino acid code in mRNA.
- Takes place in cytoplasm.
- Occurs on ribosomes when a tRNA molecule with three bases (anticodons) specific for a particular amino acid binds to the complementary mRNA codon.
- Four stages:

  > 1. Amino acid activation.
  > 2. Initiation of polypeptide chain formation begins with the amino acid, methionine.
  > 3. Chain elongation.
  > 4. Chain termination. Three codons, UAA, UGA and UAG, are signals for chain termination.

4. Post-translational modification of proteins
- Gives the mature protein functional activity and includes peptide cleavage and covalent modifications, such as glycosylation, phosphorylation, carboxylation and hydroxylation of specific residues.
- A newly synthesized protein is directed to appropriate destination, e.g. cytoplasm or cell membrane, by conserved amino acid sequence motifs, e.g. the signal peptide, and moieties added by post-translational modification.

GENETIC CODE
- Each DNA strand codes for the synthesis of many polypeptides. A segment of DNA that codes for one polypeptide chain is called a gene.

GENETICS AND MOLECULAR MEDICINE

- Genetic information is encoded by a sequence of bases in a non-overlapping code. Three bases (a *triplet*) specify one amino acid. There are 4^3, or 64, possible trinucleotide sequences of the four nucleotides in mRNA.
- The genetic code is degenerate, i.e. some amino acids are coded for by more than one triplet codon. AUG is the codon for chain initiation and for the amino acid methionine.
- Coding sequences (*exons*) are interrupted by sequences of unknown function (*introns*).
- Single base or point mutations may involve base transitions, transversion, deletion or insertion.

CONTROL OF PROTEIN SYNTHESIS

In eukaryotes, this may occur by modification of DNA, or at the level of transcription and translation.
1. Regulation by induction–derepression
2. Regulation by repression.

Possible faults in protein biosynthesis (Fig. 1.5)

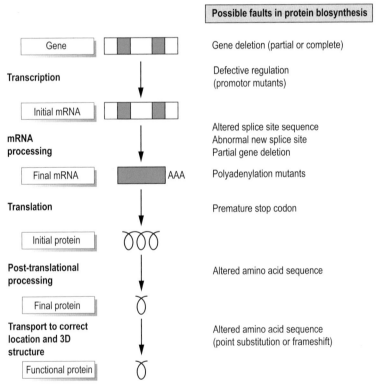

Fig. 1.5 **Faults in protein synthesis.**

> **Inhibitors of protein synthesis**
> **Antibiotics**   Rifampicin, streptomycin, tetracycline, chloramphenicol, erythromycin.
> **Pyrimidine analogues**   5-Fluorouracil, cytosine arabinoside, idoxuridine.
> **Purine analogues**   Mercaptopurine, adenine arabinoside, thioguanine.
> **Alkylating agents**   Cyclophosphamide, chlorambucil, bleomycin.
> **Others**   Vincristine, bleomycin, methotrexate, doxorubicin, etoposide, hydroxyurea, cisplatin.

CELL CYCLE (see p. 242)

- Replication of DNA occurs during the S phase of the cell cycle (i.e. DNA synthetic phase). This is preceded by G_1 (the first gap phase), when the cells prepare to duplicate their chromosomes. After the S phase, there is a second gap phase (G_2), during which cells prepare to divide. Cell division occurs during the mitotic (M) phase.

RECOMBINANT DNA TECHNOLOGY

APPLICATIONS (Fig. 1.6)

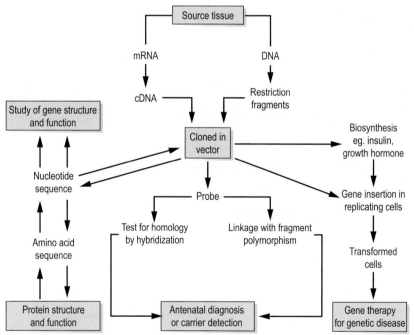

Fig. 1.6 Applications of gene analysis.
Modified from Emery's elements of medical genetics, 10th edn. Churchill Livingstone.

BASIC TECHNIQUES OF GENE ANALYSIS

DNA can be extracted using standard techniques from any tissue containing nucleated cells, including blood and chorionic villus material.

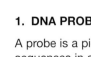

1. DNA PROBE HYBRIDIZATION

A probe is a piece of single-stranded DNA which is used to detect homologous sequences in a sample of genomic DNA. If the probe is radiolabelled, its location after binding can be identified by exposure to X-ray film.

There are three main sources of **gene probes**:
1. Complementary DNA (cDNA), i.e. DNA that is complementary to mRNA.
2. Cloned cDNA.
3. DNA fragments prepared from genomic DNA.

2. GENE MAPPING

Restriction enzymes

Examples: *Eco*RI, *Hpa*II, *Ala*I, *tog*I

- These are bacterial enzymes that recognize specific DNA sequences and cleave DNA at these sites. Each enzyme has its own recognition sequence and will cut genomic DNA into a series of fragments that can be analysed.
- The enzymes are named according to their organism of origin, e.g. *Eco*RI is derived from *E. coli*.
- Because DNA is negatively charged, the DNA fragments can be ordered according to their size by electrophoresis in an agarose gel. It is possible to build up restriction enzyme maps of areas of the genome using different restriction enzymes that cleave DNA within or outside the gene of interest.

Preparation of and uses of a gene probe (Figs 1.7 and 1.8)

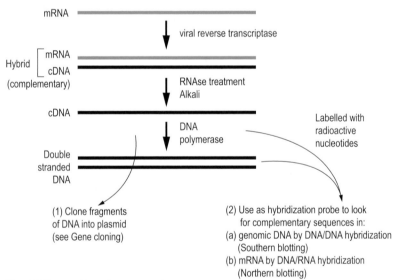

Fig. 1.7 Preparation of a gene probe.

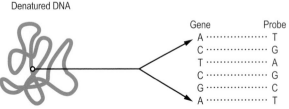

Fig. 1.8 Gene probe.

Restriction fragment length polymorphisms (RFLPs)

- Variations in non-coding DNA sequences are extremely frequent throughout the genome, and when they affect restriction enzyme cleavage sites, DNA fragments of different sizes will result. These variations are called restriction fragment length polymorphisms.
- If they occur in or near the gene of interest they provide potential linkage markers for following mutant genes through families.
- Since the development of methods for analysing microsatellite markers, RFLPs are not routinely used in genetic linkage studies because southern blotting requires more DNA per sample, and is less well suited to high throughput of samples than the polymerase chain reaction (PCR).
- A restriction map is a diagram depicting the linear arrangement of restriction enzyme cleavage sites on a piece of DNA, and provides a means of characterizing DNA.

Other markers

- Polymorphic genetic markers: any Mendelian characteristic used to follow the transmission of a segment of chromosome through a pedigree.
- Other markers used in gene mapping include:
  (i) *Dinucleotide repeats:* usually CA repeated many times, the number varying as a polymorphism can be detected by PCR.
  (ii) *Variable number tandem repeats:* VNTRs; arrays or repetitive DNA sequences which vary in number and can be detected by blotting.
  (iii) *Microsatellites:* stretches of DNA consisting of 2, 3 or 4 nucleotides – a marker that is well suited to genetic linkage analysis.
  (iv) *Single nucleotide polymorphisms* (SNPs): variations in one base pair which are randomly scattered throughout the genome and provide a virtually limitless source of markers to explore the variation in the human genome.

Southern and Northern blot technique

- A method of transferring DNA fragments that have been size-fractionated by gel electrophoresis to a nylon membrane such that the relative positions of the DNA fragments are maintained. The DNA is then usually visualized on an autoradiograph following hybridization with a specific DNA or RNA probe.
- Useful for detection and size determination of specific restriction fragments in a DNA digest, e.g. detection of a sickle cell globin gene (Fig. 1.9).
- **Northern blotting** is analogous to Southern blotting except that the molecules of RNA rather than DNA are separated by electrophoresis.

3. GENE CLONING

- The insertion of foreign DNA into bacterial plasmids, bacteriophages or cosmids (see Note).
- Used in the preparation of **Gene libraries**, which are large collections of clones that together encompass all the DNA in the genome (genomic libraries) or all the sequence expressed as mRNA in the tissue from which the library was prepared (cDNA library). Such libraries can be screened to identify clones that contain a particular insert of interest, and large amounts can be made for detailed molecular analysis.

> **Note:** *Plasmids*: Closed circular extrachromosomal DNA molecules which replicate autonomously in bacteria. *Bacteriophages*: Viruses that multiply in bacteria. *Cosmids*: Artificial vectors which are hybrids between a bacteriophage and a plasmid.

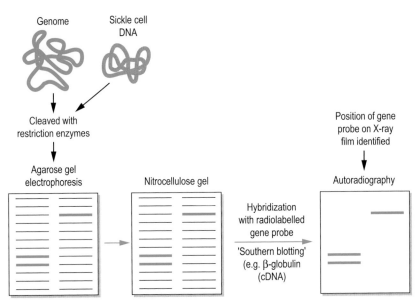

Fig. 1.9 Southern blotting.

The cloning of DNA into a plasmid (Fig. 1.10)

Essential requirements
1. A method of specifically cutting and then religating DNA.
2. A source of carrier DNA (e.g. plasmid).
3. A transfer method (e.g. conjugation).
4. A method of selecting the recombinant (e.g. antibiotic resistance).
5. A method of detecting the product of the cloned gene, e.g. enzyme-linked immunoabsorbent assay (ELISA).

4. GENE SEQUENCING

The identification and localization of new genes has been greatly enhanced by the development of methods for the large-scale sequencing of whole genomes in bacteria (e.g. *E. coli, H. pylori*), yeasts and nematodes (*C. elegans*).

Tools used
1. *Expressed sequence tags (ESTs)*: short sequences of cDNA clones which are available on public databases. Currently about 50% of all human genes are represented and this figure will rapidly increase until all human coding sequence has been identified and can be characterized.
2. *Sequence-tagged sites (STSs)*: ESTs which have been assigned a map location by PCR (see below) of various genomic resources.
3. *Bioinformatics*: a variety of computational methods is now available for rapid comparison of raw sequence data, so that eventually the evolutionary relationship between all genes from bacteria to human will be understood.
4. *Gene targeting*: homologous genes in a variety of organisms can be simultaneously inactivated and the phenotype observed to give clues to the function of the gene product. A 'knockout mouse' is one in which a particular gene has been inactivated such that the animal will no longer

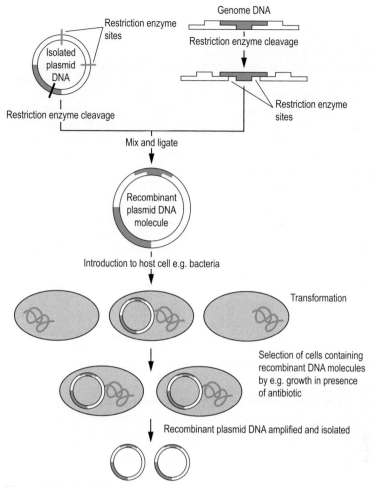

Fig. 1.10 Cloning DNA into a plasmid.

produce the protein corresponding to that gene. This allows the modelling of particular human diseases in which a naturally occurring mouse mutant does not exist.

5. *Transgenic analysis*: the insertion of a foreign (usually human) gene into another organism, such as a mouse, to look at its effect on phenotype. Mutations can be systematically introduced to alter the protein function and the gene can be expressed under the control of tissue-specific promoters to look at function in particular cell types.

The Human Genome Project

Three main scientific objectives:

1. The creation of genetic maps.
2. The development of physical maps. Consists of 30 000 sequence-tagged site (STS) markers distributed at intervals of 10 000 bases along the genome.
3. Determination of the complete sequence of human DNA, and the functional importance and structure of the 80 000 genes contained within the genome.

Uses of recombinant cloned DNA

1. Isolation and sequencing of individual genes.
2. Preparation of probes for studying function of isolated genes, e.g. gene mapping using Southern blot technique.
3. As gene probes for rapid diagnosis of certain bacterial, viral and parasitic illnesses, in addition to diagnostic pathology, e.g. classification of lymphomas.
4. Pharmaceutical production of large quantities of proteins, such as human insulin, growth hormone, somatostatin, tissue-plasminogen activator (t-PA), erythropoietin, G-CSF and GM-CSF, interferon and hepatitis B vaccine.
5. Carrier detection, especially X-linked recessive disorders; presymptomatic diagnosis of autosomal dominant disorders and prenatal diagnosis of all categories of mendelian disorders (see Note).
6. Potential correction of genetic defects (i.e. gene therapy).

> **Note:** Some diseases for which genetic prediction using DNA analysis is currently available are: haemophilia A and B; sickle cell disease; thalassaemia (α and β); muscular dystrophy (Duchenne and Becker's); triplet repeat disorders; adult polycystic disease; phenylketonuria; cystic fibrosis; glucose-6-phosphate-dehydrogenase deficiency; and familial hypercholesterolaemia.

Gene microarray analysis or Gene expression profiling

A molecular technique made possible by the sequencing of the human genome and availability of probes for expressed human genes. It allows a quantitative comparison of the expression of thousands of human genes on a single chip or slide (the 'microarray') in, for example, normal and malignant B cells.

Antisense technology

Antisense suppression is where the expression of a protein is inhibited by the annealing of a complementary RNA or synthetic oligonucleotide to a sequence within the mRNA, so blocking or reducing the efficiency of translation. Can be used to block the expression of some genes in tissue culture, but the technique is limited by difficulties in controlling the stringency of mRNA/DNA annealing.

5. POLYMERASE CHAIN REACTION (PCR)

This is an amplification reaction in which a small amount of a DNA template is amplified to provide enough to perform analysis (prenatal diagnosis, detection of an infectious organism or the presence of a mutated oncogene).

The crucial feature of PCR is that to detect a given sequence of DNA it only needs to be present in one copy (i.e. one molecule of DNA). It is therefore an extremely sensitive technique.

Outline of the procedure (Fig. 1.11)

- A small sample of DNA is placed in a tube.
- Two oligonucleotides are added. These have sequences matching two sequences of the DNA that flank the region of interest.
- A thermostable DNA polymerase is added.
- The mixture is heated to just below 100°C and the DNA dissociates into two single strands (Fig. 1.11).
- The solution is allowed to cool and the single strands bind to the oligonucleotides, which are in excess.
- The oligonucleotide now acts as a primer for DNA polymerase and is extended to form a new double-stranded molecule.

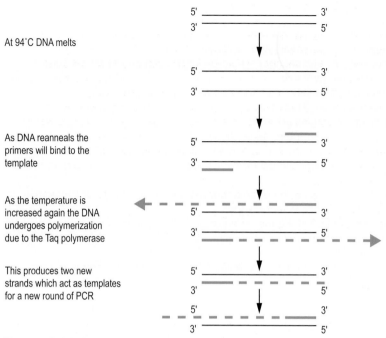

At 94°C DNA melts

As DNA reanneals the primers will bind to the template

As the temperature is increased again the DNA undergoes polymerization due to the Taq polymerase

This produces two new strands which act as templates for a new round of PCR

Fig. 1.11 Polymerase chain reaction.

- The cycle is repeated, with the amount of DNA doubling each time.
- *Reverse transcriptase PCR (RT-PCR):* A modification of PCR that is used to study gene expression. The viral enzyme RT can use RNA as a template for the production of a strand of DNA. The product of this reaction is then used for PCR as above. It is used to detect very small amounts of mRNA.

Application to molecular genetics
1. Analysis of restriction fragment length polymorphisms.
2. Analysis of messenger RNA.
3. Amplification of fragments for identification by Southern blotting.
4. Assessment of genetic polymorphism in linkage analysis.
5. DNA sequencing.
6. Site-directed mutagenesis.

Application to medicine
1. Diagnosis of infections, e.g. mycobacteria, HIV, meningococcus, herpes simplex.
2. Forensics (hair, blood, semen).
3. Quantification of gene expression (where mRNA template is first reverse transcribed into a cDNA equivalent before amplification (RT-PCR)).
4. Prenatal diagnosis from chorionic villus sampling, of known genetic mutations, e.g. cystic fibrosis, Duchenne muscular dystrophy.
5. Detection of minimal residual tumour (e.g. *bcr-abl* in chronic myeloid leukaemia) and mutations in malignant tumours to assess prognosis.
6. Investigation of evolution of pathogens, e.g. HIV, HCV.
7. Tissue typing by PCR and detection of genetic variants, especially of MHC (major histocompatibility complex) class II alleles.

GENE THERAPY

Addition, insertion or replacement of a normal gene or genes.

- **Strategies:** two potential gene therapy strategies:
  1. *Germline*: genetic changes would be introduced into every cell type including the germline.
  2. *Somatic cell*: genetic modifications are targeted specifically at the diseased tissue. At present only somatic cell strategies are allowed. Germline strategies are considered unethical as genetic changes would be transmitted to future generations.
- **Techniques** (still mostly experimental) include the following:
  1. Treatment of a genetic defect by insertion of a normal gene (e.g. in cystic fibrosis).
  2. Blockade of expression of an abnormal gene (e.g. the *BCL2* leukaemia gene) with antisense technology.
  3. The introduction of a gene for an enzyme that converts a prodrug into a cytotoxic metabolite (e.g. thymidine kinase to convert 5-fluorocytosine into 5-fluorouracil).
- **Vector systems:** the means by which DNA is delivered to the target cells and is one of the major difficulties to overcome. Two main system types:
  1. Physical (i.e. non-viral), e.g. liposomes.
  2. Viral, which may integrate into the genome (retroviral-, lentiviral- and adenoviral-associated vectors) or be maintained as an episome (adenoviral).

Conditions for which gene therapy has been attempted
1. Adenosine deaminase immune deficiency
2. Thalassaemia
3. Sickle cell disease
4. Phenylketonuria
5. Haemophilia A
6. Cystic fibrosis
7. Duchenne muscular dystrophy.

CHROMOSOMAL ABNORMALITIES (Table 1.3)

Account for 50% of all spontaneous miscarriages and are present in 0.5–1% of all newborn infants.

Table 1.3 Types of chromosome mutations

Numerical	
Aneuploidy (gain or loss of >1 chromosome)	Monosomy
	Trisomy (gain of 1 homologous chromosome)
	Tetrasomy (gain of 2 homologous chromosomes)
Polyploidy (addition of >1 complete haploid chromosomes)	Triploidy
	Tetraploidy
Structural (Fig. 1.12)	
Translocations	e.g. Burkitt's lymphoma (translocation from chromosome 8 to 14), Philadelphia chromosome
	Reciprocal
	Robertsonian
Deletions (loss of >1 nucleotide)	e.g. Wilms' tumour (deletion from chromosome 11)
Insertions (addition of >1 nucleotide)	
Inversions	
Different cell lines (mixploidy)	
Mosaicism	
Chimaerism	

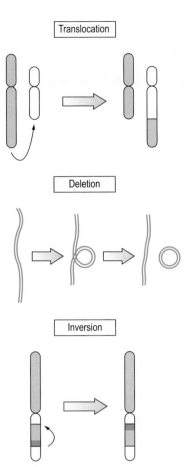

Fig. 1.12 Structural chromosome mutations.

AUTOSOMAL DISORDERS

Chromosomes 21, 18, 13, 5.

1. TRISOMIES

(a) Down's syndrome
Trisomy 21, mongolism. Incidence strongly affected by maternal age (see Note):
- – 1:1200 live births (mothers under 30 years)
- – 1:100 live births (mothers aged 39 years)

Note: Maternal age also affects birth rates of: hydrocephalus, anencephaly, achondroplasia (paternal age also); i.e. increased frequency with age.

Causes
- Non-dysjunction (94% of cases). Sporadic incidence related to maternal age.
- Mosaicism (2% of cases). Less marked physical or intellectual dysfunction.
- Robertsonian translocation (4% of cases). Abnormalities in parents' chromosomes.

Clinical features
- Mental retardation, short stature, hypotonia and characteristic craniofacial abnormalities (flat occiput, oval face, epicanthic folds, Brushfield spots, macroglossia), simian palmar creases.
- Associated anomalies, e.g. congenital heart disease (atrial septal defect, patent ductus arteriosus and Fallot's tetralogy), tracheo-oesophageal fistulae, duodenal atresia, leukaemia and hypothyroidism.

(b) Edward's syndrome
Trisomy 18.

Clinical features
- Mental retardation, craniofacial abnormalities (prominent occiput, low-set ears, micrognathia). 'Rocker bottom' foot deformity. Cardiac abnormalities.

(c) Patau's syndrome
Trisomy 13.

Clinical features
- Mental retardation, cleft palate and lip, polydactyly and microphthalmia.

2. DELETIONS

(a) 'Cri du chat' syndrome
Partial deletion of short arm of chromosome 5.

Clinical features
- Mental retardation, spasticity, high-pitched cry, craniofacial abnormalities (micrognathia, low-set ears, epicanthic folds).

(b) Prader–Willi syndrome and Angelman syndrome
Deletion of chromosome 15.

Clinical features
- Prader–Willi (paternal inheritance): neonatal hypotonia, facial obesity, low IQ, short stature and genital hypoplasia.
- Angelman (maternal inheritance): hypertonia, ataxic gait, prominent jaw, deep-set eyes, absent speech and mental retardation ('happy puppet syndrome').

PHILADELPHIA CHROMOSOME

This is an *acquired* chromosomal abnormality present in 85% of cases of chronic myeloid leukaemia, due to the deletion of the long arm of chromosome 22 with translocation, usually on to chromosome 9. It persists during remission, and the prognosis is worse if absent. Also reported to occur in myelofibrosis and polycythaemia rubra vera.

SEX CHROMOSOME DISORDERS

Present in 25–30% of early abortions and 7% of deaths in first year of life. Incidence 1:550 live births.

(a) Turner's syndrome (ovarian dysgenesis)
Karyotype 45 XO, i.e. no sex chromatin body.
Incidence 1:2000 live female births.

Causes
- Non-disjunction of sex chromosomes.
- Mosaicism (XO/XX, XO/XY or XO/XXX).

Clinical features
- Phenotypically female, short stature, wide carrying angle, webbing of neck, short metacarpals (retarded bone age), sexual infantilism (lack of breast development with widely spaced nipples, scanty pubic and axillary hair).
- Primary amenorrhoea (occasional menstruation occurs in mosaicism), high gonadotrophin levels, low oestrogen level.
- Slight intellectual defect.
- Associated anomalies include coarctation of the aorta and renal abnormalities.

(b) Noonan's syndrome
Karyotype 45 XY.

Clinical features
- Similar features to Turner's syndrome but phenotypically male.
- Complete absence of testicles, cryptorchidism.
- Gonadal function may be normal.

(c) Testicular feminization syndrome (androgen insensitivity)
Karyotype 46 XY, i.e. one sex chromatin body.

Clinical features
- Main cause of male pseudohermaphroditism. (The most common cause of female pseudohermaphroditism is congenital adrenal hyperplasia.)
- Inadequately virilized due to target organ failure.
- Phenotypically female, well-developed breasts and female contours but lacking body hair, with small, blind vaginas. No uterus or fallopian tubes. Gonads are testes, producing testosterone.

(d) Kleinfelter's syndrome (seminiferous tubule dysgenesis)
Karyotype 47 XXY, XXXYY or XXYY, i.e. one or two sex chromatin bodies. Incidence: 1:400–600 male births.

Clinical features
- Tall, thin men with bilateral gynaecomastia and infertility due to hypogonadism (small, azoospermic testes).
- Increased incidence of mental subnormality.
- High urinary gonadotrophins with 17-ketosteroid content.

(e) 47 XYY
Incidence: 1:2000 live female births.
- Tall, aggressive males with increased tendency to psychiatric illness. More common in prison communities. Fertility normal.

(f) Fragile X syndrome
- Most common inherited cause of mental retardation.
- Associated with a fragile site on the long arm of the X chromosome, and shows modified X-linked inheritance.
- There is an expansion of the molecular level of the CGC triplet repeat, which can exist as a premutation or a full mutation.
- Affected males are moderately to severely mentally retarded; carrier females can show mild mental retardation.

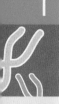
(g) Chromosomal breakage syndromes
- Rare, autosomal recessive disorders caused by underlying defects in DNA repair.
- Characterized by increased chromosome breakage in cultured cells, and an increased tendency to leukaemia and lymphoma.

(h) Triple X syndrome
Karyotype 47 XXX
- Intelligence normal or mildly impaired.
- Fertility normal.

SINGLE-GENE ABNORMALITIES

- Follow Mendelian patterns of inheritance.
- Approximately 6000 disorders. Affect from 1:10 000 to 1:100 000.
- Mutations may be inherited or occur spontaneously.
- Result from substitution (point mutation), deletion, insertion, inversion and triplet repeat expansion (unstable dynamic expansion, see p. 27).
- Online Mendelian Inheritance in Man (OMEM) web page is a regularly updated source of information (http://www.ncbi.nlm.nih.gov).
- Autosomal dominant.
- Autosomal recessive.
- X-linked dominant.
- X-linked recessive.

Unusual patterns of inheritance can be explained by phenomena such as genetic heterogeneity, mosaicism, anticipation and mitochondrial inheritance.

Table 1.4 Proportions of genes in common among different relatives		
Degree of relationship	Examples	Proportion of genes in common
First	Parents to child, sib to sib	1/2
Second	Uncles or aunts to nephews or nieces, grandparents to grandchildren	1/4
Third	First cousins, great-grandparents to great-grandchildren	1/8

AUTOSOMAL DOMINANT INHERITANCE

Approximately 1500 conditions described (generally 'structural-type' disorders), for example:

Achondroplasia
Adult polycystic kidney disease*
Charcot–Marie–Tooth syndrome
Ehlers–Danlos and Marfan's syndromes*
Erythropoietic protoporphyria (see Note)
Facioscapulohumeral muscular dystrophy
Familial adenomatous polyposis*
Familial hypercholesterolaemia*
Gardner's syndrome
Gilles de la Tourette syndrome
Hepatic porphyrias

Hereditary haemorrhagic telangiectasia
Hereditary sensory and motor neuropathy*
Hereditary spherocytosis
Huntington's chorea*
Myotonic dystrophy*
Neurofibromatosis type I and II*
Osteogenesis imperfecta (Table 1.5)
Retinitis pigmentosa*
Retinoblastoma
Tuberous sclerosis*
Von Hippel–Lindau disease*
Von Willebrand's disease.

Note: An exception is congenital erythropoietic porphyria which has an autosomal recessive inheritance.

*Autosomal disorders showing a delayed age of onset or exhibiting reduced penetrance in which linked DNA markers or specific mutational analysis can be used to offer presymptomatic diagnosis.

Table 1.5 Types of osteogenesis imperfecta

Type	Inheritance	Severity	Colour of sclerae
I	Autosomal dominant	Mild	Blue
II	New mutation	Lethal in perinatal period	Blue
III	Autosomal recessive	Fractures at birth	White
IV	Autosomal recessive	Marked fragility	White

Summary

1. Both sexes are equally affected.
2. Heterozygotes are phenotypically affected, i.e. no carrier condition.
3. 50% of children are affected (Fig. 1.13).

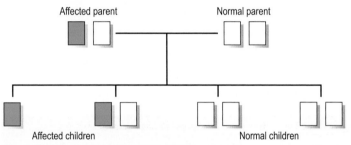

Fig. 1.13 Autosomal dominant inheritance.

4. Risk remains the same for each successive pregnancy.
5. Can exhibit variable expressivity (i.e. range of phenotypes, e.g. tuberous sclerosis can be asymptomatic with harmless kidney cysts, or fatal in next generation due to brain malformation) and reduced penetrance (e.g. Huntington's disease – 100% penetrance).
6. Can exhibit anticipation (i.e. occurrence of disease with a progressively earlier age of onset in successive generations, e.g. in triplet repeat expansion diseases).
7. Rare, and generally less severe than autosomal recessive.
8. High new mutation rate.

AUTOSOMAL RECESSIVE INHERITANCE

Approximately 1000 conditions described (generally 'metabolic-type' disorders), for example:

Agammaglobulinaemia
Albinism
α_1-Antitrypsin deficiency
Congenital adrenal hyperplasia
Congenital erythropoietic porphyria
Cystic fibrosis
Friedreich's ataxia
Haemoglobinopathies (e.g. sickle cell disease and thalassaemias)
Infantile polycystic disease
Limb-girdle muscular dystrophy
Most inborn errors of metabolism (e.g. galactosaemia, glycogen storage diseases, homocystinuria, phenylketonuria, lipidoses and mucopolysaccharidoses)
Werdnig–Hoffman disease
Wilson's disease
Xeroderma pigmentosa.

Summary
1. Both sexes are equally affected.
2. Only manifests in homozygous state. Heterozygotes are phenotypically unaffected, i.e. carrier state exists.
3. When both parents carry the gene, 1:4 children are affected and 2:4 children are carriers (Fig. 1.14).

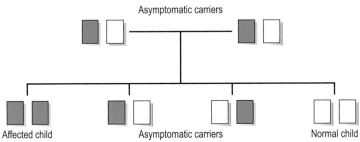

Asymptomatic carriers

Affected child   Asymptomatic carriers   Normal child

Fig. 1.14 Autosomal recessive inheritance.

4. Asymptomatic carriers produce affected children. Those with the disease do not usually have affected children unless they marry a carrier, i.e. increased risk of disease among offspring of consanguineous marriages.
5. Variable expressivity less of a problem than with autosomal dominant inheritance.
6. For ethnic associations see Table 1.6.

Table 1.6 Ethnic associations with autosomal recessive diseases	
Disease	*Ethnic groups*
β-Thalassaemia	Mediterraneans, Thais, Blacks, Middle East populations, Indians, Chinese
Sickle cell disease	US and African Blacks, Asian Indians, Mediterraneans (especially Greeks) and Middle East populations
Tay–Sachs disease	Ashkenazi Jews
Gaucher disease	Ashkenazi Jews
Bloom syndrome	Ashkenazi Jews
Adrenogenital syndrome	Eskimos
Severe combined immunodeficiency	Apache Indians
Cystic fibrosis	Caucasians
Albinism	Hopi Indians

SEX-LINKED DOMINANT INHERITANCE

Rare, e.g. vitamin D-resistant rickets (X-linked).

Summary
1. Affects both sexes, but females more than males.
2. All children of affected homozygous females are affected.
3. Females pass the trait to half their sons and half their daughters.
4. All daughters of affected males are affected, but none of their sons.

SEX-LINKED RECESSIVE INHERITANCE

Approximately 200 conditions described (almost exclusively X-linked), for example:

Adrenoleucodystrophy
Becker's muscular dystrophy
Colour blindness
Complete testicular feminization
  syndrome
Duchenne muscular dystrophy
  (Table 1.7)
Fabry's disease
Glucose-6-phosphate dehydrogenase
  deficiency
Haemophilia A (VIII) and B (IX)

Hunter's syndrome
Ichthyosis
Immunodeficiencies:
  agammaglobulinaemia and severe
  combined immunodeficiency
Lesch–Nyhan syndrome
  (hypoxanthine guanine
  phosphoribosyl transferase
  deficiency)
Nephrogenic diabetes insipidus
Wiscott–Aldrich syndrome.

Table 1.7 Inheritance in muscular dystrophies		
Muscular dystrophy	*Inheritance*	*Presentation*
Duchenne	X-linked recessive	Most common, presents early
Becker	X-linked recessive	Milder, presents later
Limb-girdle (Erb)	Autosomal recessive	Less common
Facioscapulohumeral-peroneal	Autosomal dominant	Long course
Distal myopathy (Welander)	Autosomal dominant	Late onset
Ocular myopathy	Autosomal dominant	Retinopathy or dysphagia may also be present

Summary

1. Affected cases are usually males carrying the gene and homozygous females (rare).
2. Half the sons of carriers are affected, and half the daughters are carriers.
3. No male-to-male transmission: condition is transmitted by carrier women who produce affected boys, normal boys, carrier girls and normal girls with equal frequency (Fig. 1.15).
4. Affected males can have only normal sons and carrier daughters.
5. Affected cases have affected brothers and affected maternal uncles.
6. Abnormalities used in carrier detecting of X-linked disorders (Table 1.8).

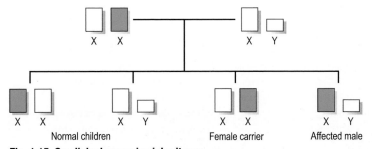

Fig. 1.15 Sex-linked recessive inheritance.

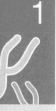

GENETICS AND MOLECULAR MEDICINE

Table 1.8 Abnormalities used in carrier detection of X-linked disorders

Disorder	Abnormality
Clinical	
Ocular albinism	Mosaic retinal pigmentary pattern
Retinitis pigmentosa	Mosaic retinal pigmentation, abnormal electroretinogram
Alport syndrome	Haematuria
Biochemical	
Haemophilia A	Reduced factor VIII activity:antigen ratio
Haemophilia B	Reduced levels of factor IX
G6PD deficiency	Erythrocyte G6PD activity reduced
Lesch–Nyhan syndrome	Reduced hypoxanthine-guanine phosphoribosyl transferase activity in skin fibroblasts
Vitamin D-resistant rickets	Serum phosphate level reduced
Duchenne muscular dystrophy	Elevated serum creatine kinase level
Becker muscular dystrophy	Elevated serum creatine kinase level

MITOCHONDRIAL GENETIC DISORDERS

- The mitochondrial genome is circular and approximately 16.5 kb in length.
- It encodes genes for the mitochondrial respiratory chain and for some species of transfer RNA.
- Mitochondrial genetic disorders are mostly rare and complex neurological conditions, e.g. mitochondrial encephalopathy, lactic acidosis and stroke-like episodes (MELAS) (Table 1.9).
- Mitochondrial DNA (mtDNA) mutates 10 times more frequently than nuclear DNA. As there are no introns, a mutation will invariably affect a coding sequence.
- Maternal inheritance: no mitochondria are transferred from spermatozoa at fertilization.
- Normal and mutant mtDNA may coexist within one cell (heteroplasmy).
- Poor genotype–phenotype correlation. The proportion of mitochondria with a mutation in their DNA and mutational heterogeneity are possible reasons for the range of phenotypic severity seen.

Table 1.9 More common mitochondrially inherited disorders

Disorder	Features
MELAS	**M**itochondrial **E**ncephalopathy, **L**actic **A**cidosis, **S**troke-like episodes, diabetes mellitus
MERRF	**M**yoclonic **E**pilepsy, **R**agged-**R**ed **F**ibres in muscle, ataxia, sensorineural deafness
NARP	**N**europathy, **A**taxia, **R**etinitis **P**igmentosa, developmental delay, lactic acidosis
Chronic progressive external ophthalmoplegia	Ptosis, ophthalmoplegia
Leber's hereditary optic neuropathy	Visual loss, neurodegenerative features
Hypertrophic cardiomyopathy with myopathy	HOCM, muscle weakness
Diabetes with deafness	Diabetes mellitus, sensorineural deafness
Aminoglycoside-induced deafness	Deafness induced by use of aminoglycoside antibiotics
Pearson syndrome	Pancreatic insufficiency, pancytopenia, lactic acidosis

DYNAMIC/UNSTABLE MUTATIONS: TRIPLET OR TRINUCLEOTIDE REPEAT DISEASES

A number of mainly neurological genetic diseases are caused by a mutation that is an expansion of a repetitive sequence of three nucleotides. This arrangement (triplet amplification) appears to be prone to instability and has therefore become known as a dynamic mutation.

- Conditions include Huntington's disease, myotonic dystrophy, fragile X syndrome (four main variants), Friedreich's ataxia, X-linked spinobulbal muscular atrophy (SBMA), neuronopathy (Kennedy syndrome), spinocerebellar ataxia (at least seven variants) and Machado–Joseph disease.
- Mutant alleles arise from a population with repeats at the upper end of normal range which are prone to instability.
- Disease severity worsens with an earlier age of onset in successive generations (genetic anticipation).
- The length of the expansion continues to increase as cells divide throughout life (somatic instability).
- Trinucleotide repeats either lie in the 5′ non-coding region of genes, where they disrupt gene transcription because they cause steric hindrance of RNA polymerase, or they code for the amino acid glutamine (CAG) and appear to produce a toxic protein which forms intracellular inclusion bodies.

MOLECULAR BASIS OF SINGLE-GENE DISORDERS

Autosomal dominant

Achondroplasia　　Disorder of skeletal development due to mutations in the fibroblast growth factor receptor type 3. Almost all patients have mutations at the same site in the protein.

Polycystic kidney disease　　Leading genetic cause of renal failure in adults and accounts for 10% of end-stage renal disease. Causative gene in the vast majority of cases (*ADPKD1*) is called *polycystin* and is believed to be involved in the establishment of epithelial cell polarity in development.

Myotonic dystrophy　　One of the trinucleotide repeat disorders (see above). The mutation is an expansion in the 3′ untranslated region of a protein kinase (dystrophia myotonica protein kinase), although the mechanism whereby this leads to the phenotype is still controversial.

Familial hypercholesterolaemia　　One of the few inborn errors of metabolism inherited as a dominant trait. Due to mutations which disrupt the synthesis, function or recycling of the low density lipoprotein receptor, there is poor uptake of LDL-bound cholesterol and high serum levels.

Marfan's syndrome　　Results from mutations in a gene called *fibrillin*, the protein product of which is the major component of extracellular microfibrils and is widely distributed in connective tissue throughout the body.

Neurofibromatosis (NF1)　　The progressive accumulation of nerve sheath tumours is caused by mutations in a tumour supressor gene called *neurofibromin*; a GTPase-activating protein (GAP) which enhances the inactivation of growth-promoting signals. 30–50% are due to new mutations. NF2 is a different disorder which is characterized by the development of bilateral acoustic neuromas.

Familial breast cancer　　Mutations in at least two genes (*BRCA-1* and 2) give rise to familial breast cancer, often in association with ovarian tumours.

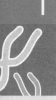

Autosomal recessive

α₁-Antitrypsin deficiency   One of the most common hereditary diseases affecting Caucasians. The prime function of the enzyme is to inhibit neutrophil elastase and it is one of the serpin superfamily of protease inhibitors.

Cystic fibrosis   The defective gene encodes a protein called the cystic fibrosis transmembrane conductance regulator (CFTR), which is involved in the regulation of ion flux through chloride channels and in mucin production. The opening of the protein is mediated by ATP binding. Over 70% of the mutations in Caucasians are due to a deletion of three nucleotides (encoding a phenylalanine residue) at position 508 (ΔF 508).

Wilson's disease   Due to mutations in a copper-binding protein, which is probably important for binding copper to the transport protein, caeruloplasmin.

X-linked

Duchenne dystrophy   A genetic disease due to mutations in a protein called *dystrophin*, which is part of a large complex of membrane-associated proteins, defects in most of which can cause forms of muscular dystrophy. Out-of-frame deletions lead to the production of a nonsense protein which is completely without functionality. In-frame deletions lead to the formation of a truncated protein with partial function, and to the milder *Becker dystrophy*.

PRENATAL AND POSTNATAL DIAGNOSIS

PRENATAL: INDICATIONS

1. Women aged over 35 years.
2. Raised maternal serum alphafetoprotein (see box).

Causes
1. Anencephaly
2. Open spina bifida
3. Incorrect gestational age
4. Intrauterine fetal bleed
5. Threatened miscarriage
6. Multiple pregnancy
7. Congenital nephritic syndrome
8. Abdominal wall defect.

---

3. Strong family history of neural tube defects, e.g. previous affected child.
4. Strong family history of chromosomal abnormality.
5. Carriers of X-linked recessive diseases who have decided to terminate male fetuses.
6. Known carriers of prenatally diagnosable biochemical disorders, e.g. creatine kinase in Duchenne muscular dystrophy, phenylalanine tolerance test in phenylketonuria, alphafetoprotein in neural tube defects.
7. Conditions for which genetic prediction using DNA analysis is available, e.g. α- and β-thalassaemia, cystic fibrosis, fragile X syndrome, haemophilia A, Huntington's disease, muscular dystrophy (Duchenne and Becker), myotonic dystrophy, spinal muscular atrophy.

Standard techniques

1. Non-invasive maternal screening
• Screening for infections that cause congenital malformations (TORCH screen).

- Triple test (serum αFP, hCG and oestradiol) for Down syndrome and neural tube defects at 16 weeks.
- Ultrasound for structural abnormalities at 18 weeks.

2. *Invasive: amniocentesis, chorionic villus sampling, fetoscopy.*

Amniocentesis

- For neural tube defects, chromosome abnormalities, metabolic disorders, molecular defects.
- Performed at about 16 weeks gestation.
- Risk to fetus approximately 1%.

Chorionic villus sampling

- For chromosome abnormalities, metabolic disorders, molecular defects.
- Performed at 10–12 weeks gestation.
- Involves aspiration via a cannula inserted through the cervix under ultrasound guidance.
- Chorionic villi can be used for chromosomal analysis, fetal DNA analysis and certain biochemical investigations.
- Risk of causing miscarriage is approximately 2–3%.

Fetoscopy

- Preferred at 16–20 weeks.
- Blood for chromosome abnormalities, haematological disorders, congenital infections.
- Liver for metabolic disorders and skin for hereditary skin disorders.

POSTNATAL DIAGNOSIS

Guthrie test

- Performed between 6th and 14th day of life.
- Screens routinely for phenylketonuria, TSH level and histidinaemia. Also: galactosaemia, glucose-6-phosphate dehydrogenase deficiency and hyperleucinaemia (maple syrup urine disease).

MULTIFACTORIAL OR POLYGENIC INHERITANCE (Table 1.10)

Table 1.10 Mendelian versus multifactorial inheritance

Mendelian	Multifactorial
Gene results in disease	May have many contributing genes, but do not develop disease if less than threshold
All or nothing	Additive with a varying phenotype
Risk does not increase through life	May acquire increasing liability through life

- Observed phenotype is due to the additive effect of many different gene loci. Environmental factors may be involved.
- The genetic liability of individuals to develop a disease of multifactorial aetiology has a normal distribution, and the condition occurs when a certain threshold is exceeded (Fig. 1.16).
- Risk of phenotype increases if:
  - Previous offspring affected
  - First-degree relative affected
  - Relatives severely affected.

Examples

(i) Congenital malformations
Neural tube defects:
- Spina bifida (2 per 1500 births)
- Anencephaly (2 per 1000 births); risk after first, second and third affected child is 1:20, 1:8 and 1:4, respectively
Congenital heart disease (6 per 1000 births)
Cleft lip ± cleft palate (1 per 1000 births)
Pyloric stenosis (3 per 1000 births; M:F ratio = 5:1)
Congenital dislocation of hip (1 per 1000 births; M:F ratio = 1:8)
Hirschsprung's disease (M:F ratio = 3:1).

(ii) Common adult diseases
- Insulin dependent diabetes mellitus (40% concordance for IDDM in monozygotic twins; 98% are HLA-DR3 or -DR4 and -B8. Only 50% of non-diabetics have these alleles
- Schizophrenia (heritability is 85% (see below))

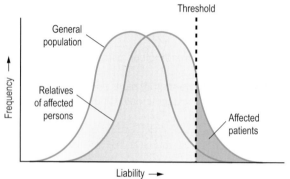

Fig. 1.16 Threshold effect in multifactorial inheritance.

- Manic depression
- Breast cancer (a small proportion of cases are due to single-gene mutations: *BRCA-1* and *BRCA-2*).
- Rheumatoid arthritis
- Epilepsy
- Multiple sclerosis
- Peptic ulcer (heritability is 37%, and 50% of affected families have increased pepsinogen)
- Glaucoma
- Essential hypertension (heritability is 62%)
- Ischaemic heart disease
- Asthma (heritability is 80% and is associated with HLA-A$_2$)
- Alzheimer's disease (about 10% inherit Alzheimer's disease as a monogenic autosomal dominant, and a proportion of these arise from mutations in the amyloid precursor protein on chromosome 21).

Heritability
- Estimates of the heritability of a condition provide an indication of the relative importance of genetic factors in its causation.
- Estimated from the degree of resemblance between relatives expressed in the form of a correlation coefficient.

- Estimates of heritability of some common diseases:
  - Schizophrenia 85%
  - Asthma 80%
  - Cleft palate 76%
  - Pyloric stenosis 75%
  - Ankylosing spondylitis 70%
  - Hypertension 62%
  - Congenital hip dislocation 60%
  - Peptic ulcer 37%
  - Congenital heart disease 35%

POPULATION GENETICS

The Hardy–Weinberg principle

- Mathematical equation that is the basis of population genetics. The frequency of the alleles within a population remain constant from one generation to the next.

> - *Assumptions:*
>   1. Population is large
>   2. Mating is random
>   3. Mutation rate remains constant
>   4. Alleles are not selected for (i.e. they confer no reproductive or survival advantage)
>   5. There is no migration in or out of population.

- *Factors which disturb this equilibrium*:
  1. Non-random mating
  2. Change in the number of mutant alleles in the population
  3. Selection for or against a particular genotype, small population size and migration
  4. *Genetic drift* (i.e. in small populations, one allele may be transmitted to a high proportion of offspring by chance, resulting in marked changes in gene frequency between two generations)
  5. *Founder effect* (occurs in small isolated populations that breed among themselves. If one of the original founders had a certain disease, this will remain over-represented in successive generations).
- Closely associated loci in the same chromosome are linked if genes at these loci segregate together more than 50% of meioses. The *lod score* is a mathematical indication of the relative likelihood that two loci are linked. A lod score >3 is confirmation of linkage.

Ethnic groups and genetic disease (Table 1.11)

Table 1.11 Ethnic groups and genetic disease	
Population with high frequency	*Associated disease*
Scandinavians	α_1-Antitrypsin and lecithin cholesterol acyl transferase (LCAT) deficiency, congenital nephrotic syndrome
Northern Europeans	Cystic fibrosis
Ashkenazi Jews	Tay-Sachs disease, Gaucher's disease
Sephardic Jews and Armenians	Familial Mediterranean fever
Eskimos	Congenital adrenal hyperplasia and pseudocholinesterase deficiency
Mediterranean races	β-Thalassaemia, glucose-6-phosphate dehydrogenase deficiency and familial Mediterranean fever
Chinese	Glucose-6-phosphate dehydrogenase deficiency
Africans	Haemoglobinopathies especially sickle cell disease, α- and β-thalassaemias
South African whites	Porphyria variegata

Heterozygotic advantage

- When a serious autosomal recessive disorder has a relatively high incidence in a large population, this is likely to be due to heterozygote advantage.
- For example, for sickle cell disease in tropical Africa and β-thalassaemia and G6PD deficiency in the Mediterranean, there is good evidence that heterozygote advantage results from reduced susceptibility to *Plasmodium falciparum* malaria.
- *Mechanism:* red cells of heterozygotes with sickle cell can more effectively express malarial or altered self antigens, which will result in more rapid removal of parasitized cells from the circulation. In Americans of African origin who are no longer exposed to malaria, it would be expected that the frequency of the sickle cell allele would gradually decline. Predicted rate of decline is so slow that it will be many generations before it is detectable.

Genetic variations in drug metabolism (see p. 344)

ONCOGENESIS

REGULATION OF GENE EXPRESSION

- 80 000 genes in the human genome.
- Each cell typically expresses 16 000–20 000 genes.
- Expression is regulated by transcription factors; proteins which bind to DNA at the 5′ end of genes (the promoter) and initiate transcription of genes (Fig. 1.17).
- Some genes have a fundamental biological role and will be expressed in all cells at all times ('housekeeping genes').

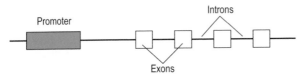

Fig. 1.17 Promoter, introns and exons.

THE SOMATIC EVOLUTION OF CANCER

- Cancer cells are a clonal population of cells. The malignant phenotype arises from the accumulation of mutations in multiple genes.
- It is a combination of three types of genetic mutation (inherited, spontaneous and environmentally determined) which leads to cancer. Therefore cancer evolution is a complex, multifactorial process.
- Most tumours show visible abnormalities of chromosome banding on light microscopy, suggesting that as tumours develop they become more bizarre and more prone to genetic error.
- In contrast to other types of genetic disorders, for most cancers the genetic mutations are not inherited but arise in somatic cells during adulthood as a result of exposure to environmental carcinogens. Multiple mutations are usually involved.
- These mutations (inherited and acquired) commonly involve three types of genes: oncogenes, tumour suppressors and genes involved in DNA-repair mechanisms (Fig. 1.18).

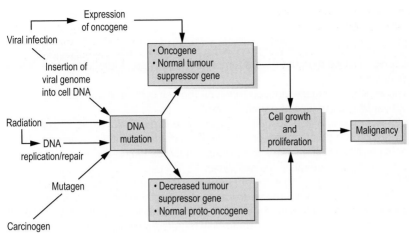

Fig. 1.18 Pathways to malignancy.

Multistage process of carcinogenesis

Development of cancer involves a minimum of two 'hits'. Persons at risk of familial cancer inherit the first 'hit' in the germ cell, the second 'hit' occurring in somatic cells in mitosis. In persons with sporadically occurring cancer, both 'hits' occur in somatic cells.

ONCOGENES

- Oncogenes, when expressed, lead to loss of growth control by a dominant gain of function mutation (i.e. only one copy needs to be mutated for cancer to occur).
- **Protooncogenes** or cellular oncogenes (c-onc), found in the normal human genome and expressed in normal tissue, have a central role in the signal-transduction pathways that control cell growth and differentiation (Fig.1.18).
- May be growth factors, growth factor receptors, intracellular signalling transduction factors (e.g. GTP-binding proteins, postreceptor tyrosine kinases and cytoplasmic factors), DNA-binding nuclear proteins and cell cycle factors.

Examples
- **ras** is a small G-protein which is one of the most commonly mutated genes in solid tumours. It acts to promote cell growth and division.
- **c-myc** is a transcription factor which commits the cell to go into mitosis. DNA-binding nuclear protein is overexpressed in Burkitt's lymphoma because of a translocation which juxtaposes it to the immunoglobulin heavy-chain promoter.
- In the Philadelphia chromosome in CML, a **bcr-abl** fusion gene product is created by a translocation. This protein is a postreceptor tyrosine kinase which is not under normal regulatory influences.

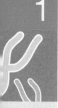

TUMOUR SUPPRESSOR GENES AND INHERITED FAMILY CANCER SYNDROMES (Table 1.12)

- In contrast to oncogenes, these exert a **recessive** effect, such that both copies must be mutated before tumorigenesis occurs. Mutation results in loss of function.
- These genes normally function to inhibit the cell cycle and therefore, when activated, lead to loss of growth control.
- **p53** is a protein which occupies a pivotal role in the cell cycle as it stops progress through the cycle, preventing DNA damaged through wear and tear being replicated. It encodes a transcription factor, the normal function of which is to downregulate the cell cycle.
- p53 is also a central regulator of apoptosis. Inactivation of p53 is the primary defect in the **Li–Fraumeni syndrome** (a dominantly inherited monogenic cancer syndrome characterized by breast carcinoma, sarcomas, brain and other tumours). It is the most commonly mutated gene in tumours, and over 50% of bladder, breast, colon and lung cancers have the p53 mutations clustered in a conserved region of exons 5–10. This is in contrast to the location of p53 mutation in hepatocellular carcinoma.

Genetic cancer syndromes

About 5% of colorectal and breast cancer cases are as a result of an inherited cancer susceptibility gene. Many tumour types have been studied for loss of heterozygosity of chromosome 13 and elsewhere, to identify the location of tumour suppressor genes. Over 20 have been identified; retinoblastoma, p53 and adenomatous polyposis coli genes have been cloned.

- *Retinoblastoma* is the commonest malignant eye tumour in childhood. All of the bilateral and 15% of the unilateral cases are inherited as an autosomal dominant trait. The gene for this trait is localized to the proximal long arm of chromosome 13 (13q14).
- *Familial adenomatous polyposis (FAP)* is inherited as an autosomal dominant disorder. More than 90% of patients with FAP develop bowel cancer. There is an interstitial deletion of a region of the long arm of chromosome 5 (5q21).
- *Colorectal carcinoma.* Allele loss on chromosome 18q is seen in over 70% of colorectal cancers. The candidate gene for this region is called **d**eleted in **c**olorectal **c**arcinoma (DCC). It is expressed in normal colonic mucosa, but is either reduced or absent in colorectal carcinomas.
- *Li-Fraumeni syndrome* (a dominantly inherited monogenic cancer syndrome characterized by breast carcinoma, sarcomas, brain and other tumours). Inactivation of p53 is the primary defect.

Table 1.12 Some familial cancers due to tumour suppressor mutations		
Tumour	*Gene*	*Locus*
Retinoblastoma, osteosarcoma	RB1	13q14
Familial adenomatous polyposis	APC	5q31
Li–Fraumeni syndrome	TP53	17p13
von Hippel–Lindau syndrome	VHL	3p25–26
Multiple endocrine neoplasia type II	RET	10q11.2
Breast–ovarian cancer	BRCA1	17q21
Breast cancer	BRCA2	13q12–13
Wilms' tumour	WT1	11p13
Neurofibromatosis I	NF1	17q12–22
Colorectal, pancreatic or oesophageal cancers	DCC	18q21

MISMATCH REPAIR GENES

- Seen in hereditary non-polyposis coli (HNPCC): an autosomal dominant disorder. Associated with the presence of new, rather than loss of, alleles in DNA from tumour tissue. This phenomenon is known as microsatellite instability or replication error. Individuals who inherit a mutation in one of the mismatched repair genes for HNPCC are heterogeneous for a loss of function mutation leading to an increased mutation rate and increased risk of developing malignancy.
- HNPCC accounts for less than 5% of colon cancer, but 15% of colorectal cancers exhibit microsatellite instability.

APOPTOSIS (see also p. 105)

This is the morphological description of cells undergoing '*programmed cell death*', a process whereby unwanted cells are removed by the activation of specific genetic pathways.

Features
- Cell shrinkage
- Compaction of chromatin
- Nuclear blebbing, but mitochondrial pathology preserved (unlike necrosis)
- Cell fragmentation and formation of apoptotic bodies
- Phagocytosis
- Energy-dependent process (in contrast to necrosis).

Functions of apoptosis
1. Elimination of cells in embryological development (e.g. motor neurons)
2. Induction of tolerance to self antigens by removal of autoreactive T lymphocytes
3. Removal of virally infected cells
4. Removal of cells which have undergone DNA damage.

Principal mediators
p53   A tumour supressor gene which inhibits mitosis and drives apoptosis in cells in which DNA has been damaged. Mutation correlates with poor prognosis in tumours.
bcl-2   A strong negative regulator of apoptosis. If it is overexpressed in tumours, cells have a prolonged survival.
fas   (CD95) A cellular receptor which, when activated, is directly coupled to the activation of intracellular proteases which lead to apoptosis.
caspases   Present in all cells and, unless inhibited, lead to the morphological changes of apoptosis.

Diseases of excess and insufficient apoptosis

Excess
- Neurodegeneration, e.g. Alzheimer's and Parkinson's disease
- HIV disease ($CD4^+$ cells die through programmed cell death).

Insufficient
- Cancer
- Autoimmunity.

Cell senescence or ageing

- May be associated with repetitive DNA sequences, called telomeres, that are found at the end of chromosomes. They are not replicated in the same way as chromosomal DNA, but are synthesized by the enzyme *telomerase*.
- Cell ageing is associated with shortening of telomeres, possibly due to the absence of telomeres in somatic cells.

IMMUNOGENETICS

THE MAJOR HISTOCOMPATIBILITY COMPLEX

- The major histocompatibility complex (MHC) in humans is located on the short arm of chromosome 6, and carries the genes determining the histocompatibility antigens, termed human leucocyte antigens (HLA), specific to each individual.
- Responsible for tissue rejection and some other immunological functions.
- Several distinct loci code for the major histocompatibility antigens (HLA-A, -B, -C, -DR, -DQ, and -DP antigens) and some complement components (Fig. 1.19).

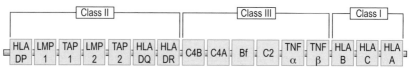

Fig. 1.19 HLA loci and their genes.
HLA = human leucocyte antigen, LMP = latent membrane protein, TAP = transporter associated with antigen processing, TNF = tumour necrosis factor.

- Each locus has several alleles: (57 alleles at the A locus, 111 at the B, 34 at the C and 228 at the D locus).

3 classes of MHC gene products:
1. Class I antigens are coded for by HLA-A,-B,-C genes. They are present on all nucleated cells, and determine graft rejection.
2. Class II antigens are coded for by HLA-D, -DR, -DP and -DQ genes. They are only present on monocytes/macrophages, B lymphocytes and occasionally activated T lymphocytes. They act as receptors for the presentation of antigen to helper T cells (immune response genes).
3. Class III antigens are associated with certain complement components (e.g. C2, C4 and C3b receptor). Not involved in either immune response or graft rejection.

- I region: A region of the MHC where immune response (Ir) genes are located and plasma membrane (Ia) molecules are encoded.
- Ir genes: Genes that control the ability of helper T cells to develop a specific immune response to antigen.
- Ia: Histocompatibility antigen found primarily on B cells, but also on some macrophages and T cells.

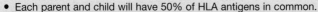

- Each parent and child will have 50% of HLA antigens in common.
- Non-identical siblings have:
  - 1:4 chance of sharing all four HLA antigens
  - 2:4 chance of sharing two antigens
  - 1:4 chance of sharing no antigens.

CLASSIFICATION OF DISEASES ASSOCIATED WITH HLA

Certain diseases are associated with particular HLA antigens (Table 1.13). This may be due to:

1. Linkage disequilibrium (i.e. allelic association) with an unidentified disease susceptibility gene, e.g. an immune response gene.
2. Reflect the function of the specific HLA antigen.

Table 1.13 Diseases associated with HLA

HLA antigen	Disease	Relative risk*
A3	Haemochromatosis	9
B5	Behçet's disease	6
B27	Ankylosing spondylitis	90
	Reiter's syndrome	37
	Psoriatic arthritis	4
	Acute anterior uveitis	3
DR2	Multiple sclerosis	4
	Pernicious anaemia	1.7
	Narcolepsy	1.4
	Juvenile-onset diabetes mellitus	4
DR3	Dermatitis herpetiformis	15
	Coeliac disease	11
	Sjogren's syndrome	10
	1° biliary cirrhosis	8
	Chronic active hepatitis	7
	Addison's disease	6
	Systemic lupus erythematosus	6
	Grave's disease	4
	Hashimoto's thyroiditis	3.5
	Insulin-dependent diabetes mellitus	3
	Myasthenia gravis	2
DR4	Insulin-dependent diabetes mellitus	6
	Rheumatoid arthritis	4
DR5	Pernicious anaemia	9
DR7	Coeliac disease	5

*Relative risk is the factor of increased risk for developing the disease among individuals with the HLA antigen. If there is no association, the relative risk is 1.

2

MICROBIOLOGY

**PROCARYOTIC PATHOGENIC
  BACTERIA** 40
Classification of Gram-positive and
  Gram-negative bacteria 40
Bacterial characteristics, diseases and
  reservoirs of infection 41
  Gram-positive rods (Table 2.3) 42
  Gram-positive cocci (Table 2.4) 44
  Gram-negative pyogenic cocci
    (Table 2.5) 46
  Gram-negative bacilli (Tables 2.6–2.9)
    47
  Gram-negative bacteria
    (Tables 2.10–2.12) 54
Endotoxins and exotoxins 58
Antibacterial chemotherapy 58
  Spectra of activity and sites of action
    58
  Bactericidal and bacteriostatic drugs
    61
  Antibiotic resistance 61

VIRUSES 62
Structure of the virion 62
RNA-containing viruses 62
  Important RNA viruses 63
DNA-containing viruses 69
Human slow virus infections 70

Oncogenic viruses 71
Important serological tests 71
  Hepatitis B serology 71
  HIV serology 72
  Syphilis serology 72
Spectra of activity and sites of action of
    antiviral drugs 73

FUNGI 74
Important fungal infections 74
Antifungal chemotherapy 74

PARASITES 75
Important parasitic infections 75
  Plasmodial infection 77
Antiparasite chemotherapy 78

OTHER PATHOGENS 79
Common opportunistic pathogens 79
Zoonoses 79
Alert organisms 79
Incubation periods 80

IMMUNIZATION 81
Vaccines 81
Immunization schedule 82
  Contraindications 83
  Travel vaccines 84
Sterilization and disinfection 84

Table 2.1 Comparison of bacteria, rickettsiae, chlamydiae and viruses

Characteristics	Bacteria	Rickettsiae	Chlamydiae	Viruses
1. Obligate intracellular parasite	–	+	+	+
2. Contains both DNA and RNA	+	+	+	–
3. Visible with light microscope	+	+	–	–
4. Contains muramic acid in cell wall	+	+	+	–
5. Independent metabolic activity	+	+	+	–
6. Synthesizes ATP	+	+	–	–
7. Susceptible to antibacterial antibiotics	+	+	+	–

PROCARYOTIC PATHOGENIC BACTERIA

CLASSIFICATION OF GRAM-POSITIVE AND GRAM-NEGATIVE BACTERIA
(Fig. 2.1)

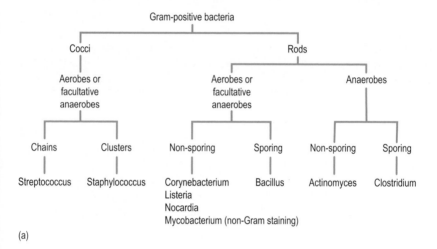

(a)

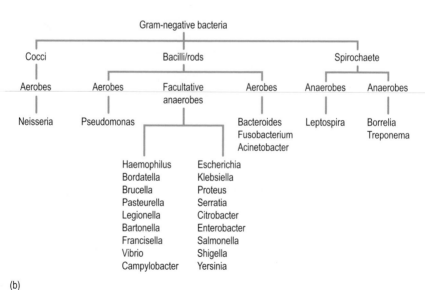

(b)

Fig. 2.1 Classification of bacteria.

General characteristics

In general:

- All cocci are Gram-positive   Exceptions: Neisseria
- All rods are Gram-negative   Exceptions: Bacillus, Clostridia and Corynebacterium
- All pathogens are   Exceptions: Clostridia and Bacteroides
  facultative anaerobes   (obligate anaerobes)
- Encapsulated bacteria   *Strep. pneumoniae, K. pneumoniae, N. meningitidis, H. influenzae*
- Gram-resistant organisms   Mycobacteria and Nocardia (wax-like outer layer)
     Mycoplasma (no cell wall)
     Rickettsia, Coxiella, Chlamydia (intracellular bacteria)
     Treponema and Borrelia

Bacterial virulence mechanisms: EAT ICE

- **E**nzyme-mediated tissue damage
- **A**dherence
- **T**oxin-induced local and systemic effects (endotoxins and exotoxins)
- **I**nvasion
- **C**irculation from and spread from primary infection site
- **E**vasion of host immune response.

Bacteria producing enzymes

Staph. aureus: β-lactamase, coagulase, catalase, hyaluronidase, DNAase
Strep. pyogenes: streptolysin, streptokinase, hyaluronidase, DNAase
N. gonorrhoea: β-lactamase
E. coli: β-lactamase
Cl. perfringens: phospholipase.

Table 2.2 Lactose-fermenting characteristics of bacteria

Lactose fermenters	Non-lactose fermenters
Escherichia coli	Salmonella
Klebsiella	*Shigella dysenteria*
Shigella sonnei	*Shigella flexneri*
	Shigella boydi
	Proteus
	Yersinia

BACTERIAL CHARACTERISTICS, DISEASES AND RESERVOIRS OF INFECTION

Bacterial characteristics, the diseases produced in humans and the reservoirs of infection are presented in Tables 2.3–2.12.

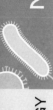

Table 2.3 Gram-positive rods

Genus and species	Characteristics	Diseases produced in humans	Reservoirs of infection
Corynebacterium			
C. diphtheria	• Aerobic, non-spore-forming • Catalase +ve • Non-haemolytic • Toxin production	• Diphtheria (non-invasive infection) • Diphtheria can cause prosthetic device infections	• Nasopharynx of case or carrier
Listeria			
L. monocytogenes	• Aerobic • Haemolytic • Often in pairs	• Meningoencephalitis, chiefly in neonates and immunocompromised patients	• Widely distributed in animals and humans
Bacillus			
B. anthracis	• Aerobic, spore-forming	• Cutaneous and pulmonary anthrax	• Anthrax in animals (cattle and sheep) • Occasional human infection
B. cereus	• Enterotoxins	• Food poisoning	• Contaminated fried rice
Clostridium			
Cl. welchii (perfringens)	• Anaerobic, spore-forming • α-Haemolytic toxin	• Food poisoning and gas gangrene • Sometimes associated with diabetes	• Soil and intestinal flora of humans and animals
Cl. oedematiens and Cl. septicum	• Anaerobic, spore-forming	• Gas gangrene	• Soil and dust • Faeces of humans and animals
Cl. tetani	• Anaerobic, spore-forming	• Tetanus	• Intestinal flora of humans and animals • Soil and dust
Cl. botulinum	• Anaerobic, spore-forming • Heat-labile neurotoxin	• Botulism • Mild watery diarrhoea	• Soil and dust • Badly canned food
Cl. difficile	• Anaerobic, spore-forming • Toxigenic strains produce exotoxins A and B* • Non-toxigenic strains are not usually pathogenic	• Pseudomembranous colitis	• Commonest enteropathogen in hospital patients • Source of infection may be endogenous, exogenous from the environment or directly from a carrier • Carriage rates in healthy volunteers vary from 0 to 15%. Spores can be found on the hands of patients and staff, as well as on beds and floors

*__Toxin A__ is an enterotoxin, thought to bind to mucosal receptors which enter the cell and cause fluid secretion and mucosal damage. __Toxin B__ is a cytotoxin which also binds to specific membrane receptors, but is 1000 times more potent in tissue cultures than toxin A.

MICROBIOLOGY

Table 2.3 (Cont'd)

Genus and species	Characteristics	Diseases produced in humans	Reservoirs of infection
Actinomyces A. israelii	• Anaerobic • Branching filaments	• Actinomycosis, abscess in cervicofacial region, (occasionally in abdomen and chest) usually after surgery or trauma	• Commensal in mouth
Nocardia N. asteroides	• Anaerobic • Branching filaments • Weak acid-fast	• Opportunistic infection • Pulmonary and systemic nocardiosis • Brain abscess, mycetoma and other skin infections, mostly in immunocompromised patients	• Saprophytic in soil
Mycobacterium M. tuberculosis (human type) and M. bovis (bovine type)	• Aerobic • Rod-shaped • Acid- and alcohol-fast (requires Lowenstein–Jensen medium for culture)	• Pulmonary TB • TB of lymph nodes, intestine, bones and joints • Meningitis and genitourinary infection	• Lungs of humans, cattle and birds
M. leprae	• Cannot be cultured in vivo	• Leprosy	
Atypical mycobacteria M. ulcerans	• Colonies often pigmented	• Skin ulcers (tropics)	
M. kansasii M. malmehoens M. xenopi	• Some grow slowly and others rapidly	• Lung disease	
M. marinum	• May exhibit unusual temperature requirements	• Granulomatous skin lesions associated with cleaning fish tanks and swimming pools	
M. cheloni		• Cutaneous abscesses; occasionally disseminated infection in the immunocompromised	
M. avium–intracellulare		• Cervical lymphadenopathy in children; chest infections and disseminated/invasive infections in AIDS patients	
M. fortuitum		• Lung disease	

Table 2.4 Gram-positive cocci

Genus and species	Characteristics	Diseases produced in humans	Reservoirs of infection
Streptococcus			
Str. viridans (α-haemolysis)	• Facultative anaerobes*, some microaerophilic • In chains • Catalase –ve	• Dental abscess • Subacute bacterial endocarditis	• Commensal in mouth
Str. mutans		• ?Dental caries	
Str. pyogenes (β-haemolysis)† Lancefield Group A	• Grouped by carbohydrate antigens • In chains • Catalase –ve • Production of haemolytic exotoxins, e.g. streptokinase, hyaluronidase and DNAase	• Acute tonsillitis, wound infections, puerperal sepsis, otitis media, scarlet fever, rheumatic fever and glomerulonephritis • Skin and soft tissue infections, e.g. pyoderma, impetigo, erysipelas, acute cellulitis • Toxic shock syndrome • Necrotizing fasciitis‡	• Nose and throat of case and carrier
Lancefield Group B		• Septicaemia (without focus), meningitis • Important pathogen in neonatal period	
Lancefield Group C		• Pharyngitis, cellulitis	
Str. faecalis (Lancefield Group D) Lancefield Group G	• In short chains or pairs	• Urinary tract infections, wound infections and cholecystitis	• Commensal of large intestine
		• Cellulitis	
Str. pneumoniae (pneumococcus) (α-haemolysis)	• Diplococcus • Heavily encapsulated	• Lobar pneumonia, infections of eye and ear, purulent meningitis and sinusitis	• Commensal of upper respiratory tract
Str. milleri		• More frequent in splenectomized patients • Deep abscesses, especially liver, lung and brain	

Streptococcal haemolysis

α (incomplete) haemolysis):   S. pneumoniae, S. viridans and some enterococci
β (complete) haemolysis):   S. pyogenes (group A), S. agalactiae (group B)
γ (no haemolysis):   Some enterococci

* Facultative organisms can grow with or without air.
† Streptolysin-O is an oxygen-labile haemolysin. Anti-streptolysin-O (ASO) appears within 1–2 weeks of infection, reaches a maximum at 3–5 weeks and disappears within 6–12 months.
‡ Several factors predispose to infection, including penetrating injuries, surgical procedures, cuts, burns, varicella infection, and childbirth.

Table 2.4 (Cont'd)

Genus and species	Characteristics	Diseases produced in humans	Reservoirs of infection
Staphylococcus			
Staph. aureus (β-haemolysis) (see box below)	• Coagulase +ve (most strains) and catalase –ve • In clumps • Phage typing identifies virulent strains • Six types of enterotoxin are known (see Table 2.5)	• Superficial infections, including boils and carbuncles, scalded skin syndrome in neonates, toxic epidermal necrolysis (Ritter–Lyell disease) and toxic shock syndrome, wound infections, osteomyelitis, bronchopneumonia, endocarditis, vascular catheter infections, septicaemia, pseudomembranous colitis, and food poisoning	• Colonizes nose and perineum of carriers • Contaminated salads and milk
Staph. saprophyticus (epidermis, albus and micrococcus)	• Coagulase +ve and catalase –ve • In clumps	• Infection of indwelling cannulae, other prosthetic device infections, endocarditis, and urinary tract infections	• Contaminated salads and milk

Toxin production associated with *Staph. aureus*

Toxin*	Effect
Enterotoxins (A–E)	Released into foods resulting in food poisoning, Act as superantigens
Exfoliative or epidermolytic toxins A and B	Scalded skin syndrome, producing peeling of layers of epidermis
Haemolysins α, β, γ and δ	Cytolytic; lyses erythrocytes
Leucocidins	Lyse leucocytes and macrophages
Toxic shock syndrome toxin-1 (TSST-1)	Vascular collapse, rash with desquamation. Acts as a superantigen
Coagulase	Clots plasma
Fibrinolysin	Digests fibrin
Hyaluronidase	Breaks down hyaluronic acid
DNAase	Hydrolyses DNA
Lipase	Lipolytic
Protein A	Antiphagocytic

* Toxin production varies between strains of *Staph. aureus*.

Table 2.5 Gram-negative pyogenic cocci

Genus and species	Characteristics	Diseases produced in humans	Reservoirs of infection

Neisseria
N. meningitides (meningococcus)
	• Both aerobic
	• Both diplococcus
	• Need enriched medium and CO_2 for culture
	• Serogroups A and C are commonest worldwide
		• Acute meningitis
		• Septicaemia
			• Commensal in nasopharynx (carriage rate in general population is approx. 25%)
			• Transmission is via respiratory route
			  – More common in the winter weather, and has two peaks of incidence, in infancy and teenage years
			  – Predisposing factors are influenza infection, smoking and complement C5 and C9 deficiencies

N. gonorrheae (gonococcus)	• In the UK, group B is the most common	• Gonorrhoea, ophthalmia neonatorum, suppurative urethritis in the male, acute cervicitis in the female, pelvic inflammatory disease, suppurative arthritis and endocarditis	
Moxarella catarrhalis	• Aerobic non-motile • Cocci or short bacilli arranged in pairs	• Otitis media and sinusitis in children. Infective exacerbation of COPD in adults, pneumonia in elderly	

MICROBIOLOGY

Table 2.6 Gram-negative bacilli: Parvobacteria

Genus and species	Characteristics	Diseases produced in humans	Reservoirs of infection
Haemophilus H. influenzae	• Facultative anaerobe • Encapsulated • Needs factors V and X for growth	• Chronic bronchitis, bronchopneumonia, acute epiglottis and purulent meningitis in children	• Commensal in nasopharynx
H. parainfluenzae		• Exacerbations of chronic lung disease	
H. aegyptius (Koch–Weeks bacillus)	• Aerobic	• A form of conjunctivitis	• Conjunctiva of a case
H. ducreyi	• Aerobic	• Genital ulcers, chancroid	
Bordetella Bord. pertussis	• Very fragile • Small coccobacillus • Needs Bordet–Gengou agar and CO_2 for culture	• Whooping cough	• Nasopharynx of a case

Brucella
(i) Br. abortus
 	
(ii) Br. melitensis
(iii) Br. suis
(iv) Br. canis
	• Non-sporeforming, aerobic
	• All are small coccobacilli
	• Need CO_2 for culture
		• Brucellosis	• Disease in
			  (i) goats, sheep (most common worldwide; Mediterranean countries)
			  (ii) cattle (worldwide)
			  (iii) pigs (Denmark and USA)
			  (iv) dogs
			• Secondary human infection
			• Consumption of unpasteurized milk

Table 2.6 (Cont'd)

Genus and species	Characteristics	Diseases produced in humans	Reservoirs of infection
Pasteurella *P. multocida*	• Aerobic	• Wound sepsis following a bite	• Dogs and cats
Legionella *L. pneumophila*	• Fastidious organism • Exotoxin • Demonstrated with difficulty in tissues, using a silver stain	• Nosocomial pneumonia • Pontiac fever	• Air-conditioning units
Francisella *F. tularensis*	• Pleomorphic • Capsulated	• Tularaemia (ulceroglandular and oculoglandular form) (Fever, tonsillitis, headaches, hepatosplenomegaly, lymphadenopathy)	• Plague-like disease of rodents, widespread in USA and occasionally in Europe • Acquired by handling animal carcasses
Eikenella *E. corrodens*	• Slow growing • Facultative anerobe	• Human bite infections • Infective endocarditis (HACEK organisms)	
Gardnerella *G. vaginitis*	• Facultative anaerobes	• Bacterial vaginosis • Asymptomatic vaginal carriage in 60% of women	
Streptobacillus *S. moniliformis*		• Rat-bite fever	

Table 2.7 Gram-negative bacilli: Vibrios

Genus and species	Characteristics	Diseases produced in humans	Reservoirs of infection
Vibrio			
V. cholerae (classic and Eltor types)	• Aerobic, curved, motile rods	• Cholera (non-invasive infection)	• Human cases and carriers • Endemic disease in India and Bangladesh
V. parahaemolyticus	• Salt-dependent • Haemotoxins	• Food poisoning	• Warm seawater; seafood, especially shellfish
V. vulnificus		• Wound infection, tissue necrosis and septicaemia	• Contaminated seawater or raw oysters
Aeromonas			
A. hydrophilia	• Aerobic, facultative anaerobe • Motile	• Usually in patients with other serious disease; occasionally isolated from blood, CSF and wounds; diarrhoeal disease; complications of use of medicinal leeches in plastic surgery	
Campylobacter			
C. fetus subspecies	• Microaerophilic	• Acute bloody diarrhoea	• Disease in wide range of animals
Helicobacter pylori (discovered in 1984)	• Spiral organism • Invasive tests require endoscopy (histology, culture and urease-based tests) • Non-invasive H. pylori antibody tests are >85% sensitive	• Peptic ulcer disease • Role in gastric carcinoma and lymphoma	• 50% prevalence in Western countries (higher in developing countries) • Prevalence increases with age • Transmission is thought to occur by the faecal–oral or oral–oral route, and is associated with close contact and poor sanitation

Table 2.8 Gram-negative bacilli: the enterobacteriae (non-spore-forming rods)

Genus and species	Characteristics	Diseases produced in humans	Reservoirs of infection

Escherichia
E. coli
	• Aerobic
	• Lactose fermenter
	• Many antigenic types
	• Enterotoxins
		• Urinary tract and wound infections, peritonitis, cholecystitis, septicaemia, neonatal meningitis
		• Gastroenteritis caused by E. coli:
		  Enterotoxigenic (ETEC) Infantile gastroenteritis and traveller's diarrhoea
		  Enteroaggregative (EAggEC) Infant diarrhoea
		  Enteropathogenic (EPEC) Infant diarrhoea
		  Enteroinvasive (EIEC) Dysentery
		  Enterohaemorrhagic (EHEC) see below
			• Commensal in large bowel
			• Contaminated meat, milk and water

E. coli 0157:H7 (first described in 1983)	• Serotype is designated by somatic (O) and flagellar (H) antigens • Produces shigella-like toxin • Vascular damage may lead to leakage of toxins, e.g. lipopolysaccharide, into circulation, which may initiate complications	• Asymptomatic infection • Non-bloody or bloody diarrhoea • Haemolytic–uraemic syndrome in approx 6% of cases • Thrombotic thrombocytopenic purpura	• Contaminated ground beef, raw milk and water
Klebsiella K. aerogenes	• Aerobic • Lactose fermenter • Heavily encapsulated	• Urinary tract and wound infections, otitis media and meningitis	
K. pneumoniae		• Pneumonia	• Saprophytic in water; also commensal in respiratory tract and intestine of humans and animals

Table 2.8 (Cont'd)

Genus and species	Characteristics	Diseases produced in humans	Reservoirs of infection
Morganella M. morganii	• Lactose fermenter	Urinary tract infection, other forms of sepsis	• Moist environments in hospital • Human and animal intestine
Providencia P. stuartii P. rettgeri P. alcalifaciens		Urinary tract infection, other forms of sepsis	• Moist environments in hospital • Human and animal intestine
Serratia S. marcescens	• Lactose fermenter	Wide range of nosocomial infections	• Moist environments in hospital • Human and animal intestine
Citrobacter C. freundii	• Lactose fermenter	Wide range of nosocomial infections	• Moist environments in hospital • Human and animal intestine
Enterobacter E. aerogenes E. cloacae	• Lactose fermenter	Wide range of nosocomial infections	• Moist environments in hospital • Human and animal intestine
Proteus Pr. mirabilis and other species	• Aerobic • Non-lactose fermenters • Swarming growth on agar medium	• Urinary tract and wound infections	• Commensal in large bowel • Occasionally pathogenic
Salmonella S. typhi* and S. paratyphi A, B and C	• Aerobic • Non-lactose fermenters • Enterotoxins	• Typhoid fever, septicaemia and paratyphoid fever (the enteric fevers)	• Contaminated food and water • Small bowel and gallbladder of cases and carriers
S. typhimurium		• Food poisoning	
S. enteriditis and other species		• Food poisoning	• Cattle, poultry and pigs

*Widal test.
'O' (somatic) antigen appears on the 10th day of infection; antibody titres fall soon after infection.
'H' (flagellar) antigen appears late in the disease; antibodies are more specific and persist for long periods.
'V' (surface) antigen is measure of virulence; antibodies are present in about 75% of carriers.

Table 2.8 (Cont'd)

Genus and species	Characteristics	Diseases produced in humans	Reservoirs of infection
Shigella Sh. flexneri Sh. boydii Sh. sonnei and Sh. dysenteriae	• Non-lactose fermenters • Endotoxin and exotoxin production	• Bacillary dysentery	• Human cases and carriers
Pseudomonas Burkholderia[†] and Stenotrophomonas Ps. aeruginosa	• Aerobic • Non-lactose fermenting • Produces pigments: fluorescein and pyocyanin	• Hospital-acquired infections, pneumonia in ventilated patients, urinary tract and wound infections and septicaemia	

B. pseudomallei [†]	• Diagnosed by blood or pus cultures and serology
	• Resistant to aminoglycosides
	• Used to be classified as member of Pseudomonas group
		• 4 presentations of melioidosis
		  – acute
		  – subacute
		  – chronic
		  – subclinical
		• Pulmonary involvement is commonest site
		• May be chronic with suppurative abscesses at several sites
			• Endemic in South-East Asia (Thailand, Southern China), Central and South America, and Northern Australia
			• Direct contact with contaminated soil or water
			• Sporadic cases occur in temperate climates among travellers to endemic areas

B. cepacia[†]	• Slow growing on conventional solid media	• Lower respiratory tract colonization and infection in cystic fibrosis patients	• Environmental bacillus
S. maltophilia	• Used to be classified as member of Pseudomonas group	• Hospital-acquired infections, often multiply antibiotic-resistant	• Also found in human intestines

[†]Several of the human pathogens formerly classified in the genus Pseudomonas have been reclassified.

Table 2.9 Gram-negative bacilli: the anaerobes

Genus and species	Characteristics	Diseases produced in humans	Reservoirs of infection
Yersinia Y. pestis Y. pseudotuberculosis Y. enterocolitica	• Aerobic	• Bubonic plague, pneumonic plague • Gastroenteritis (invasive infection), mesenteric adenitis	• Rats: fleas transfer infection to man
Bacteroides* B. fragilis and other species	• Anaerobic, non-spore-forming	• Appendicitis, peritonitis, wound infection, brain abscess, septicaemia and postoperative bacteraemic shock	• Commensal in intestine of man and animals • Present in vaginal flora and mouth
Fusobacterium F. fusiforme	• Anaerobic, non-spore-forming	• 'Vincent's' angina, gingivitis and stomatitis are associated with this organism and Borr. vincenti	• Commensal in mouth and intestine
Acinetobacter	• Strict anaerobes	• Hospital-acquired infections • Hospital outbreaks, especially in intensive care units, e.g. ventilator-associated pneumonia, catheter-related septicaemia. Readily colonizes wards and specialist units, e.g. burns units	

*Other non-sporulating anaerobes associated with human disease in addition to Bacteroides, include Actinomyces (pugesi), Propionibacterium (acne, opportunistic infection of prosthetic devices or intravascular lines) and Peptostreptococcus (aspiration pneumonia, sinusitis, brain abscess, intra-abdominal sepsis).

Table 2.10 Gram-negative bacteria: the spirochaetes

Genus and species	Characteristics	Diseases produced in humans	Reservoirs of infection
Borrelia			
Borr. vincenti	• Aerobic • Long with loose spirals	• 'Vincent's' infections of gums or throat	• Commensal of mouth
Borr. recurrentis	• Anaerobic	• European relapsing fever	• Louse-borne
Borr. duttoni	• Anaerobic	• West African relapsing fever	• Tick-borne
Borr. burgdorferi	• Anaerobic	• Lyme disease	• Tick-borne
Treponema			
Tr. pallidum	• Anaerobic • Short with tight spirals, and motile	• Syphilis	• Infected human cases • Sexually transmitted
Tr. pertenue	• Anaerobic	• Yaws	
Tr. carateum	• Anaerobic	• Pinta	
Leptospira			
Lepto. ictero-haemorrhagica	• Anaerobic • Fine, tight spirals with hooked ends	• Weil's disease	• Rodents
Lepto. canicola	• Anaerobic	• Canicola fever	• Dogs and pigs

MICROBIOLOGY

Table 2.11 Gram-negative bacteria: the rickettsiae and bartonellae

Genus and species	Characteristics	Diseases produced in humans	Reservoirs of infection
Rickettsia	• Very small obligate intracellular bacteria • Positive Weil–Felix reaction, except *C. burnetii*		
R. prowazekii		• Epidemic typhus fever	• Louse-borne (humans, flying squirrels)
R. mooseri		• Endemic typhus	• Flea-borne (rats)
R. rickettsii		• Rocky Mountain spotted fever	• Tick-borne (rodents, dogs)
R. tsutsugamushi		• Scrub typhus	• Mite-borne (mites, rodents)
R. typhi		• Endemic marine typhus	• Flea-borne (rats, mice)
R. conorii		• Boutonneuse fever	• Tick-borne (rodents, dogs)
R. africae		• African tick-bite fever	• Tick-borne (rodents)
Coxiella			
C. burnetii	• Typical rickettsia	• Q fever (atypical pneumonia, meningoencephalitis, endocarditis)	• Disease in cattle, sheep and goats • No vector
Bartonella			
B. bacilliformis		• Parasitises blood cells • Oroya fever (fever, rashes, lymphadenopathy, hepatosplenomegaly, cerebellar syndrome, retinal haemorrhages, haemolysis, oedema) • Verruga peruana (benign skin eruption with haemangioma-like skin nodules)	• Infected humans. Found only in South America and transmitted by sandfly vectors (Andes, Peru, Ecuador, Colombia, Thailand)
B. henselae		• Cat scratch fever • Bacillary angiomatosis	• Louse-borne, cat fleas
B. quintana		• Trench fever • Bacillary angiomatosis	

Table 2.11 (Cont'd)

Genus and species	Characteristics	Diseases produced in humans	Reservoirs of infection
Ehrlichia	• Obligate intracellular bacteria	• Fever, headache, abdominal pain, conjunctivitis, lymphadenopathy, jaundice, rash, confusion	• Tick-borne
E. chaffeensis	• Attacks monocytes	• Human monocytic ehrlichiosis	• USA: humans, deer and dogs
E. phagocytophilia (the 'HGE' agent)	• Attacks neutrophils	• Human granulocytic ehrlichiosis • Causes T-cell dysfunction with opportunistic infections	• USA: humans, mice, dogs and deer
Mycoplasma M. pneumoniae	• Very small, obligate intracellular bacteria, with no rigid cell wall • Special enriched media for culture	• Primary atypical pneumonia, upper respiratory tract infection • CNS complications, e.g. Guillain–Barré syndrome	• Human cases and carriers • Droplet spread
Ureaplasma urealyticum	• Related genus that hydrolyses urea	• Urethritis • Endocarditis • Pelvic inflammatory disease	
M. hominis		• Pyelonephritis • Pelvic inflammatory disease • Postabortal and postpartum fever	• Colonization with genital mycoplasmas occurs through sexual contact

Table 2.12 Gram-negative bacteria: chlamydia

Genus and species	Characteristics	Diseases produced in humans	Reservoirs of infection
Chlamydia			
C. psittaci	• Very small spheres • Obligate intracellular bacteria	• Psittacosis	• Sick birds and their infectious excreta • Droplet spread

C. trachomatis	• Very small spheres
	• Obligate intracellular bacteria
	• Serotypes
	  – A, B, Ba, C
	  – D–K
	  – L1, L2, L3
		• Trachoma
		• Cervicitis, conjunctivitis, urethritis, proctitis, pneumonia
		• Lymphogranuloma venereum
		• Urethritis, pelvic inflammatory disease
		• Possible cause of opportunistic infections in the immunocompromised host (arteritis and meningitis)
			• Humans
			• Humans
			• Humans

C. pneumoniae		• Atypical pneumonia	

ENDOTOXINS AND EXOTOXINS (Table 2.13)

Table 2.13 Comparison of exotoxins and endotoxins

Characteristic	Exotoxin	Endotoxin
Produced by:	Certain Gram +ve and –ve bacteria	Gram –ve bacteria
Composed of:	Secreted polypeptide	Lipid A in lipopolysaccharide in cell wall
Stability	Heat labile	Heat stable
Antigenicity	Highly antigenic. Toxoids	Poorly antigenic
Biological actions	Inhibits protein synthesis	LPS molecule induces TNFα
Clinical effects	Various ↑ **Production of cAMP** • Anthrax toxin • Cholera toxin: secretory diarrhoea • *E. coli* enterotoxin: secretory diarrhoea • Pertussis toxin: fluid and electrolyte loss, mucus secretion in respiratory tract **Inhibition of protein synthesis** • Diphtheria toxin: cell death • *P. aeruginosa* exotoxin: cell death • Shiga toxin: watery diarrhoea, haemolytic–uraemic syndrome **Altered nerve transmission** • Tetanus toxin: flaccid paralysis • Botulinum toxin: spastic paralysis	Fever, hypotension, shock, disseminated intravascular coagulation Important in the pathogenesis of Gram –ve septic shock (endotoxic) shock, e.g. *Salmonella, E. coli, Proteus* and *Klebsiella*

ANTIBACTERIAL CHEMOTHERAPY

SPECTRA OF ACTIVITY AND SITES OF ACTION (Table 2.14 and Fig. 2.2)

Table 2.14 Antibacterial chemotherapy: spectra of activity

Antibiotic	Spectrum of activity
Penicillins (penicillinase-sensitive)	**Gram +ve cocci** • *Staph. aureus* (non-penicillinase-producing strains) • *Strep. pneumoniae, Strep. viridans* and β-haemolytic strep. **Gram –ve cocci** • *N. meningitides* and *gonorrhoeae* **Gram +ve bacilli** • *B. anthracis, Cl. tetani* **Resistant organisms** • Penicillinase-producing staphylococci **Other** • *Strep. faecalis* • *N. gonorrhoeae* (some strains) • *H. influenzae* • *E. coli* • *Klebsiella* sp. • *Proteus* sp. • *Pseudomonas aeruginosa* • *Bacteroides fragilis* • *Mycoplasma pneumonia* (lacks a cell wall)
β-Lactamase inhibitors Clavulanic acid Tazobactam Sulbactam	No intrinsic antibacterial activity, but irreversible inhibitors of most plasmid-mediated (but not chromosomally mediated) β-lactamases. When combined with a penicillin, they enable it to resist degradation
Flucloxacillin/methicillin (penicillinase-resistant)	Penicillinase-producing staphylococci[†]

Table 2.14 *(Cont'd)*

Antibiotic	Spectrum of activity
Amoxicillin/ampicillin (penicillinase-sensitive)	• Similar spectrum to penicillins • Also effective against some Gram −ve organisms, e.g. *E. coli*, *H. influenzae*, *Brucella* and *Salmonella* species
Monobactams and carbapenems Aztreonam (monobactam) Imipenem (carbapenem) Both contain β-lactam rings	• Resistant to many β-lactamases
Cephalosporins **1st generation** • Cefadoxil • Cefaloridine • Cefalexin • Cefradine **2nd generation** • Cefamandole • Cefotoxin • Cefuroxime **3rd generation** • Cefotaxime • Ceftriaxone • Ceftazidime	• 1st generation has a similar spectrum to penicillins • 2nd and 3rd generations have a broader spectrum and are active against some Gram −ve bacteria, e.g. *E. coli*, *Salmonella* and *Klebsiella* spp. • 3rd generation also active against anaerobic species, and are very resistant to β-lactamases. Less anti-staphylococcal activity. • Active against *P. aeruginosa* (ceftazidime)
Glycopeptides Vancomycin Teicoplanin	• Aerobic and anaerobic Gram +ve infections • Reserved for resistant staphylococcal infections and *Clostrium difficile*
Linezolid (oxazolidinones)	• Serious Gram +ve infections including MRSA and glycopeptide-resistant strains • Bacteriostatic
Aminoglycosides Amikacin Gentamicin Neomycin Streptomycin	• Serious Gram −ve infections, e.g. *E. coli*, *Pseudomonas*, *H. influenzae* • Some strains of *Staph. aureus* • Low activity against anaerobes, streptococci and pneumococci • *Mycobacterium tuberculosis* (streptomycin/amikacin)
Quinolones Ciprofloxacin Ofloxacin Levofloxacin Nalidixic acid	• Broad spectrum • Broad spectrum • More active against pneumococci, but less against *P. aeruginosa* • Gram +ve bacteria
Tetracycline (longer-acting analogues are demeclocycline and doxycycline) Minocycline	• Broad spectrum against Gram +ve and −ve bacteria and intracellular pathogens • *Brucella*, *Chlamydia*, *Mycoplasma* and *Rickettsia* (Q fever) However, *Proteus*, *Pseudomonas* and many *Staph.* and *Strep.* strains are resistant
Chloramphenicol	• Typhoid and paratyphoid infections • *H. influenzae* meningitis • *Klebsiella* sp. • *Rickettsia* sp. • *Chlamydia* sp.

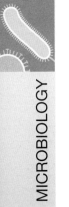

Table 2.14 (Cont'd)	
Antibiotic	*Spectrum of activity*
Macrolides Erythromycin Clarithromycin Azithromycin	• Similar spectrum to penicillins • *Mycoplasma* sp. • Diphtheria carriers • *Legionella pneumophila* • *Chlamydia* sp. • *Campylobacter* sp. Erythromycin: most Gram +ve bacteria and spirochaetes Clarithromycin/azithromycin: *H. influenzae*, atypical mycobacteria and *H. pylori*
Antifolates Sulphonamides/co-trimoxazole/ trimethoprim	• Severe urinary tract infections and chronic bronchitis • *Salmonella* infections • *Brucella* sp. • *Pneumocystis carinii* • *Toxoplasma gondii*
Rifampicin	• Gram +ve and –ve bacteria • *Mycobacterium tuberculosis*
Lincosamides Clindamycin Metronidazole Tinidazole Nitrofurantoin Polymixins Colistin	• Similar to the macrolides; Gram +ve cocci, including penicillin-resistant staphylococci and many anaerobes • Antiprotozoal • Anaerobic bacteria • Gram +ve bacteria and *E. coli* • Gram –ve bacteria, including *Pseudomonas aeruginosa*
Streptogramins Quinupristin Dalfopristin	• Bactericidal • All Gram –ve bacteria and vancomycin-resistant • *Enterococcus faecium*

† Most strains of *Staph. aureus* are sensitive to cloxacillin, cephalosporins and gentamicin; 50% of strains in the community and 85% in hospitals are resistant to benzylpenicillin.

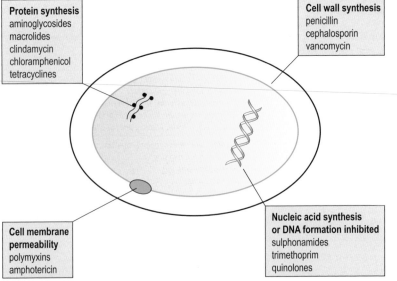

Protein synthesis
aminoglycosides
macrolides
clindamycin
chloramphenicol
tetracyclines

Cell wall synthesis
penicillin
cephalosporin
vancomycin

Cell membrane permeability
polymyxins
amphotericin

Nucleic acid synthesis or DNA formation inhibited
sulphonamides
trimethoprim
quinolones

Fig. 2.2 Sites of action of antibacterials.

BACTERICIDAL AND BACTERIOSTATIC DRUGS (Table 2.15)

> **Bactericidal drugs** kill bacteria; these are preferable if the host is immunocompromised.
> **Bacteriostatic drugs** stop bacterial division; bacteria are eliminated by the host's defences.

Table 2.15 Bactericidal and bacteriostatic drugs

Bactericidal	Bacteriostatic
Penicillins	Tetracyclines
Cephalosporins	Chloramphenicol*
Aminoglycosides	Sulphonamides
Nitrofurantoin	Trimethoprim
Co-trimoxazole	PAS
Erythromycin	Novobiocin
Metronidazole	Clindamycin
Isoniazid, pyrazinamide	Metronidazole
Quinolones (ciprofloxacin, norfloxacin)	Quinolones
Rifampicin	Ethambutol

*Bactericidal against some bacteria, e.g. *Strep. pneumoniae, H. influenzae.*

> **Drugs in combination**
> In general:
> - The combination of a bacteriostatic drug with a bactericidal drug results in *antagonism,* e.g. penicillin with chloramphenicol or tetracycline.
> - Bactericidal drugs in combination tend to be *synergistic,* e.g. aminoglycosides with penicillin.
> - Synergism is unusual when two bacteriostatic drugs are used in combination.

ANTIBIOTIC RESISTANCE

- Natural resistance
- Acquired resistance arises either by:
  1. Emergence of pre-existent resistant mutant pathogens (e.g. penicillinase-resistant) through selective pressure, or by
  2. New mutation through several possible mechanisms.
     (a) *Transformation* – direct uptake of genetic material liberated from another cell.
     (b) *Conjugation* – genetic exchange between two bacterial strains with transfer of a *resistance (R) factor or plasmid* (DNA packages) which is dependent on cell-to-cell contact, e.g. development of gentamicin resistance.
     (c) *Transduction* – transfer of genetic material from one cell to another by means of a *viral vector or bacteriophage,* e.g., development of penicillin resistance by *Staph. aureus*
     (d) *Transfection* – infection of a cell with isolated DNA or RNA from a virus of virus vector.
- Enzyme-mediated resistance is the most important form of acquired resistance seen in clinical isolates, and is generally plasmid-mediated.
- Plasmid gene responsible for resistance may form a transposon. This is capable of 'hopping' from the plasmid to the chromosome, e.g. spread of

β-lactamase genes from plasmids of enteric bacteria to *Haemophilus* and *Neisseria* species.

* Hospital multiple-resistant organisms include *E. coli*, *Klebsiella* and methicillin-resistant *Staph. aureus* (MRSA), which also has variable resistance to the aminoglycosides.

VIRUSES

STRUCTURE OF THE VIRION (Fig. 2.3)

Virion

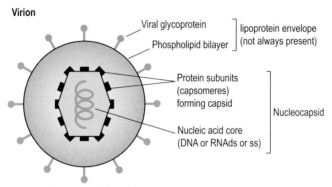

Fig. 2.3 Structure of the virion.

RNA-CONTAINING VIRUSES (Table 2.16)

Table 2.16 RNA-containing viruses		
RNA-containing viruses	*RNA genome*	*Main diseases produced in humans*
Picornaviruses	ss linear	
A. Enteroviruses:		Usually subclinical
Polio (3 types)		• Poliomyelitis, aseptic meningitis
Coxsackie A (23 types)		• Aseptic meningitis, herpangina, conjunctivitis
Coxsackie B (6 types)		• Pleurodynia, myocarditis, aseptic meningitis and encephalitis
Enterovirus 70		• Pandemic conjunctivitis
Enterovirus 72		
ECHO (31 types)		• Aseptic meningitis, conjunctivitis
B. Hepatovirus		• Hepatitis A
C. Rhinoviruses (>100 serotypes)		• Common cold
Orthomyxoviruses and paramyxoviruses	ss linear	
Influenza A, B, C, parainfluenza		• Upper respiratory tract infections, influenza, Reye's syndrome
Mumps		• Mumps, occasionally meningitis
Measles		• Measles, encephalomyelitis, subacute sclerosing panencephalitis
Respiratory syncytial virus (RSV)		• Bronchiolitis
Reoviruses	ds linear	
Reovirus		• Upper respiratory tract infections
Rotavirus		Infantile diarrhoea

Table 2.16 *(Cont'd)*

RNA-containing viruses	RNA genome	Main diseases produced in humans
Coronavirus	ss linear	• Severe acute respiratory syndrome (SARS)
Togaviruses	ss linear	
Alphaviruses		• Encephalitides in the US (St Louis, Western and Eastern equine viruses)
Rubivirus		• Rubella
Arenaviruses	ss circular	
Lassa fever		• Lassa fever
Lymphocytic choriomeningitis		Aseptic meningitis in humans
Filoviruses	ss linear	• Marburg and Ebola fever
Retroviruses*	ss circular	
Human immunodeficiency virus (HIV) 1 and 2		• HIV disease, AIDS (see p. 118) Spectrum of HIV-related neurological disease
Human T-cell lymphotrophic virus (HTLV) HTLV-I		• Adult T-cell leukaemia, HTLV-associated myelopathy, tropical spastic paraparesis (HAM/TSP), HTLV-associated uveitis (HAU)
HTLV-II		• T-cell hairy leukaemia
Rhabdoviruses	ss linear	
Rabies		• Rabies
Calciviruses, astroviruses and small round viruses (SRVs)	ss linear	
Hepatitis E		• Hepatitis
Norwalk virus		• Gastroenteritis
Astrovirus		• Gastroenteritis
Bunyaviruses	ss linear	• California encephalitis • Hanta virus
Flaviviruses	ss linear	• Dengue fever • Hepatitis C • St Louis encephalitis • Yellow fever

ds, double-stranded; ss, single-stranded.
*Retroviruses:
Unlike other RNA viruses, their genomes are replicated through DNA intermediates, using a unique enzyme called reverse transcriptase.

Summary:
Double-stranded RNA – reovirus
Positive single-stranded RNA – picornaviruses, togavirus
Negative single-stranded RNA – orthomyxovirus, paramyxovirus, arenavirus, rhabdovirus, bunyavirus.

IMPORTANT RNA VIRUSES

Hepatitis C (HCV)

• Positive stranded RNA virus of over 9000 nucleotides. It is classified into two major genotypes which demonstrate a geographical variation in distribution. The genotype affects pathogenicity and response to medical therapy.
• Present in 0.5–8% of blood donors.

- The most common forms of transmission are through contaminated blood products (most common cause of post-transfusion hepatitis) and intravenous drug use, but also sexual contact and vertical transmission.
- Acute infection is often asymptomatic; 25% suffer an icteric illness; 60% of patients have a chronic course; 20% will develop cirrhosis after 20 years, and 15% of these will develop hepatocellular carcinoma.
- Diagnosis uses second- and third-generation antibody assays. The polymerase chain reaction can also be used to detect the presence of hepatitis C RNA. Quantitative assays are available for assessing the level of viraemia. A vaccine has not been developed.
- Interferon α and ribavirin are the treatment of choice. Overall 50% of patients will demonstrate a response by 6 months.

Hepatitis D (HDV)
- Defective RNA virus which can only replicate in HBV-infected cells.
- Transmission is by infected blood and sexual intercourse.
- HDV accentuates HBV infection, resulting in more severe liver disease.
- Diagnosis is by HDV antibody (or rarely antigen) detection.
- No vaccines available at present.

Hepatitis E (HEV)
- 27.34 nm diameter unenveloped, single-stranded RNA virus.
- True incidence unknown, but approximately 2% of blood donors are seropositive.
- Most outbreaks and sporadic cases have occurred in developing countries, e.g. China, India, Pakistan and Mexico. Hepatitis E can also be transmitted vertically and by the faecal–oral route. No animal hosts have been identified.
- Incubation period is 2–9 weeks. The majority of cases experience a self-limiting hepatitis. Severe fulminant hepatitis may occur in pregnant women.

Viral haemorrhagic fever
- Filoviruses:
  - Marbury and Ebola.
- Bunyaviruses:
  - Hanta
  - California encephalitis
  - Rift Valley encephalitis
  - Crimean–Congo haemorrhagic fever.
- Arenaviruses:
  - Lassa
  - Lymphocytic choriomeningitis
  - Argentinian haemorrhagic fever
  - Bolivian haemorrhagic fever
  - Venezuelan haemorrhagic fever.
- Incubation period 5–17 days.
- *Clinical features*: purpura, mucosal haemorrhages and multiorgan failure.
- May be asymptomatic or mild disease.

Dengue fever
- Transmitted by *Aedes aegyptii* mosquito.
- Incubation period 7 days.
- *Clinical features*: fever, headache, arthralgia, retro-orbital pain, backache and generalized macular rash. In dengue shock syndrome: mucosal haemorrhage, thrombocytopenic and hypovolaemic shock.

Human immunodeficiency virus (HIV)

- HIV-I (formerly HLTV-III) is a retrovirus containing single-stranded RNA.
- The proviral genome consists of the *gag*, *pol* and *env* genes (Table 2.17 and Fig. 2.4), at least five regulatory genes and long terminal redundancies (LTRs) at each end.
- See also page 118.

Table 2.17 Principal components of HIV	
Genes	*Products*
Structural	Glycoprotein viral envelope
env	• gp160 (gp120 + gp41)
gag	• Core proteins (p24, p17, p15)
Enzymes	
pol	• Reverse transcriptase, protease, integrase, ribonuclease
Regulatory	
tat	
rev	• Activating and regulatory proteins
nef	

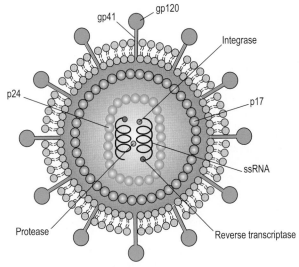

Fig. 2.4 Structure of the genome.

Stages in the life cycle (Fig. 2.5)

1. *Attachment and fusion:* binding of viral gp120/gp41 to CD4 and a chemokine coreceptor (7 transmembrane domain G-protein coupled) is required for HIV infection of cells:
   - Macrophage-tropic (M-tropic) or R5 strains replicate in macrophages and CD4 T cells and use the CCR5 chemokine coreceptor.
   - T-lymphocyte-tropic (T-tropic) or X4 strains use the CXCR4 chemokine coreceptor.
2. *Formation of HIV provirus:* viral reverse transcriptase (RT) synthesizes a complementary DNA from the viral genome, forming an RNA-DNA hybrid. Enzyme then degrades the RNA strand and synthesizes a complementary

MICROBIOLOGY

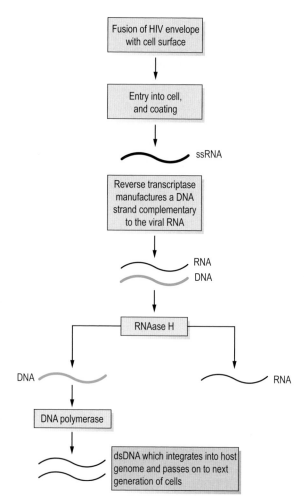

Fig. 2.5 HIV life cycle.

DNA strand, forming a double-strand viral DNA. RT has no proofreading function and copying errors commonly occur during this stage.

3. *Viral integrase* allows integration of viral DNA into host nuclear DNA, forming provirus.
4. Activation of infected T cells promotes *transcription of proviral DNA* into RNA progeny.
5. Nef protein is required for *HIV activation*.
6. Synthesis of viral proteins is followed by *budding of virions* at the cell membrane.

Chemokine receptor mutations
Homozygous 32 base-pair deletion in CCR5 gene (Δ-32 allele) associated with apparent resistance to HIV infection in highly HIV exposed but uninfected persons. Heterozygote mutation in CCR5 and CXCR4 associated with slower rate of disease progression in infected individuals. Chemokine receptor antagonists are in development as potential HIV therapies.

Site of action of main classes of HIV drugs (Fig. 2.6)
1. Nucleoside reverse transcriptase inhibitors (NRTIs)
2. Non-nucleoside reverse transcriptase inhibitors (NNRTIs)
3. Protease inhibitors (PIs)
4. Fusion inhibitors.

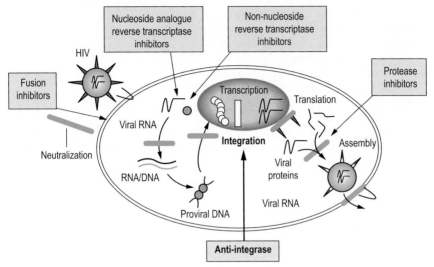

Fig. 2.6 HIV life cycle: potential antiviral targets.

Pathogenesis
- HIV infects CD4 helper cells and other cells that express CD4 (macrophages, dendritic cells in skin and microglial cells in brain), and a chemokine coreceptor. Chronic low-level infection of macrophages acts as the major reservoir for HIV in the body. Cytolytic and latent infection in T cells.
- Immune system abnormalities: change in the cytokine profile; decreased macrophage activity; hypergammaglobulinaemia; decreased CD4 and CD8 proliferation.
- Factors preventing HIV immune control:
  1. Viral 'sanctuary sites' in e.g. brain, genital tract, lymph nodes
  2. Viral latency
  3. Genetic mutation
  4. Serology (p. 72).

Epidemiology
Acquisition of infection:
- The major routes of transmission of HIV-1 are sexual contact, intravenous exposure to blood and blood products, and vertical transmission during pregnancy.
- The median time from infection to development of AIDS in the absence of antiretroviral therapy is 10 years. Rate of disease progression depends on a number of factors including route of transmission, age of infection, symptomatic primary infection, plasma viral load (with viral load <5000 copies/ml, risk of progression to AIDS in 5 years is 8%, and 62% if viral load >36 000 copies/ml), and CD4 count.
- HIV-2 has the same transmission routes as HIV-1 but a lower transmission rate and slower rate of progression; 45% sequence homology with HIV-1; and found mainly in West Africa.

Clinical stages

1. Primary infection:
   - 25–65% have an illness at seroconversion. Usually a mild mononucleosis-like illness 2 weeks–3 months after exposure, with fever, maculopapular rash, sore throat, lymphadenopathy, night sweats and diarrhoea. May include mouth and genital ulcers and neurological features such as encephalopathy, meningitis or myelopathy.
2. Asymptomatic infection – variable duration (1–10 years):
   - CD4 cell counts usually $>350 \times 10^6$/l.
   - Low level of viral load.
3. Symptomatic disease:
   - Viral replication increases and CD4 count declines.
   - Malaise, weight loss, fever, night sweats and development of opportunistic infections.
4. AIDS:
   - Usually correlates with a decrease in the CD4 cell count to $<200 \times 10^6$/l (Table 2.18).

Table 2.18 AIDS indicator diagnoses

Type	Specific disease
Bacterial infection	• *Mycobacterium avium-intracellulare* complex (MAC) infection, disseminated • Extrapulmonary tuberculosis *(Mycobacterium tuberculosis)* • *Salmonella* septicaemia, recurrent
Viral infection	• Cytomegalovirus disease • Herpes simplex virus infection, chronic or disseminated • Progressive multifocal leukoencephalopathy (JC virus)
Fungal infection	• Candidiasis of the oesophagus, trachea or lungs *(Candida albicans)* • Cryptococcal meningitis *(Cryptococcus neoformans)* • Histoplasmosis *(Histoplasma capsulatum)* • *Pneumocystis carinii* pneumonia
Protozoal infection	• Cryptosporidiosis, chronic with diarrhoea *(Cryptosporidium* spp.) • Toxoplasmosis of the brain *(Toxoplasma gondii)*
Neoplasia	• Cervical cancer (invasive) • Kaposi's sarcoma • Primary lymphoma of the brain • Other non-Hodgkin's lymphomas
Other	• HIV wasting syndrome

A diagnosis of AIDS is made for HIV-infected patients who manifest any of these diseases, regardless of their T-cell count.

Human T-cell leukaemia viruses (HTLV-I)

- Identified in 1980.
- Unique 3′ region (PX region) crucial in host gene activation.
- Endemic in Southern Japan, the Caribbean, Central and South America and parts of Africa.
- Cause of adult T-cell leukaemia (ATL) in 1–4% over a lifetime; associated myelopathy or tropical spastic paraparesis (HAM TSP) (0.02–5%) in 4th decade; lymphadenopathy; hepatosplenomegaly; skin lesions; hypercalcaemia. Blood contains abnormal lymphocytes with lobulated nuclei ('flower cells').

DNA-CONTAINING VIRUSES (Table 2.19)

Table 2.19 DNA-containing viruses		
DNA-containing viruses	*DNA genome*	*Main diseases produced in humans*
Herpesviruses	ds linear	
Alpha subfamily		
Herpes simplex (HSV) I and II		Stomatitis, cold sores, keratoconjunctivitis, genital herpes, neonatal herpes, aseptic meningitis and encephalitis
Varicella-zoster (VZV)		Chicken pox, herpes zoster
Gamma subfamily		
Epstein–Barr virus (EBV)		Infectious mononucleosis, also possible Burkitt's lymphoma and nasopharyngeal carcinoma
Human herpesvirus 7 (HHV-7)		Roseola infantum, febrile convulsions
Human herpesvirus 8 (HHV-8)		Kaposi's sarcoma, primary effusion lymphoma (HIV related), multicentre Multicentric Castleman's disease (HIV related)
Beta subfamily		
Cytomegalovirus		Cytomegalic inclusion disease, pneumonitis, retinitis and colitis, intrauterine infection
Human herpesvirus 6 (HHV-6)		Roseola infantum, mononucleosis with cervical infection, encephalitis in transplant patients
Hepadnaviruses	ds partially circular	
Hepatitis B		Hepatitis
Adenoviruses (41 serotypes)	ds linear	Possible vector gene therapy Upper respiratory tract infections, epidemic keratoconjunctivitis, diarrhoea
Papovaviruses	ds linear	
Papillomavirus		Warts
Polyoma (BK and JC) viruses		Progressive multifocal leucoencephalopathy
Poxviruses	ds linear	
Variola		Smallpox
Vaccinia		Vaccinia (used in vaccines)
Molluscum contagiosum		Molluscum contagiosum
Orf		Pustular dermatitis
Parvoviruses	ss linear	
Parvovirus B19		Erythema infectiosum ('fifth disease'), haemolytic and aplastic crises, arthropathy, abortion
ds, double-stranded; ss, single-stranded.		

DNA-containing viruses: the HHAPPP(Y) viruses

Herpesviruses,   **P**apovaviruses,
Hepadnaviruses,   **P**ox viruses,
Adenoviruses,   **P**arvoviruses.
All DNA viruses are double-stranded except Parvoviruses.

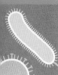

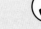

Comparison of DNA and RNA viruses
In general:
- **All DNA viruses** are **double-stranded** (except parvovirus) and naked (except for herpesvirus, poxvirus and hepadnavirus).
- **All RNA viruses** are **single-stranded** (except reovirus) and enveloped (except for picornavirus and reovirus).

HUMAN SLOW VIRUS INFECTIONS (Table 2.20)

Table 2.20 Human slow virus infections

Virus/agent	Disease
Measles	Subacute sclerosing panencephalitis (SSPE)
Papovavirus (JC virus)	Progressive multifocal leucoencephalopathy (PML)
	HIV encephalopathy
Rubella	Progressive rubella panencephalitis (PRP)
Retrovirus	Acquired immune deficiency syndrome (AIDS)
Prion disease	Kuru
	Creutzfeldt–Jakob disease (CJD) and its variant form
	Gerstmann–Sträussler–Scheinker disease (GSS)
	Fatal familial insomnia
?Measles virus	Multiple sclerosis

Prion diseases (transmissible spongiform encephalopathies)
Prion protein:
- Proteinaceous infectious particle; virus-like particle, but with no nucleic acid content (conformationally altered forms of a normal protein).
- Exceptionally resistant to heat and other inactivating agents.
- Prion protein occurs in a normal form (PrPc) and an abnormal form (PrPSc) which forms aggregates and causes disease. PrPSc can bind to PrPc on cell surfaces and convert the normal form to the abnormal form.
- The pathogenic prion-related protein (PrP) is encoded by the PRNP gene on chromosome 20. It is protease-resistant and accumulates in the brain. In the familial forms, mutations of the PRNP gene are found.
Clinical features:
- Rare.
- Long incubation periods (1–30 years).
- Protracted, severe progressive course; always fatal.
- Present classically with rapidly progressive neurodegeneration, cognitive impairment, ataxia, myoclonus and motor dysfunction.
- May be genetic, sporadic or infectious. Iatrogenic transmission of CJD has been well documented following human growth hormone therapy, transplantation of infected tissue or by contact with contaminated medical devices. How CJD is transmitted from cattle with bovine spongiform encephalopathy remains controversial.
- No antibody or immune response.
- Histologically these diseases resemble amyloidoses, in which the host-encoded protein acquires a β-sheet conformation producing amyloid, which accumulates and causes vacuolar degeneration of neurons, and gliosis with no inflammation.

ONCOGENIC VIRUSES (Table 2.21)

- May possess either RNA or DNA.
- Invasion of the host cell results in recombination with the host genome, causing permanent infection of the cell. These transformed cells differ from normal cells in that they have lost their capacity for contact inhibition.
- The RNA viruses become integrated by an RNA-dependent DNA polymerase (reverse transcriptase).

Table 2.21 Oncogenic viruses

Virus	Disease
Poxvirus	Molluscum contagiosum
Hepatitis B	Liver cancer
EBV	Burkitt's lymphoma (in malaria-infested parts of Africa), and other lymphomas in immunosuppression; nasopharyngeal carcinomas (S. China)
Human papilloma virus (HPV)	Skin warts (serotypes 1–4) Anogenital warts or condylomata acuminata (serotypes 6, 11) Laryngeal papillomas (serotypes 6, 11) Cervical intraepithelial neoplasia (CIN) (serotypes 16, 18)
HTLV-I	Adult T-cell leukaemia (ATLL)
HHV-8	Kaposi's sarcoma
Adenovirus, SV40	Malignant neoplasms in mice

IMPORTANT SEROLOGICAL TESTS

1. HEPATITIS B SEROLOGY (Table 2.22 and Fig. 2.7)

Hepatitis B (HB)
- Part double-stranded, 42-mm enveloped particle with inner 27-mm core particle (Dane particle).
- Three viral antigens:
  1. Surface antigen (HBsAg) leading to production of HBsAb.
  2. Core antigen in Dane particles (HBcAg) leading to production of HBcAb.
  3. DNA polymerase-associated 'e' antigen (HBeAg) is formed as the result of the breakdown of core antigen released from infected liver cells. Marker of infectivity.
- Whole particle and surface antigen present in serum, saliva and semen.

Table 2.22 Interpretation of hepatitis B serum antigen and antibody markers

HBsAg	Anti-HBs	Anti-HBc	Interpretation
+	–	–	Early acute disease – patient is considered infectious
+		+	Acute disease or chronic carrier – patient is considered infectious
–	+	+	Convalescing from the disease or immune
–	+	+	Immune via disease or vaccination
–	–	+	Recent disease. Serum taken after HBsAg disappeared and before anti-HBs – patient is considered infectious

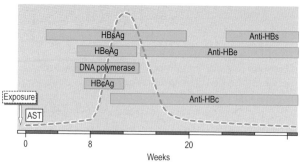

Fig. 2.7 **Timing of virological events in acute hepatitis B.**

2. HIV SEROLOGY

- Serum antibody to HIV may appear between 2 weeks and 1 year after infection (most commonly 1–3 months after infection).
- An enzyme-linked immunoabsorbent assay (ELISA) is used to screen for HIV antibody. When a positive test is obtained, it should be confirmed with a Western blot or further Elisa assay.
- The Western blot measures patient antibody to specific HIV proteins (see p. 119). Combining these two tests, the false-positive rate is 1 in 135 200.
- Detection of RNA viral load in plasma along with the CD4 count is important in monitoring disease progression and response to antiretroviral therapy.

3. SYPHILIS SEROLOGY

Non-treponemal tests (VDRL and RPR)

These detect an antibody-like substance (anticardiolipin antibody which is not a specific antitreponemal antibody) which appears more commonly and in high titre in treponemal disease. Relatively insensitive in primary/late syphilis.

1. Venereal disease research laboratory (VDRL) test: antibody detected by a flocculation reaction.
2. Rapid plasma reagin (RPR).

Treponemal tests

These are more specific.

1. Treponema pallidum haemagglutination test (TPHA).
2. Treponema pallidum immobilization test (TPI).
3. Fluorescent treponemal antibody absorption test (FTA-ABS): most sensitive test for syphilis; positive early in the disease.

Interpretation of results

- If treatment is early in primary infection, then serological tests may remain negative.
- If treated during the secondary stage when serology is usually positive, non-treponemal tests revert to negative within a year, but treponemal tests usually remain positive for years.
- Treatment in the late stages may not affect the serological reactions.
- Non-treponemal tests positive and treponemal tests negative: classic biological false-positive reaction, such as with acute viral illness, collagen vascular disease, pregnancy, leprosy and malaria.
- False-positive treponemal tests: genital herpes, psoriasis, rheumatoid arthritis, SLE.

SPECTRA OF ACTIVITY AND SITES OF ACTION OF ANTIVIRAL DRUGS (Table 2.23 and Fig. 2.8)

- Aciclovir and related compounds are characterized by their selective phosphorylation in herpes-infected cells via a viral thymidine kinase (TK) (rather than a host kinase).
- Phosphorylation yields a triphosphate nucleotide that inhibits viral DNA polymerase and viral DNA synthesis.
- These drugs are selectively toxic to infected cells, because in the absence of viral TK, the host kinase activates only a small amount of drug.

Table 2.23 Drugs used for main viral infections (see Fig. 2.8)

Influenza (A, B)	Hepatitis (HBV, HCV)	Human papilloma virus (HPV)	Cytomegalovirus (CMV)	Herpes simplex viruses (HSV-1, HSV-2)	Varicella zoster virus (VZV)
A: Amantadine Rimantadine A & B: Oseltamivir Ribavirin Zanamivir	B: Lamivudine Adefovir Tenofovir B & C: Interferons (IFNs) C: IFNs + ribavirin	Cidofovir IFNs	Cidofovir Fomivirsen Foscarnet Ganciclovir	Aciclovir Famciclovir Foscarnet Idoxyuridine Valaciclovir	Aciclovir Ara-A Cidofovir Famciclovir Valaciclovir

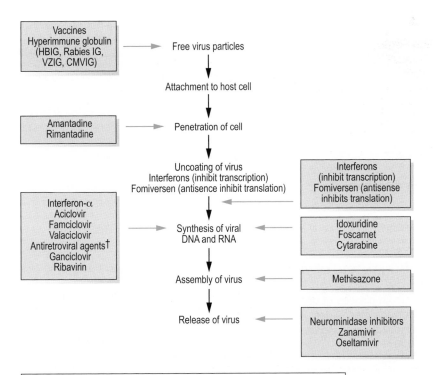

Fig. 2.8 Sites of action of antivirals.

†Nucleoside reverse transcriptase inhibitors (NRTI) e.g. ZDV, ddl, ddc, 3TC, d4T
Non-nucleoside reverse transcriptase inhibitors (NNRTI) e.g. nevaripine, delavirdine

MICROBIOLOGY

FUNGI

IMPORTANT FUNGAL INFECTIONS (Table 2.24)

Table 2.24 Important fungal infections	
Genus	*Main diseases produced in humans*
Dermatophytes	
Epidermophyton	• Tinea of foot, groin and nail
Microsporum	• Tinea of head and body
Tricophyton	• Tinea of head, body and nails ('athlete's foot')
Malassezia	• Pityriasis versicolor
Pathogenic yeasts	
Candida (similar to yeasts but can also form long, non-branching filaments)	• Candidiasis, oral thrush, oesophagitis, vulvovaginitis and skin disease • Causes septicaemia with endocarditis and meningitis in immunocompromised persons
Torulopsis	• Oropharyngitis, vulvovaginitis, septicaemia and endocarditis
Cryptococcus	• Meningitis, lung, skin and bone infection
Dimorphic fungi (i.e. grow as moulds and yeasts)	
Blastomyces dermatidis	• N. American blastomycosis (especially Mississippi and Ohio valleys): primary infection of lungs, and sometimes skin
Paracoccidioides brasiliensis	• S. American blastomycosis • Less commonly Central America
Coccidioides immitis	• Coccidioidomycosis: usually a benign infection of the lungs; rarely disseminated spread. Occurs in USA from California to Texas, Central and S. America
Histoplasma capsulatum	• Acute or chronic pulmonary infection • Disseminated histoplasmosis with granulomata especially in lymphoreticular organs. Meningitis and endocarditis may also occur. Found in Eastern and Central USA
Histoplasma capsulatum duboisii	• African histoplasmosis
Miscellaneous fungal infections	
Aspergillus	• Primary infection usually of the lung: asthma. • Systemic infection: aspergillosis
Mucor and rhizopus	• Phycomycosis: local infection of nose, paranasal sinuses, lungs and gastrointestinal tract may lead to systemic infection and meningitis
Penicillium marneffei	• Penicilliosis found in South-East Asia and southern China
Sporothrix schenckii	• Sporotrichosis; worldwide distribution

ANTIFUNGAL CHEMOTHERAPY

Four main classes of drugs:
1. Polyene macrolides
2. Imidazole antifungals
3. Triazole
4. Others.

1. **Polyene macrolides** (amphotericin B and nystatin):
   - Bind to membrane ergosteral altering membrane integrity.
   - Amphotericin is a broad-spectrum antifungal used in serious systemic infections.
   - Nystatin is used to suppress oral and vaginal candida.

2. **Imidazoles** (clotrimazole, miconazole and ketoconazole):
   – Inhibit fungal lipid synthesis in cell membranes.
   – Used for candidiasis and dermatophyte infections and systemic mycoses (ketoconazole).
3. **Triazoles** (fluconazole, itraconazole, voriconazole):
   – Fluconazole: active against *Candida* species, *cryptococcus* neoformans.
   – Itraconazole: active against moulds e.g. Aspergillus and dimorphic fungi, e.g. Histoplasma and Blastomyces.
   – Voriconazole: active against both yeasts and fungi.
4. **Others:**
   (a) *Allylamines* (terbinafine):
       – Dermatophyte infections.
   (b) *Flucytosine*:
       – Potent inhibitor of DNA synthesis.
       – Adjunct to amphotericin in cryptococcal meningitis.
   (c) *Griseofulvin*:
       – Interferes with microtubule formation or nuclear acid synthesis.
       – Used for widespread and intractable dermatophyte infection where topical therapy has failed.
   (d) *Candins* (echinocandins, caspofungins):
       – Depresses cell wall formation by inhibiting glycan synthesis.
       – Used for treatment of candidiasis and aspergillosis.

- *Amphotericin B* is the drug of choice for all agents listed, except for candida (nystatin).
- *Griseofulvin* is the drug of choice for dermatophytes but is ineffective against aspergillus.
- *Ketoconazole* is recommended for blastomycosis, coccidioidomycosis and candida.
- *Miconazole* is recommended for coccidioidomycosis, cryptococcus and candida.
- *Fluconazole* is used to treat candidiasis and cryptococcal meningitis.
- *5-Flucytosine* is used mainly in the treatment of cryptococcus in combination with amphotericin B.

PARASITES

IMPORTANT PARASITIC INFECTIONS (Table 2.25)

Table 2.25 Important parasitic infections		
Genus	*Mode of infection*	*Main disease produced in humans*
Taenia solium (pork tapeworm)	Via ingestion of ova	• Enteritis
Enterobius vermicularis (threadworms)	Via ingestion of ova	• Pruritus ani
Ascaris lumbricoides (roundworms)	Via ingestion of ova	• Enteritis, pneumonitis, ileal and biliary obstruction, acute cholangitis
Toxocara canis	Via ingestion of ova	• Visceral larvae migrans, toxocariasis (hepatosplenomegaly, chorioretinitis and CNS mass lesions)
Echinococcus granulosa	Via ingestion of ova	• Pulmonary and hydatid disease
Entamoeba histolytica	Via ingestion of cyst	• Amoebiasis, amoebic liver abscess
Naegleria and Acanthamoeba	Via ingestion of cyst	• Meningitis

Table 2.25 (Cont'd)

Genus	Mode of infection	Main disease produced in humans
Coccidia	Via ingestion of cyst	
Cryptosporidium parvum	Via ingestion of cyst	• Cryptosporidiosis, severe protracted diarrhoea in AIDS
Isospora belli	Via ingestion of cyst	
Cyclospora cayetanensis	Via ingestion of cyst	
Microsporidia		
Enterocytozoon bieneusi		• Severe protracted diarrhoea in AIDS
Encephalitozoon intestinalis cuniculi		• Severe protracted diarrhoea and eye disease in AIDS patients
Giardia lamblia	Via ingestion of cyst	• Giardiasis, malabsorption
Toxoplasma gondii	Via ingestion of cyst	• Widespread, usually asymptomatic infection, encephalitis in immunocompromised Also intrauterine infection
Trichinella spiralis	Via ingestion of larvae	• Trichinosis (myalgia and eosinophilia)
Taenia saginata (beef tapeworm)	Via ingestion of larvae	• Enteritis
Taenia solium	Via ingestion of larvae	• Enteritis and cysticercosis (focal • lesions in skeletal and cardiac muscle, subcutaneous tissue and brain)
Diphyllobothrium latum	Via ingestion of larvae	• Enteritis and vitamin B$_{12}$ deficiency
Ancylostoma duodenale (hookworm)	Via larval penetration of skin	• Enteritis and iron deficiency anaemia
Schistosoma mansoni	Via cercarial penetration of skin	• Enteric schistosomiasis, hepatic fibrosis (S. America, Caribbean, Africa and Middle East)
Schistosoma japonicum	Via cercarial penetration of skin	• Enteric schistosomiasis, precancerous bladder inflammation (Far East)
Schistosoma haematobium	Via cercarial penetration of skin	• Haematuria
Plasmodium falciparum, vivax and ovale	Via bite of arthropod vector	• Malaria, blackwater fever (falciparum)
Leishmania (Old World)		
L. donovani	Sandfly	• Visceral leishmaniasis (Africa, Asia)
L. tropica	Sandfly	• Cutaneous leishmaniasis
L. major	Sandfly	(Africa, Asia, Mediterranean)
Leishmania (New World)		
L. braziliensis	Sandfly	• 'Espundia' cutaneous and mucosal leishmaniasis (Latin America)
L. mexicana	Sandfly	• Cutaneous (Mexico, Central America, Texas)
L. chagasi	Sandfly	• Visceral (Latin America)
Onchocerca volvulus	Black Fly	• Onchocerciasis ('river blindness'), skin nodules
Wuchereria bancrofti	Mosquito	• Lymphadenitis and elephantiasis
Brugia malayi	Mosquito	
Loa loa	Fly	• Calabar swellings, subconjunctival adult worms
Trypanosoma		
T. rhodiense	Tsetse fly	• Sleeping sickness
T. gambiense	Tsetse fly	
T. cruzi	Reduvid bug	• Chagas' disease
Trichomonas vaginalis	Via direct contact	• Silent venereal infection in females • and males, or acute vaginitis in • females and acute urethritis in males
Pneumocystis carinii	Via inhalation	• Pneumonitis in premature infants and immunosuppressed adults (e.g. AIDS)

PLASMODIAL INFECTION (Table 2.26)

Table 2.26 Plasmodial infection in humans		
Species	Fever cycle (h)	Clinical condition
Plasmodium falciparum malaria	36–48	Malignant tertian
Plasmodium malariae	72	Quartan malaria
Plasmodium ovale	36–48	Benign tertian malaria
Plasmodium vivax	36–48	Benign tertian malaria

Life cycle of *Plasmodium* species (Fig. 2.9)

1. The Anopheles mosquito is the intermediate host. It is infected by blood-borne gametocytes from humans.
2. These develop in the mosquito and sporozoites are formed which pass into the blood stream when a human is bitten.

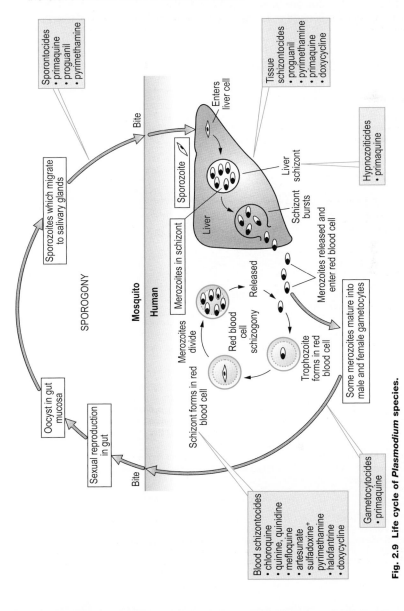

Fig. 2.9 Life cycle of *Plasmodium* species.

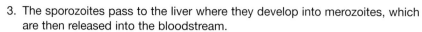

3. The sporozoites pass to the liver where they develop into merozoites, which are then released into the bloodstream.
4. These are taken up by the erythrocytes where they develop and divide (schizogony). This coincides with the clinical attack of malaria following rupture of erythrocytes, and is the phase most susceptible to treatment.
5. Some gametocytes are formed and are released into the blood where they can reinfect the mosquito.

Prophylaxis

- Suppressive prophylaxis involves the use of blood schizontocides to prevent acute attacks.
- Tissue schizontocides against the sporozoite are used to prevent the parasite becoming established in the liver.

Treatment

- Blood schizontocides are used for acute attacks.
- A hypnozonticide is used to kill dormant liver forms to prevent relapsing malaria.

ANTIPARASITE CHEMOTHERAPY (Table 2.27)

Table 2.27 Antiparasite chemotherapy

Organism	Drug
Nematodes (roundworms)	Mebendozale
Trichinella spiralis	Mebendozale
Enterobius vermicularis	Mebendozale
Ancylostoma duodenale	Mebendozale
Ascaris lumbricoides	Mebendozale, piperazine
Strongloides stercoralis	Thiabendazole, albendazole
Cestodes (tapeworms)	Niclosamide, praziquantel
Taenia saginata	Niclosamide, praziquantel
Taenia solium	Niclosamide
Echinococcus granulosa	Albendazole
Diphyllobothrium latum	Niclosamide, praziquantel
Trematodes (blood flukes)	
Schistosoma mansoni, japonicum and haematobium	Praziquantel
Protozoa	
Entamoeba histolytica	
Giardia lamblia	– Metronidazole, Tinidazole
Trichomonas vaginalis	
Plasmodium spp.	– **4-Aminoquinolines**, e.g. chloroquine, block nucleic acid synthesis by the malarial parasites in their erythrocyte forms. Used as suppressive treatment and for clinical attack
	– **Diaminopyridamines**, e.g. pyrimethamine, inhibit dihydrofolate reductase and so block the synthesis of folic acid. Effective against the erythrocyte form and formation of sporozoites
Toxoplasma gondii	– Pyrimethamine and sulphadiazine
Pneumocystis carinii	– Trimethoprim and sulphamethoxazole, pentamidine
Wucheria bancrofti	
Loa loa	
Brugia malayi	– Diethylcarbamazine, praziquantel, ivermectin
Onchocerca volvulus	
Dracunculus medinensis	– Metronidazole
Trypanosomiasis	– Suramin, pentamidine and melasoprol (for CNS disease)
Leishmaniasis	– Sodium stibogluconate, pentamidine

OTHER PATHOGENS

COMMON OPPORTUNISTIC PATHOGENS (Table 2.28)

Table 2.28 Common opportunistic pathogens

Bacteria	*Staphylococcus aureus*
	Coagulase-negative staphylococci
	Mycobacterium avium-intracellulare
	Enterobacteriaceae
Fungi	*Candida* species
	Aspergillus species
	Histoplasma species
	Isospora species
	Cryptococcus neoformans
	Pneumocystis carinii
Protozoa	Toxoplasma, cryptosporidiosis
Parasites	*Strongyloides stercoralis*
Viruses	Herpes simplex viruses
	Cytomegalovirus
	Varicella zoster virus
	Epstein–Barr virus

ZOONOSES (Table 2.29)

Table 2.29 Zoonoses

Bacteria	Rickettsiae/Chlamydiae	Viruses	Parasitical
Anthrax	Psittacosis	Dengue fever	Babesiosis
Brucellosis	Q fever	Encephalitides*	Cryptosporidiosis
Listeriosis	Rocky Mountain spotted fever	Haemorrhagic fevers	Cysticercosis
Plague		Rabies	Larva migrans
Salmonellosis		Yellow fever	Schistosomiasis
Tularaemia			Taeniasis
			Trichinosis
			Toxoplasmosis

*e.g. St Louis, Venezualan, Californian, Western equine

ALERT ORGANISMS (Table 2.30)

Table 2.30 Healthcare-associated 'ALERT' organisms

Bacteria	Viruses	Fungi
MRSA and glycopeptide-resistant *Staph. aureus*	RSV, influenza, parainfluenza	Aspergillus in bone marrow transplant units
Vancomycin-resistant enterococci	Rotaviruses, Norwalk-like virus	
Verocytotoxin-producing *E. coli*	Varicella zoster virus	
Multiresistant coliforms	HIV, hepatitis B and C	
C. difficile		
Strep. pyogenes		
Penicillin-resistant pneumococci		

INCUBATION PERIODS (Tables 2.31–2.32)

Table 2.31 Incubation of common infections

Incubation period	Disease
Short: 1–7 days	Anthrax Diphtheria Gonorrhoea Meningococcus Influenza Cytomegalovirus Group A streptococci (erysipelas) Scarlet fever Bacillary dysentery
Intermediate: 7–14 days	Measles Lassa fever Whooping cough Malaria Tetanus Typhus fever Typhoid Poliomyelitis
Long: 14–21 days	Brucellosis Amoebiasis Chickenpox Rubella Mumps
Very long: >21 days	Hepatitis: A (2–6 weeks) B (2–6 months) C (6 weeks–6 months)

Table 2.32 Food poisoning incubation periods

Organism	Incubation period (h)	Food
Short		
Scombrotoxin	Up to 1 hour	Fish
Bacillus cereus	0.5–6.0	Rice
Staphyloccus aureus	1–6	Meat
Intermediate		
Vibrio parahaemolyticus	6–36	Seafood
Clostridium perfringens	12–24	Meat
Clostridium botulinum	12–36	Processed food
E. coli	12–72	Food or water
Salmonellae	18–48	Meat, eggs, poultry
Yersinia enterocolitica	24–36	Milk
Small round structured viruses	36–72	Any food
Longer		
Rotavirus	1–7 days	Food or water
Shigella	2–3 days	Any food
Cryptosporidium	4–12 days	Water
Campylobacter jejuni	2–5 days	Milk, water
Giardia lamblia	1–4 weeks	Water

VACCINES

Vaccines in clinical use are shown in Table 2.33, and live attenuated and killed vaccines are compared in Table 2.34.

Table 2.33 Vaccines in clinical use

Live attenuated bacteria	Bacillus Calmette–Guérin (BCG)
Live attenuated viruses	Measles ⎫ Mumps ⎬ i.e. MMR Rubella ⎭ Polio (oral/Sabin) Varicella zoster Yellow fever Typhoid (Ty21a)
Whole killed, organism	Rabies Polio (Salk) Pertussis Typhoid Cholera Influenza*
Subcellular fragment Inactivated toxin (toxoid) Capsular polysaccharide Surface antigen	Diphtheria Tetanus Cholera (new) Meningococcus (group A and C) Pneumococcus (23 capsular types), Haemophilus influenzae b (Hib) Typhoid (new) Hepatitis B recombinant-DNA-based

*Non-live subunit trivalent preparation with two A and one B subunits. Vaccination is recommended for all groups at risk, e.g. patients with diabetes, renal failure, and the immunosuppressed.

Table 2.34 Differences between live attenuated and killed vaccines

Factor	Live attenuated	Killed
Immunity	Strong; localized Usually appropriate type Usually good memory May induce 'herd' immunity	May be weak May be inappropriate (e.g. antibody vs CMI) Memory variable (poor with polysaccharides)
Boosting	Usually not required	Often required
Adjuvant	Not required	Usually required
Safety	Unsafe in immunocompromised, may revert to virulence	Usually safe if properly inactivated
Storage	Depends on 'cold chain'	Usually no problem
Side-effects	Egg hypersensitivity (some viruses)	Toxicity (e.g. pertussis?)

IMMUNIZATION SCHEDULE

The ages at which immunization should take place, as recommended in the UK, are shown in Table 2.35.

Table 2.35 Recommended UK immunization schedule

Recommended age	Vaccine
Neonatal	BCG (infants of Asian mothers or with family history of active TB)
2-months	Diphtheria-tetanus-pertussis (DPT)—1st dose
	Oral polio vaccine (OPV)—1st dose
	Haemophilus influenzae b (Hib) vaccine
	Meningococcal
3 months	DPT—2nd dose
	OPV—2nd dose
4 months	DPT—3rd dose
	OPV—3rd dose
1–2 years	Measles/mumps/rubella (MMR)
3–5 years or at	DT—booster
school entry	OPV—booster
	MMR booster
10–13 years	BCG (for tuberculin –ve)*
11–13 years	Rubella (girls only)
13–18 years	Rubella for seronegative women of child-bearing age
(on leaving	Influenza† and Hepatitis B for individuals in high
school)	risk groups (see box below)
	Polio and tetanus booster
	Diphtheria booster with low-dose vaccine

*Other indications: contracts of known BCG cases; neonates born in households where there is active TB; immigrants from countries with a high prevalence of TB, and their children, wherever born; health workers at risk of exposure, e.g. lab. workers and veterinary staff.
†Indications: the elderly, especially those in long-term residential accommodation; children in residential accommodation who have reached the age of 4 years; those with chronic heart, lung and renal disease, or diabetes; medical, nursing and ambulance staff.

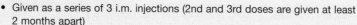

Hepatitis B vaccination
- Given as a series of 3 i.m. injections (2nd and 3rd doses are given at least 2 months apart)
- Hbs Ab response in 95–99%. Booster dose is given to 50% with non-protective antibody titres (increased risk with immunocompromised, haemodialysis patients, aged ≤ 40 years and smokers)

Indications in low prevalence areas
1. Homosexual men
2. Intravenous drug users
3. Patients with clotting disorders
4. Chronic renal failure patients on dialysis
5. Health care workers
6. Partners of infectious Hep and Ag patients
7. Persons with multiple sexual partners
8. Infants born to Hbs Ag-positive mothers (at birth)

Contraindications to recombinant vaccine
Allergies to yeast or to components of vaccine

CONTRAINDICATIONS

Contraindications to immunization

1. Febrile illness, intercurrent infections
2. Hypersensitivity to egg protein contraindicates influenza vaccine; previous anaphylactic reaction to egg contraindicates influenza and yellow fever vaccines.

No live vaccine

No live vaccine should be used in cases of:

1. Immunodeficiency
2. Immunosuppression
3. High dose of corticosteroids
4. Malignancy, e.g. lymphoma, leukaemia, or Hodgkin's disease
5. Pregnancy.

Non-contraindications

The following are *not* contraindications to immunization:

1. Family history of any adverse reactions following immunization
2. Family history of convulsions
3. Previous history of pertussis, measles, rubella or mumps infection
4. Prematurity
5. Stable neurological conditions, e.g. cerebral palsy or Down's syndrome
6. Asthma, eczema or hay fever
7. History of jaundice after birth
8. Over the age recommended in immunization schedule
9. Recent or imminent surgery
10. Replacement corticosteriods.

Preparations for passive immunization

Normal or specific immunoglobulin

- Measles, hepatitis A and B, chickenpox, tetanus, rabies, rubella and mumps.
- All used for prophylaxis and postexposure treatment (within 72 hours) except hepatitis A.

Antitoxins

- Diphtheria, gas gangrene and botulism.
- All used for prophylaxis and postexposure treatment.

TRAVEL VACCINES (Table 2.36)

Table 2.36 Travel vaccines

Vaccine	Booster interval (years)	No. of doses	Time interval between 1st and 2nd doses	Time interval between 2nd and 3rd doses
Hepatitis A (Havrix)	5–10	3	2–4 months	6–12 months
Hepatitis B	2–5	3	1 month	5 months
Japanese encephalitis	1–4	3	1–2 weeks	2–4 weeks
Meningococcus	3	1		
Polio	5–10	3	>6 weeks	>6 weeks
Tetanus	5–10	3	4 weeks	4 weeks
Tick typhus	5–10	3	1–3 months	9–12 months
Typhoid s.c. (Vi)	3	1		
Rabies	10	3	7–28 days	6–12 months
Yellow fever	10	1		

STERILIZATION AND DISINFECTION

- *Sterilization*: the process by which all viable microorganisms, including spores, are removed or killed.
- *Disinfection*: the process by which most, but not all viable microorganisms are removed or killed.
- *Pasteurization*: the process used to eliminate pathogens in foods such as milk. Spores are unaffected.

The characteristics of some agents used in sterilization and disinfection are presented in Table 2.37.

Table 2.37 Agents used in sterilization and disinfection

Group	Example	Bactericidal Gram-negative	Bactericidal Gram-positive	Sporicidal	Fungicidal	Viricidal	Mycobactericidal	Uses
Alcohols	70% ethyl alcohol	+	+	–	–	–	–	Skin antiseptic
Aldehydes	Formaldehyde	+	+	+	+	+	+	Fumigation
	Glutaraldehyde	+	+	+	+	+	+	Disinfection of fibreoptic endoscopes
Biguanides	Chlorhexidine	–	+	–	–	–	–	Hand wash; skin antiseptic
Halogens	Hypochlorites Chlorine	+	+	±	+	+	–	General environmental cleaning; blood spills; treating water
	Iodine	+	+	±	+	+	–	With alcohol, used for skin preparation; hand wash and skin ulcers
Phenolics	Phenol (carbolic acid)	±	+	–	–	–	+	Absorbed by rubber; too irritant for general use
	Hexachlorophane	–	+	–	–	–	–	Powder form for skin application, skin disinfection
	Chloroxylenols (Dettol)	–	±	–	–	–	–	
Quaternary ammonium compounds	Cetrimide	±	+	–	±	–	–	Skin disinfection
	Benzalkonium chloride	±	+	–	+	–	–	Preservative of topical preparation/ antimicrobial plastic catheters

+, yes; –, no; ±, intermediate.

3

IMMUNOLOGY

GLOSSARY   88

**THE IMMUNE RESPONSE
   SYSTEM**   92
Innate and adaptive immunity   92
Cells and molecules involved in the
   immune response   93
   Antigen-recognition lymphoid cells
      (B and T lymphocytes)   93
   Granulocytes   98
   Macrophages   98
   Dendritic cells   98
   Natural killer cells   99
   Cytokines   99
   Accessory molecules   103
   Other molecules   104
   Apoptosis   105

IMMUNOGLOBULINS   105
Properties, functions and reactions   105
Structure of immunoglobulin
      molecule   108
Clinical considerations   109
   Paraprotein   109
   Macroglobulins   110
   Cryoglobulins   110
   Cold agglutinins   110
   Monoclonal antibodies   110

COMPLEMENT   111
The complement system   111
Complement pathways   111
Complement deficiencies   112

HYPERSENSITIVITY   112
Classification   112

IMMUNODEFICIENCY   115
Primary immunodeficiency   115
   B-cell disorders   115
   T-cell disorders   116
   Combined B- and T-cell disorders   116
   Neutrophil disorders   117

Secondary immunodeficiency   118
   Hypogammaglobulinaemia   118
   T-cell deficiency   118
   Hypergammaglobulinaemia   119

AUTOIMMUNE DISEASE   120
Explanatory theories for breakdown in
      self tolerance   121
Autoantibodies   121
   Antinuclear antibodies   122

BLOOD GROUP IMMUNOLOGY   123
ABO group   123
Rhesus (CDE) group   124
   Rhesus incompatibility   124
Minor blood group system   124

TRANSPLANTATION IMMUNOLOGY
      124
Terminology   124
Graft rejection and survival   125
Stem cell transplantation   126
Graft versus host disease
      (GVHD)   126
Xenotransplantation   127

TUMOUR IMMUNOLOGY   127
Tumour-associated antigen   127
Tumours of the immune system   128

IMMUNOLOGICAL ASSAYS   129
1. Agglutination assays   129
   Coombs' antiglobulin test   129
2. Complement fixation tests   129
3. Immunofluorescence tests   130
   Flow cytometry   130
4. Immunoenzyme assays   130
5. Radioimmunoassay   131
6. Immunodiffusion   131

Adaptive immunotherapy	The transfer of immune cells for therapeutic benefit.
ADCC, antibody-dependent cellular cytotoxicity	A cytotoxic reaction in which the Fc receptor-bearing killer cells recognize target cells via specific antibodies.
Adhesion molecules	Cell surface molecules involved in cell–cell interaction or the binding of cells to extracellular matrix, where the principal function is adhesion rather than cell activation, e.g. integrins and selectins.
Adjuvant	Any foreign material introduced with an antigen to enhance its immunogenecity, e.g. killed bacteria, (mycobacteria), emulsions (Freund's adjuvant) or precipitates (alums).
Alloantibody	Antibody raised in one individual and directed against an antigen (primarily on cells) of another individual of the same species.
Allogeneic	See page 124.
Allotypes	The protein of an allele which may be detectable as an antigen by another member of the same species. Plasma proteins are an example of antigenically dissimilar variants.
Alternative pathway	The activation pathways of the complement system involving C3 and factors B, D, P, H and I, which interact in the vicinity of an activator surface to form an alternative pathway C3 convertase.
Anaphylatoxins	Complement peptides (C3a and C5a) which cause mast cell degranulation and smooth muscle contraction.
Anchor residues	Certain amino acid residues of antigenic peptides are required for interaction in the binding pocket of MHC molecules.
Antigenic peptides	Peptide fragments of proteins which bind to MHC molecules and induce T-cell activation.
APCs (antigen-presenting cells)	A variety of cell types which carry antigen in a form that can stimulate lymphocytes.
Apoptosis	Programmed cell death: a mode of cell death which occurs under physiological conditions and is controlled by the dying cell itself ('cell suicide').
Autologous	Originating from the same individual.
β_2-microglobulin	A polypeptide which constitutes part of some membrane proteins including the class I MHC molecules.
Bcl-2	A molecule expressed transiently on activated B cells which have been rescued from apoptosis.
CD markers (cluster of differentiation)	Used as a prefix (and number). Cell surface molecules of lymphocytes and platelets that are distinguishable with monoclonal antibodies, and may be used to distinguish different cell populations.

Cell adhesion molecules (CAMs)	A group of proteins of the immunoglobulin supergene family involved in intercellular adhesion, including ICAM-1, ICAM-2, ICAM-3, VCAM-1, MAd CAM-1 and PECAM.
Class I/II restriction	The observation that immunologically active cells will only operate effectively when they share MHC haplotypes of either the class I or class II loci.
Class switching	The process by which B cells can express a new heavy chain isotype without altering the specificity of the antibody produced. This occurs by gene rearrangement.
Clonal selection	The fundamental basis of lymphocyte activation in which antigen selectively causes activation, division and differentiation only in those cells which express receptors with which it can combine.
Collectins	A group of large polymeric proteins including conglutinin and mannose-binding lectin (MBL) that can opsonize microbial pathogens.
Colony-stimulating factors (CSFs)	A group of cytokines which control the differentiation of haemopoetic stem cells.
Constant regions	The relatively invariant parts of the immunoglobulin heavy and light chains, and the α, β, γ and δ chains of the T-cell receptor.
Co-stimulation	The signals required for the activation of lymphocytes in addition to the antigen-specific signal delivered via their antigen receptors. CD28 is an important costimulating molecule for T cells and CD40 for B cells.
Defensins	A group of small antibacterial proteins produced by neutrophils.
Dendritic cells	Derived from either the lymphoid or mononuclear phagocyte lineages. A set of cells present in tissues, which capture antigen and migrate to lymph nodes and spleen, where they are particularly active in presenting the processed antigen to T cells.
Domain	Segments or loops on heavy and light chains formed by intrachain disulphide bonds. Each immunoglobulin domain consists of about 110 amino acids.
Epitope	Part of an antigen that binds to an antibody-combining site or a specific T-cell surface receptor, and determines specificity. Usually about 9–20 amino acids in size.
Fas ligand	The ligand that binds to the cell surface molecule Fas (CD95) which is normally found on the surface of lymphocytes. When Fas ligand binds to its receptor, cell death (apoptosis) is triggered.
Genetic restriction	Describes the phenomenon where lymphocytes and antigen-presenting cells interact more effectively when they share particular MHC haplotypes.
Gut-associated lymphoid tissue (GALT)	Accumulations of lymphoid tissue associated with the gastrointestinal tract.

Haplotype	A set of genetic determinants coded by closely linked genes on a single chromosome.
Hapten	A substance of low molecular weight which is not itself immunogenic, but which can bind to an antibody molecule and produce a new antigenic determinant.
Helper (T$_H$ cells)	A functional subclass of T cells which can help generate cytotoxic T cells and cooperate with B cells in the production of antibody responses. Helper cells recognize antigen in association with class II molecules.
Heterologous	Originating from a different individual or different inbred line.
Heterophile antigen	Antigen which occurs in tissues of many different species and is therefore highly crossreactive, e.g. Paul–Bunnell antigen which reacts with both sheep and beef erythrocytes.
HLA	See page 36.
Idiotype	Unique antigenic determinant on the antigen-binding region of an immunoglobulin molecule.
Hypervariable regions	Amino acid sequences within the variable regions of heavy and light immunoglobulin chains and of the T-cell receptor which show the most variability and contribute most to the antigen-binding site.
Immunoglobulin subclass	Immunoglobulin of the same class that is detectable in the constant heavy chain region, and differs in electrophoretic mobility and antigenic determinant, and function, e.g. IgG1, IgG2, IgG3 and IgG4.
Immunoglobulin supergene family (IgSF)	Molecules which have domains homologous to those seen in immunoglobulins, including MHC class I and II molecules, the T-cell receptor, CD2, CD3, CD4, CD8 ICAMs, VCAM and some of the Fc receptors.
Intercellular adhesion molecules	Cell surface molecules found on a variety of leucocytes and non-haematogenous cells which interact with leucocyte functional antigen (LFA-1); e.g. ICAM-1 (CD54), ICAM-2 (CD102) and ICAM-3 (CD50).
Integrins	One of the 'families' of adhesion molecules, some of which interact with cell adhesion molecules, and others with components of the extracellular matrix.
Isologous	Originating from the same individual or member of the same inbred strain.
Isotype	The class or subclass of an immunoglobulin common to all members of that species. Each isotype is encoded by a separate immunoglobulin constant region gene sequence that is carried by all members of a species.
Killer (K) cells	Type of cytotoxic lymphocyte that is able to mediate antibody-dependent cellular cytotoxicity (ADCC).
Langerhans' cells	Antigen-presenting cells of the skin which emigrate to local lymph nodes to become dendritic cells; they are very active in presenting antigen to T cells.

Lectin pathway	A pathway of complement activation, initiated by mannose-binding lectin (MBL) which intersects the classical pathway.
Leucocyte functional antigens (LFAs)	A group of three molecules (LFA-1 (CD11a/CD18), LFA-2 (CD2) and LFA-3 (CD58)), which mediate intercellular adhesion between leucocytes and other cells in an antigen non-specific fashion.
Linkage disequilibrium	The association of two linked alleles more frequently than would be expected by chance.
Memory cells	Long-lived lymphocytes which have already been primed with antigen but have not yet undergone terminal differentiation into effector cells. They react more readily than naïve lymphocytes when restimulated with the same antigen.
Mixed lymphocyte reaction (MLR)	Proliferative response when lymphocytes from two genetically different (i.e. allogeneic) persons are mixed in cell culture. A vital test in matching donor and recipient prior to bone marrow transplantation.
Mucosa-associated lymphoid tissue (MALT)	Lymphoid tissue associated with the bronchial tree, gastrointestinal tract and other mucosa.
Natural killer (NK) cell	Type of cytotoxic lymphocyte that has the intrinsic ability to recognize and destroy virally infected cells and some tumour cells. Specializes in killing cells that express little or no MHC molecule.
NfkB	A transcription factor which is widely used by different leucocyte populations to signal activation.
Perforin	A granule-associated molecule of cytotoxic cells, homologous to complement C9. It can form pores on the membrane of a target cell.
Reactive oxygen/ nitrogen intermediates (ROIs/RNIs)	Bactericidal metabolites produced by phagocytic cells, including hydrogen peroxide, hypophalites and nitric acid.
Selectins	Three adhesion molecules, P-selectin (CD62P), E-selectin (CD62E), and L-selectin (CD62L) involved in slowing leucocytes during their transit through venules.
Superantigens	Antigens (often bacterial, e.g. staphylococcal enterotoxins) which bind to the MHC outside the peptide-binding groove and stimulate all or most of the T cells bearing particular T-cell receptor V regions. Antigens must normally be processed in order to trigger the T-cell receptor. Superantigens are not processed but bind directly to class II and Vβ.
Suppressor (TS) cell	Functionally defined populations of T cells which reduce the immune responses of other T cells or B cells, or switch the response into a different pathway to that under investigation.
Syngeneic	Genetically identical or closely related, so as to allow tissue transplant.

TAP transporters	A group of molecules which transport proteins and peptides between intracellular compartments.
T-cell receptor (TCR)	The T-cell antigen receptor consists of either an αβ dimer (TCR-2) or a γδ dimer (TCR-1) associated with the CD3 molecular complex.
T-dependent antigens	Require recognition by both T and B cells to produce an immune response.
T-independent antigens	Can directly stimulate B cells to produce specific antibody.
Titre	The highest dilution of a given substance, e.g. antibody, that will still produce a reaction with another substance, e.g. antigen.
Toll receptors	A group of evolutionarily ancient cell surface molecules, e.g. the IL-1 receptor, some of which are involved in transducing signals for inflammation.
Transforming growth factors (TGFs)	A group of cytokines, identified by their ability to promote fibroblast growth, that are also immunosuppressive.
Tumour necrosis factor (TNF)	See page 101.

THE IMMUNE RESPONSE SYSTEM

INNATE (NON-SPECIFIC) AND ADAPTIVE (ACQUIRED) IMMUNITY
(Fig 3.1 and Table 3.1)

The innate component functions as a first line of defence and involves antigen-independent mechanisms. The adaptive component results from antigen-dependent activation, proliferation and differentiation (clonal expansion) of lymphocytes. It takes longer to mobilize but confers specificity and exhibits memory. The two are functionally interrelated in several critical ways, e.g. through cytokines and complement components.

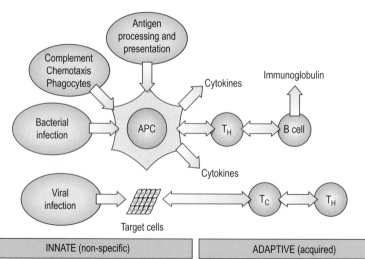

Fig. 3.1 Innate and acquired immunity.
APC = antigen presenting cells, T_H = helper T cells, T_C = cytotoxic T cells.

Table 3.1 Differences between the innate and adaptive immune response systems

Innate (non-specific system)	Adaptive (acquired system)
Components	**Components**
1. Anatomical and physiological barriers	1. Cell-mediated response effected by T cells
2. Inflammatory response with leakage of antibacterial serum proteins (acute-phase proteins) and phagocytic cells	2. Humoral immune response effected by B cells
3. Phagocytosis by neutrophils and macrophages	
4. Complement system	
Properties	**Properties**
1. Rapid: responds within minutes to infection	1. Slow: response over days to weeks
2. No antigenic specificity, i.e. the same molecules and cells respond to a range of pathogens	2. Antigenic specificity i.e. each cell is programmed genetically to respond to a single antigen
3. No memory, i.e. the response does not change after repeated exposure	3. Immunological memory, i.e. on repeated exposure the response is faster, stronger and qualitatively different
4. Preformed or rapidly formed components	4. Diversity: ability to recognize and respond to a vast number of different antigens
	5. Self/non-self recognition: i.e. lack of response (tolerance) to self-antigens but response to foreign antigens

CELLS AND MOLECULES INVOLVED IN THE IMMUNE RESPONSE

1. **Antigen-recognition lymphoid cells (B and T lymphocytes)**
2. **Granulocytes**
3. **Macrophages**
4. **Dendritic cells**
5. **Natural killer cells**
6. **Cytokines**
7. **Accessory molecules**
8. **Other molecules**

1. ANTIGEN-RECOGNITION LYMPHOID CELLS (B AND T LYMPHOCYTES)

B lymphocytes (see also Immunoglobulins, p. 105).

Functions: Humoral immunity – antibody production; control of pyogenic bacteria; prevention of blood-borne infections; neutralization of toxins.

% of total lymphocytes: 12%; mainly fixed.

Site of production: Produced in germinal centre of lymph nodes and spleen.

Assessment of function: Serum specific immunoglobulin levels; specific antibodies; immunoglobulin response to pokeweed mitogen; endotoxin and EBV.

T lymphocytes

Functions: Cell-mediated immunity; protection against intracellular organisms, protozoa and fungi; graft rejection; control of neoplasms.

% of total lymphocytes: 70–80%; mainly circulating; long-lived memory cells.

Site of production: Produced in paracortical region of lymph nodes and spleen.

| *Assessment of function:* | Delayed hypersensitivity skin reactions using candida, mumps and purified protein derivative (PPD); active sensitization with dinitrochlorobenzene (DNCP); lymphocyte transformation: mitogenic response to phytohaemagglutinin (PHA) and concanavalin-A; mixed lymphocyte reaction (MLR); lymphokine release. |
| *Identified by:* | T-cell surface phenotypes identified by reaction with monoclonal Abs (Table 3.2 and Fig. 3.2). |

T cells express either $\gamma\delta$ or $\alpha\beta$ T-cell receptors. $\alpha\beta$ T cells are divided into CD4 and CD8 subsets. T cells are further subdivided into T_H1 and T_H2 on the basis of their cytokine profiles (Fig. 3.3).

Table 3.2 T-cell surface antigens and CD markers (see also Fig. 3.3)

Surface antigen	% of peripheral T cells	HLA restriction	Function
T3 (CD3)	All		
T4 (CD4)	65	Class II MHC	T_H and T_{DH} cells
T8 (CD8)	35	Class I MHC	T_S and T_C cells

CD, cluster of differentiation; MHC, major histocompatibility complex; T_H helper T cells; T_{DH}, delayed hypersensitivity T cells; T_S suppressor T cells; T_C, cytotoxic T cells (see below).

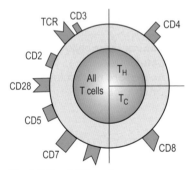

Fig. 3.2 T-cell CD markers.

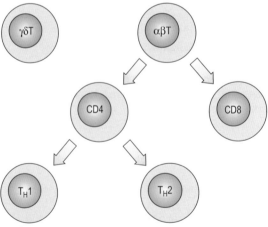

Fig. 3.3 T-cell subsets.

T-cell subpopulations

Regulatory and effector T cells
Regulatory cells:

1. **T$_H$ helper T cells CD4$^+$:** recognize antigen by means of the T-cell receptors in association with macrophage receptors. Produces cytokines and helps generate cytotoxic T cells and cooperates with B cells in production of antibody responses. Recognizes antigen in association with class II MHC molecules on the surface of antigen-presenting cells.
2. **T$_S$ suppressor T cells:** interfere with the development of an immune response of other T cells or B cells, either directly or via suppressor factors.

Effector cells:

3. **T$_C$ cytotoxic T cells CD8$^+$:** regulate the immune response and can lyse target cells, e.g. viral or tumour antigens expressing antigen peptides presented by MHC class I molecules on the surface of all nucleated cells. Interleukin-2 (IL-2) is responsible for the generation of cytotoxic T cells.
4. **T$_{DH}$ delayed hypersensitivity T cells:** release mediators that cause an inflammatory response attracting macrophages, neutrophils and other lymphocytes to the site.

Other selected important CD markers

CD28: Present in highest amounts in activated T cells. It is a T-cell costimulatory molecule which plays a major role in T cell activation.
CD45RA: An isoform of CD45 associated with active T cells that respond poorly to recall antigen.
CD45RO: An isoform associated with memory T cells. Responds well to recall antigen.
CD95: Also known as Fas, binds Fas ligand and mediates apoptosis of activated T cells.

T$_H$1 and T$_H$2 populations (Fig. 3.4)

- CD4$^+$ MHC class II-restricted T cells can also be subdivided into T$_H$1 and T$_H$2 populations based on their profiles of cytokine production.
- The **T$_H$1 profile** is associated with production of IL-2, tumour necrosis factor (TNF)-β and interferon (IFN)-γ and is driven by IL-12.
- The **T$_H$2 profile** is associated with IL-4, IL-5, IL-6 and IL-13 and is driven by IL-10.
- T$_H$1 cytokines are involved in helping cell-mediated immunity and the T$_H$2 cytokines mediate humoral immunity.
- T$_H$1 cells can downregulate T$_H$2 cells and vice versa.

T-cell antigen receptor (TCR) (Fig. 3.5)

TCR complex comprises a disulphide-linked heterodimeric glycoprotein that enables T cells to recognize a diverse array of antigens in association with MHC molecules. It consists of α and β subunits or occasionally γ and δ subunits. It is associated at the cell surface with a complex of polypeptides known collectively as CD3 which is required for activation of T cells.

- Consists of α, β subunits or, less commonly, γ or δ subunits.
- Differences in the variable regions of the TCR subunits account for the diversity of antigenic specificity among T cells.
- TCRs only recognize antigenic peptides bound to class I or class II MHC molecules.
- T cells can be divided into different subsets based on the expression of one or other T-cell receptor (TCR-1 or TCR-2).

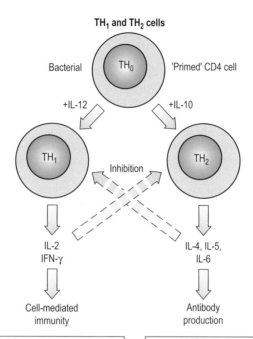

TH₁ and TH₂ cells

Bacterial ... TH₀ ... 'Primed' CD4 cell

+IL-12 ... +IL-10

TH₁ ... Inhibition ... TH₂

IL-2
IFN-γ

IL-4, IL-5,
IL-6

Cell-mediated
immunity

Antibody
production

TH₁ effects
• Reinforces early local responses
• Promotes cell-mediated cytotoxic responses
• Mediates type IV delayed type hypersensitivity

TH₂ effects
• Activates later systemic responses
• Promotes humoral antibody responses
• Promotes allergic type 1
  hypersensitivity responses
• Limits inflammatory responses

Fig. 3.4 Involvement of T$_H$1 and T$_H$2 cells in immunity.

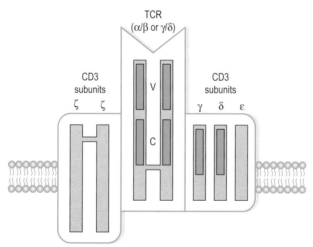

TCR
(α/β or γ/δ)

CD3
subunits
ζ   ζ

V

CD3
subunits
γ   δ   ε

C

Fig. 3.5 T-cell receptor (TCR) complex.

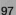

- TCR-1 cells are thought to have a restricted repertoire and to be mainly non-MHC restricted.
- TCR-2 cells express either CD4 or CD8 which determines whether they see antigen in association with MHC class II or I molecules.

T-cell recognition of an antigen
- T cells recognize antigens that originate within other cells, such as viral peptides from infected cells.
- T cells bind specifically to antigenic peptides presented on the surface of infected cells by molecules encoded by the MHC.
- The T cells use their specific receptors (TCRs) to recognize the unique combinations of MHC molecule plus antigenic peptide (Fig. 3.6).

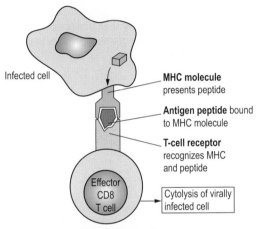

Infected cell

MHC molecule
presents peptide

Antigen peptide bound
to MHC molecule

T-cell receptor
recognizes MHC
and peptide

Effector
CD8
T cell

Cytolysis of virally
infected cell

Fig. 3.6 T-cell recognition of antigen.

Summary
- **Class I MHC pathway:** presents antigenic peptides derived from intracellular viral, foreign graft and tumour cell proteins to **CD8⁺ cells.**
- **Class II MHC pathway:** presents antigenic peptides derived from internalized microbes to **CD4⁺ cells.**

The stages in the recognition and processing of a virally infected cell by a cytotoxic CD8⁺ T cell are:
1. Entry of virus into the target cell.
2. Replication of the virus.
3. Processing of viral proteins to generate antigenic determinants which associate with MHC (HLA) class I molecules.
4. Presentation of the antigen–HLA complex for recognition by a specific CD8 cytotoxic cell, with killing of the infected cell.
5. The naïve T cells that emerge from the thymus are pre-cytotoxic T lymphocytes, and require further activation and differentiation to become the effector T cells that lyse virally infected target cells and tumour cells.

The γδ T-cell subset
- γδ TCR-expressing T cells are a minor population (> 5%) of all T cells and are a separate lineage from the αβ T cell that differentiates into CD8⁺ and CD4⁺ cells.

- The $\gamma\delta$ TCR recognizes antigen differently without processing or presentation on a MHC class I or class II molecule, e.g. non-peptide antigen such as bacterial cell wall phospholipids.
- They act as part of the first line of defence, recognizing pathogens mainly in the skin and gut.
- They can secrete cytokines, help B cells, activate macrophages and lyse virally infected cells.

2. GRANULOCYTES

- Neutrophils (PMNs): strongly phagocytic cells important in controlling bacterial infections.
- Eosinophils: weakly phagocytic: main role is in allergic reactions and destruction of parasites.
- Basophils and mast cells: non-phagocytic granulocytes that possess cell-surface receptors for IgE. Mediate allergic and antiparasitic response due to release of histamine and other mediators.

3. MACROPHAGES

Monocytes are released from the bone marrow, circulate in the blood and enter tissues, where they mature into macrophages.

Functions
1. Phagocytose microbes.
2. Secrete inflammatory mediators and complement components.
3. Present antigen associated with class II MHC and CD4$^+$ cells.
4. Secrete numerous cytokines that promote immune responses (IL-1, TNF-α, IL-6 and IL-12).

Phagocytosis of microbes by neutrophils and macrophages
1. Bacteria are opsonized by IgM, IgG, C3b and C4b, promoting their adherence and uptake by phagocytes.
2. The killing activity of neutrophils and macrophages is enhanced by highly reactive compounds: oxygen-dependent (hydrogen peroxide H_2O_2, superoxide anion, hydroxyl radicals, hypochlorous acid and nitric oxide (NO)) and oxygen-independent (acids, lysozyme–degrades, bacterial peptidoglycan, defensins (damage membranes), lysosomal proteases, lactoferrin (chelates iron). Their formation by NADPH oxidase, NADH oxidase or myeloperoxidase is stimulated by a powerful oxidative burst following bacterial phagocytosis.

---

4. DENDRITIC CELLS

Found in various tissues, e.g. Langerhans cells of the skin, peripheral blood and lymph glands.

Functions
1. Antigen-presenting cells: efficient at presenting antigen to both CD4$^+$ and CD8$^+$ cells.
2. Have phagocytic activity and release cytokines.

Antigen-presenting cells
- Include macrophages, monocytes or their derivatives (microglial cells, Kupffer cells and skin Langerhans cells).
- Characterized by their ability to phagocytose, internalize and process antigen.
- Possess Ia antigen, Fc receptors and C3b receptors and produce interleukin 1.

5. NATURAL KILLER (NK) CELLS

Functions
1. Similar function to lymphocytes – kill virus-infected cells and some tumour cells, and produce cytokines.
2. Recognition of target differs from lymphocytes – they do not bind MHC, and a carbohydrate receptor selects target. NK cells express two major classes of inhibitory receptors for MHC molecules: lectin-like receptors of the CD94 family and immunoglobulin superfamily molecules (KIRs).
3. Act rapidly, and constitute an early antiviral defence.
4. Identified by: Fc receptor for IgG.
5. Previously referred to as large granular lymphocytes (IGL) because of their appearance.

Mechanisms of NK cell killing
- Direct cytotoxicity involving contact with target cell and lysis by perforin-mediated mechanism similar to that used by T_C cells, except it is antigen independent and non-MHC restricted.
- Antibody-dependent cellular (ADCC) cytotoxicity. Binding of Fc receptors on NK cells to antibody-coated target cells initiates killing. (Neutrophils, eosinophils and macrophages also exhibit ADCC).

6. CYTOKINES (Fig. 3.7)

- Small protein signalling molecules (usually glycoproteins) of relatively low molecular weight.
- They regulate important biological processes: proliferation and differentiation, growth inhibition, apoptosis, chemotaxis and chemokinesis, resistance to viral infection, induction of cytotoxic effector cells, induction of phagocytes, promotion of intercellular adhesions and regulation of adhesion to extracellular matrix.
- Many cytokines act by causing aggregation of receptors at the cell surface, which leads to activation of second messenger system.
- The main cytokines are interferons, interleukins, tumour necrosis factor, growth factors, colony stimulating factors and chemokines.

1. Interferons (IFNs) (Table 3.3)
These glycoproteins are produced by virus-infected cells.
- Three species of interferon:
  1. Alpha-interferon (IFN-α) produced by human leucocytes
  2. Beta-interferon (IFN-β) produced by human fibroblasts
  3. Gamma-interferon (IFN-γ) produced by human T lymphocytes in response to antigenic stimulation.
- Properties:
  1. Prevent viral replication
  2. Antitumour activity
  3. Activate macrophages and natural killer (NK) cells.

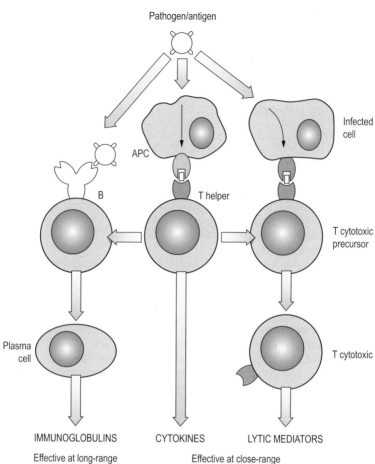

Fig. 3.7 **Interrelationship of immune cell populations.**
APC = antigen-presenting cell.

Table 3.3 Interferons (IFNs)			
Cytokine	*Immune cells*	*Induced by*	*Immunological effects*
IFN-α,-β	T and B cells, monocytes or macrophages	Mainly viruses; also some bacteria, protozoa and cytokines	Antiviral activity Stimulation of macrophages and large granular lymphocytes (LGL) Enhanced HLA (MHC) class I expression
IFN-γ	T cells and NK cells	Recognition of antigen by T-cell receptor	Antiviral activity Stimulation of macrophages and endothelium Enhanced HLA (MHC) class I and class II expression Suppression of T_H2 cells

2. Interleukins (ILs) (Table 3.4)

These cytokines stimulate proliferation of T helper and cytotoxic cells and B cells.

Interleukin-1 (IL-1) is a central regulator of the inflammatory response.

- Synthesized by activated mononuclear phagocytes.
- IL-1β is secreted into the circulation and cleaved by interleukin-1β converting enzyme (ICE).
- IL-1β levels in the circulation are only detectable in the following situations: after strenuous exercise, in ovulating women, sepsis, acute organ rejection, acute exacerbation of rheumatoid arthritis.
- Acts in septic shock by increasing the number of small mediator molecules such as PAF (platelet-activating factor), prostaglandins and nitric oxide which are potent vasodilators.
- The uptake of oxidized low density lipoproteins (LDL) by vascular endothelial cells results in IL-1 expression which stimulates the production of platelet-derived growth factor. IL-1 is thus likely to play a role in the formation of the atherosclerotic plaque.
- IL-1 has some host defence properties, inducing T and B lymphocytes, and reduces mortality from bacterial and fungal infection in animal models.

Interleukin-2 (IL-2) is also known as T-cell growth factor.

- Induces proliferation of other T lymphocytes; generates new cytotoxic cells, and enhances natural killer cells.

Table 3.4 Interleukins (ILs)

Cytokine	Immune cells	Immunological effects
IL-1α, β	Monocytes/macrophages, dendritic cells	Activation of T and B cells, macrophages, and endothelium Stimulation of acute phase response
IL-2	T_H1 cells	Proliferation and/or activation of T, B and LGL
IL-4	T_H2 cells, macrophages, mast cells and basophils, bone marrow stroma	Activation of B cells Differentiation of T_H2 cells and suppression of T_H1 cells
IL-5	T_H2 cells, mast cells	Development, activation and chemoattraction of eosinophils
IL-6	T_H2 cells, monocytes or macrophages	Activation of haemopoietic stem cells Differentiation of B and T cells Production of acute phase proteins
IL-8	T cells, monocytes, neutrophils	Chemoattraction of neutrophils, T cells, basophils Activation of neutrophils
IL-10	T_H2 and B cells, macrophages	Suppression of macrophage functions and T_H1 cells Activation of B cells
IL-12	Macrophages, dendritic cells, B cells	Suppression of macrophage functions and T_H1 cells Activation of B cells

3. Tumour necrosis factor (TNF) (Table 3.5)

- The principal mediator of the host response to Gram-negative bacteria. May also play a role in the response to other infectious organisms, and is a key cytokine in the pathogenesis of multiorgan failure.
- Activates inflammatory leucocytes to kill microbes; stimulates mononuclear phagocytes to produce cytokines; acts as a costimulator for T-cell activation and antibody production by B cells; and exerts an interferon-like effect against viruses.

Table 3.5 Tumour necrosis factor (TNF)

Cytokine	Immune cells	Immunological effects
TNF-α	Macrophages, lymphocytes, neutrophils, eosinophils,	Activation of macrophages, granulocytes, cytotoxic cells and endothelium
	NK cells	Enhanced HLA class I expression
		Stimulation of acute phase response
		Anti-tumour effects
TNF-β	T_H1 and T_C cells	Similar to TNF-α

4. Growth factors

Transforming growth factor-beta (TGF-β)
- Generally limits inflammatory response.
- Enhances IgA synthesis.
- Initiates and terminates tissue repair.
- Undergoes autoinduction.
- Released by platelets at the site of tissue injury and promotes the formation of extracellular matrix.
- Implicated in diseases of tissue fibrosis such as cirrhosis and glomerulosclerosis.

5. Colony stimulating factors (CSFs) (Table 3.6)
- These are involved in directing the division and differentiation of bone-marrow stem cells, and the precursors of blood leucocytes.

Table 3.6 Colony stimulating factors (CSFs)

Cytokine	Immune cell source	Immunological effects
GM-GSF	Many cells	Myeloid growth
G-CSF	T cells, macrophages, neutrophils	Development and activation of neutrophils
M-CSF	T cells, macrophages, neutrophils	Development and activation of monocytes/macrophages
GM-CSF	T cells, macrophages, mast cells, neutrophils, eosinophils	Differentiation of pluripotent stem cells Development of neutrophils, eosinophils and macrophages
Transforming growth factor (TGF)-β	T cells, monocytes	Inhibition of T and B cell proliferation and LGL activity
Erythropoietin*	Kidney	Erythropoiesis

*Not a typical cytokine as it has a single origin.

6. Chemokines
- Large family of cytokines that have chemoattractant properties.
- Responsible for recruiting leucocytes to inflammatory lesions, inducing release of granules from granulocytes, regulating integrin avidity and in general exhibiting proinflammatory properties.
- Chemokines are secreted by many cell types.
- The receptors for the chemokines are also family-specific (Table 3.7).

Table 3.7 Cytokine subgroups

Cytokines	Immune cell source	Immunological effects
α Subgroup CXC-type (e.g. IL-8)	Macrophage, neutrophil, endothelium, fibroblast	Attracts neutrophils and promotes their migration into tissues
β Subgroup CC-type (e.g. MIP, RANTES)	Macrophage, neutrophil, endothelium, T cell	Attracts macrophages, eosinophils, basophils and lymphocytes

Cytokine disorders

Both cytokine overexpression and underexpression or their receptors can be pathogenic:

1. Septic shock: production of IL-1, IL-6 and TNF due to endotoxin stimulation of macrophages following Gram-negative infection.
2. Toxic shock syndrome: massive release of cytokines due to superantigen stimulation of T-cells by TSST-1, a bacterial exotoxin.
3. Chagas' disease (*T. cruzi* infection): causes reduced expression of IL-2 receptor, leading to marked immune suppression.

7. ACCESSORY MOLECULES

Promote adhesion of T cells and/or signal transduction leading to T-cell activation.

Adhesion molecules (Table 3.8)

- Involved in cell–cell communication and recognition (i.e. help bind T cells to antigen-presenting cells and target cells), and control leucocyte migration (i.e. help direct T cells to sites of inflammation and lymph nodes).
- They fall into families that are structurally related:
  - **The cell adhesion molecules (CAMs)** of the immunoglobulin superfamily (antigen presentation)
  - **the cadherin superfamily** (neuromuscular interaction)
  - **integrins** (interaction between cells and the extracellular matrix)
  - **selectins** (leucocyte adhesion to endothelium during inflammation).

Table 3.8 Adhesion molecules involved in lymphocyte interactions

	Receptor on lymphocyte	Ligand on interacting cell
T cells	CD4	HLA class II
	CD8	HLA class I
	CD28	CD80
	CD2	LFA-3
	VLA-4	VCAM-1
B cells	LFA-1	ICAM-1, -2 or -3
	CD40	CD40-ligand

LFA, lymphocyte function-associated antigen; VLA, very late antigen; ICAM, intercellular adhesion molecule; VCAM, vascular cell adhesion molecule.

Coreceptor activating molecules (e.g. CD28, CTLA-4)

- Transduce signals important in regulating functional responses of T cells.

8. OTHER MOLECULES

Heat shock proteins

The *heat shock response* is a highly conserved and phylogenetically ancient response to tissue stress that is mediated by activation of specific genes. This leads to the production of specific heat shock proteins that alter the phenotype of the cell and enhance its resistance to stress. Their principal function appears to be to act as molecular chaperones for damaged protein to direct it into degradation pathways such as ubiquitination.

Free radicals

- A *free radical* is literally any atom or molecule which contains one or more unpaired electrons, making it more reactive than the native species.
- Free radical species produced in the human body are:
  - OOH$^\bullet$ (peroxide radical)   – O$_2$$^\bullet$ (superoxide radical)
  - OH$^\bullet$ (hydroxyl radical)   – NO$^\bullet$ (nitric oxide).
- The hydroxyl radical is by far the most reactive species, but the others can generate more reactive species as breakdown products.
- When a free radical reacts with a non-radical, a chain reaction ensues which results in the formation of further free radicals and direct tissue damage by lipid peroxidation of membranes (particularly implicated in atherosclerosis and ischaemic reperfusion injury within tissues).
- Free radical scavengers bind reactive oxygen species.
- Principal dietary antioxidants:
  - Vitamin E   – β-Carotene
  - Vitamin C   – Flavonoids.
- Patients with dominant familial forms of amyotrophic lateral sclerosis (motor neuron disease) have mutations in the gene for Cu–Zn SOD-1, suggesting a link between failure of free radical scavenging and neurodegeneration. Protection against heart disease and cancer may be conferred by dietary antioxidants.

Nitric oxide (NO)

NO is an important transcellular messenger molecule which is involved in a diverse range of processes.

- NO is synthesized from the oxidation of nitrogen atoms in the amino acid L-arginine by the action of *NO synthase* (NOS; Fig. 3.8).
- NO acts on target cells close to its site of synthesis, where it activates guanylate cyclase, leading to a rise in intracellular *cGMP* which acts as a second messenger to modulate a variety of cellular processes. It has a very short half-life.
- There are at least three distinct *isoforms* of NO synthase:
  1. Neuronal (constitutive) NO synthase (CNS neurotransmission, memory formation)
  2. Endothelial (constitutive) NO synthase (vasodilator tone modulation, organ-specific microcirculatory control, e.g. kidney)
  3. Macrophage (inducible) NO synthase.

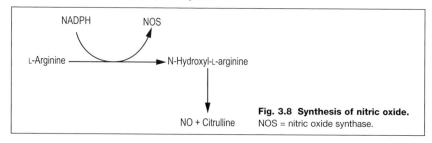

Fig. 3.8 Synthesis of nitric oxide. NOS = nitric oxide synthase.

1. Septic shock (NO is released in massive amounts and results in decreased vascular tone, cardiac output with low BP). This is because endotoxin release triggers the innate immune response when macrophages are directly activated through Toll-like receptors. Macrophage activation results in the secretion of TNF, prostaglandins and NO. There have been three main approaches to preventing septic shock:
   (i) Blocking nitric oxide production by macrophages, endothelium and smooth muscle.
   (ii) Blocking TNF with monoclonal antibodies.
   (iii) Recombinant bactericidal protein to bind to endotoxin and prevent macrophage activation. All have failed in clinical trials, probably because the innate immune response has already mediated its damage by the time symptoms develop.
2. Atherosclerosis (where NO synthesis may be impaired, leading to tonic vasoconstriction and vasospasm).
3. $1°$ and $2°$ pulmonary hypertension (inhaled NO reverses pulmonary hypertension).
4. Hepatorenal syndrome and the hypertension of chronic renal failure.
5. Glutamate-mediated excitotoxic cell death in the CNS, such as in Alzheimer's disease, and also in acute brain injury, such as stroke.
6. Tissue damage in acute and chronic inflammation (probably by interacting with oxygen-derived free radicals).
7. ARDS (adult respiratory distress syndrome).

APOPTOSIS (see also p. 35)

- Is the process of programmed cell death, and is a mechanism for the elimination of excess or damaged cells.
- Several genes have been identified that either promote *(bax, bak, bcl-Xs)* or inhibit *(bcl-2, bcl-XL, bcl-w)* apoptosis. Antiapoptotic genes could confer characteristics such as longer survival.
- It is mainly triggered through the Fas–Fas ligand interaction. Binding of Fas ligand (expressed on a killer T cell) to Fas expressed on a target cell triggers a cascade of intracellular biochemical changes in the target cell. Fas interacts with several proteins in the 'death pathway' to activate a proteolytic enzyme, caspase. The caspase proteolytic cascade then activates a cytoplasmic enzyme (caspase-activatable DNAase (CAD)) which can then migrate to the nucleus and cleave DNA into small fragments, which are the end-point of apoptosis.
- It has several important roles in shaping the adaptive immune response, e.g. after an immune response to a pathogen, redundant lymphocytes are cleared by apoptosis.
- It is also involved in some pathological processes, e.g. destruction of CD4+ cells in HIV infection; can lead to the production of autoantibodies against DNA and result in autoimmune disease; clones of B cells that have increased levels of *bcl-2* through mutations may be protected from apoptosis and develop into a B-cell malignancy.

IMMUNOGLOBULINS

PROPERTIES, FUNCTIONS AND REACTIONS

The properties and functions of the major classes of immunoglobulins are shown in Table 3.9, and the immunological reactions of IgG, IgA and IgM are summarized in Table 3.10.

Table 3.9 Properties and functions of the major classes of immunoglobulin

Ig class	Heavy chains	Molecular weight	% total Ig level	Normal plasma level	Function
IgG	γ	150 000 (monomer)	80	8–16 g/l	1. Distributed in blood and interstitial fluids 2. The major immunoglobulin of the secondary immune response* 3. The only immunoglobulin that crosses the placenta, and therefore the major protective immunoglobulin in the neonate. Most maternally transmitted IgG has disappeared by 6 months† 4. Opsonization, toxin neutralization and agglutination. Coats cells prior to killing by killer cells. Activates complement via classical pathway
IgA	α	160 000 370 000 (dimer and secretory form)	13	1.4–4 g/l	1. Principal immunoglobulin in secretions of respiratory and gastrointestinal tract and in sweat, saliva, tears and colostrum. Key defence role for mucosal surfaces 2. Polymerizes to a dimer intracellularly by binding through a cysteine-rich polypeptide (J-chain), synthesized locally by submucosal cells 3. Secreted through epithelia as the dimer bound to a secretory transport piece, synthesized locally by epithelial cells 4. When aggregated binds polymorphs and activates complement by the alternative pathway
IgM	μ	900 000 (pentamer)	6	0.5–2 g/l	1. Macroglobulin made up of five monomeric immunoglobulin subunits linked by a J-chain 2. Mainly intravascular 3. Principal immunoglobulin of the primary immune response 4. Does not cross the placenta. Fetal production of high levels of specific IgM in intrauterine infection may be of diagnostic significance, e.g. rubella 5. Agglutinates and opsonizes particulate antigens. Activates complement via the classical pathway. Blood group antibodies: IgM

* **Secondary antibody response characterized by:** 1. lowering of the threshold of immunogen; 2. shortening of the lag phase; 3. a higher rate of antibody production; 4. longer persistence of antibody production.

†**Transient disease in the newborn caused by maternal IgG:** rhesus incompatibility, autoimmune thrombocytopenia, thyrotoxicosis, myasthenia gravis, lupus erythematosus.

Table 3.9 *(Cont'd)*

Ig class	Heavy chains	Molecular weight	% total Ig level	Normal plasma level	Function
IgD	δ	170 000 (monomer)	0.1	4–40 mg/l	1. Precise functions are unknown 2. Nearly all immunoglobulin is present as cell surface receptor on human B cells and may be involved in B-cell activation
IgE	ε	185 000	0.002	0.1–1.3 mg/l	1. Immediate hypersensitivity reactions: binds to mast cells and basophils via its Fc fragment, which degranulates and releases biologically active mediators, e.g. histamine, when exposed to the appropriate antigen. Possibly of benefit in controlling certain parasitic infections 2. Serum levels correlate with severity of asthma 3. Activates various cells involved in allergic and inflammatory disease, which are activated by 2 main types of cell surface receptor: the FESR1 receptor on mast cells, basophils and eosinophils, and the FqSR2 receptor on lymphocytes. Receptor blocking monoclonal antibodies have been developed as possible asthma therapies

Table 3.10 Summary of reactions of various immunoglobulins

Reaction	IgG	IgA	IgM
Agglutination	+	+	++
Precipitation	+	+	+
Virus neutralization	+	+	+
Complement fixation	+++	–	+
Complement-dependent lysis	+	–	+++
Immune complex	+	–	+

STRUCTURE OF IMMUNOGLOBULIN MOLECULE (Fig. 3.9)

- An immunoglobulin molecule is a 4-polypeptide chain structure with two heavy and two light chains linked covalently by disulphide bonds.
- Treatment of the antibody unit with papain produces:
  - Two identical univalent *antigen-binding fragments (Fab),* each containing one antigen-binding site, and
  - One *crystallizable fragment (Fc),* which contains sites for complement fixation, reactivity with rheumatoid factors, skin and macrophage fixation and regulation of catabolism.
- *Light chains*
  - Molecular weight of approximately 23 000.
  - Two types: kappa (κ) and lambda (λ). Each immunoglobulin molecule has either two κ or two λ chains.
- *Heavy chains*
  - Molecular weight of about twice that of light chains (i.e. 50 000–75 000) and twice the number of amino acids.
  - Five classes of immunoglobulin are recognized on the basis of the Fc fragment of the heavy chain, i.e. heavy chain isotypes IgG, IgA, IgM, IgD and IgE. Heavy chain classes are also divided into subclasses of molecules, e.g. IgG1, IgG2, etc.

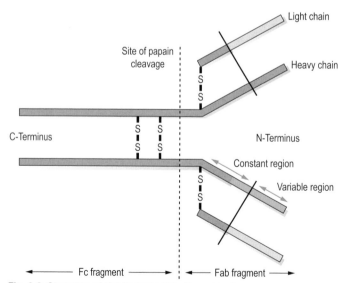

Fig. 3.9 Structure of the immunoglobulin molecule.
Fc = crystallizable fragment, Fab = antigen-binding fragment.

- Both heavy and light chains consist of two regions (Table 3.11):
  1. A *constant region* (C_H and C_L), in which the amino acid sequence of immunoglobulins of the same class is more or less identical.
  2. A *variable region* (V_H and V_L) where the amino acid sequence varies considerably from molecule to molecule and contributes to the antigen-binding site.

Table 3.11 Antigenic determinants on antibodies

Epitope class	Location	Comment on epitope
Isotype	Constant region	5 human isotopes are IgA, IgD, IgE, IgG, IgM. Each class of Ig heavy chains are identical in all members of a species
Allotype	Constant region	Vary among individuals of the same species. IgG exhibits the most allotypic difference
Idiotype	Variable region	Differ among antibodies with different antigen-binding specificities. Monoclonal antibodies have the same idiotype. Anti-idiotypic antibodies will resemble the original antigenic determinant group

Development and activation of B cells
- Direct B cell/T_H cell interaction and cytokines secreted by T_H cells are required for B cells to respond to most antigens.
- Stimulation of B cells by protein antigens induces generation of memory B cells and antibody-secreting plasma cells.
- During this clonal expansion and differentiation, the antibody affinity for antigen may change (affinity maturation), and the biological activities of the antibody can change (isotype class switching).

CLINICAL CONSIDERATIONS (see Table 3.12)

Table 3.12 Immunoglobulin products for replacement therapy

Product	Indications
Immunoglobulin replacement therapy (pooled from normal humans)	Primary immunodeficiency
High-dose immunoglobulin (pooled from normal humans)	Immunosuppressive effects used in autoimmunity
Anti-D (pooled from women with high levels of anti-D)	Prevention of haemolytic disease of the newborn
Hyperimmune immunoglobulin (pooled from humans with high titres of antibodies)	Prevention of tetanus, rabies, varicella zoster and hepatitis B
Antivenom	Treatment of snake bite
Monoclonal antibodies (raised against specific human cells in mouse hybridomas)	Used as immunosuppressants and cancer treatment

PARAPROTEIN

- A homogeneous band of one immunoglobulin, usually IgG, IgM or IgA. Its presence implies proliferation of a single clone of cells.

MACROGLOBULINS

- Globulins with a molecular weight >400 000.
- Usually IgM but may be IgM polymers.

Causes of raised macroglobulins:
- Waldenström's macroglobulinaemia, lymphoma and malignancies, diseases associated with a high ESR such as collagen disorders, sarcoidosis and cirrhosis.

CRYOGLOBULINS

- Immunoglobulins which precipitate when cooled to 4°C and dissolve when warmed to 37°C, so blood must be taken in a warm syringe and kept at 37°C until the serum has been separated.
- Three types:
  - Type (25%): monoclonal cryoglobulins (IgM, IgG or IgA).
  - Type II (25%): mixed type, monoclonal protein (often rheumatoid factor) which has bound polyclonal IgG (IgM–IgG, IgG–IgG).
  - Type III (50%): mixed polyclonal type (IgM–IgG, IgM–IgG–IgA).
- May cause Raynaud's phenomenon and cutaneous vasculitis if present in high concentrations.
- Cryoglobulinaemia: two-thirds may be associated with diseases causing a paraproteinaemia, e.g. lymphoma, myeloma, SLE, rheumatoid arthritis and chronic infection, e.g. hepatitis C. One-third are idiopathic.

COLD AGGLUTININS

- Specific IgM antibodies capable of agglutinating human red blood cells between 0°C and 4°C.
- Found in *Mycoplasma pneumoniae,* infectious mononucleosis, listeriosis and Coxsackie infections, malaria, trypanosomiasis and acquired haemolytic anaemia (Coombs test positive).

MONOCLONAL ANTIBODIES

- Myeloma cells are fused with plasma cells prepared from an immunized mouse or rat to produce a hybrid myeloma cell or 'hybridoma', which may then produce monoclonal antibodies.
- 'Humanized' antibodies (produced by enzymatic cleavage of the immunogenic mouse Fc portion) are preferable because of the potentially serious side-effects of administering mouse antibodies as therapeutic agents.

Uses
1. Lymphocyte subset determination and detection of HLA antigens.
2. Viral detection and subtyping: parasite identification.
3. Assays of peptide hormones, e.g. ACTH and PTH.
4. Identification of surface markers of cells in biopsy material, e.g. markers for transplant antigens and bacterial serotypes.
5. Histological typing of neoplasms, e.g. lymphomas, APUDomas and leukaemias.
6. Affinity chromatography to isolate and purify material, e.g. vaccines and interferon, where the amino acid sequence varies considerably from molecule to molecule.

7. Therapeutic: antitumour effect (e.g. anti-idiotype to surface immunoglobulin B-cell lymphoma), immunosuppression (e.g. treatment of graft-versus-host disease and graft rejection with OKT3) and drug toxicity (e.g. reversal of digitalis intoxication).
8. Targeting of drugs to specific tissue sites.
9. Conjugated to radioisotopes for imaging.

COMPLEMENT

THE COMPLEMENT SYSTEM

- Comprises at least nine plasma proteins and some regulatory factors, that form an enzymatic cascade and mediate several functions of the inflammatory process.
- Synthesized by macrophages or hepatocytes.
- Usually circulate in an inactive form as proenzymes.
- Heat-labile.

COMPLEMENT PATHWAYS

A cascade of sequential activation converts each proenzyme into its active state and amplifies the response. Activation may occur via two main pathways.
1. **Classical pathway.** Triggered by antigen-antibody complexes containing IgM or IgG. C1 is the initiating protein, and after binding to an Fc is able to activate C4 and C2, which in turn activate multiple C3 molecules. Constitutes a major effective mechanism for humoral immunity.
2. **Alternative pathway.** Initiated by certain antigens (lipopolysaccharide, endotoxin) and IgA complexes on cell surfaces which activate C3. Generates early innate response that does not require antibody for activation.
3. **Lectin pathway** (Fig. 3.10). Mannose-binding lectin (MBL) is a collectin that is able to bind through its lectin proteins on to carbohydrates present on bacteria. This indirectly activates the next complement components, C2 and C4.

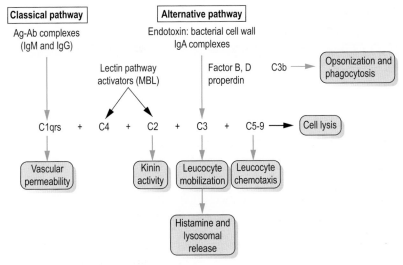

Fig. 3.10 Complement system.
MBL = mannose-binding lectin.

Summary
- The **alternative** pathway activates complement on the surface of any cell that lacks complement inhibitors.
- The **lectin** and **classical** pathways provide complement activation to molecules that have been bound by MBL or antibody.

Functions

1. Opsonization, chemotaxis and immune adherence
2. Activation of mast cells and basophils to release inflammatory mediators
3. Direct killing of microorganisms by immune cytolysis
4. Virus neutralization and processing of immune complexes.

COMPLEMENT DEFICIENCIES

- Raised levels of all complement components can occur in any inflammatory condition.
- *Low* complement levels occur in certain diseases and may correlate with disease activity, e.g. poststreptococcal glomerulonephritis, SLE nephritis, infectious endocarditis, nephritis, membranoproliferative glomerulonephritis, serum sickness, liver disease, septicaemia and disseminated intravascular coagulation.

Inherited deficiencies

Inherited deficiencies of certain groups of components are associated with characteristic clinical syndromes:

1. C1 inhibitor deficiency with hereditary angioneurotic oedema (due to uncontrolled complement activation).
2. C2, C4 deficiency (Classical pathway) with immune complex disease, e.g. Henoch–Schönlein purpura, glomerulonephritis, SLE and also streptococcal and staphylococcal infections.
3. C3 through C9 deficiency with recurrent bacterial (Neisseria) infection.
4. C5–9 deficiency with recurrent bacterial infections, especially Neisseria.
5. Decay-accelerating factor (DAF) deficiency with Paroxysmal nocturnal haemoglobinuria (PNH).

HYPERSENSITIVITY

CLASSIFICATION

See Table 3.13.

Table 3.13 Classification of hypersensitivity

Type	Mechanism	Result	Disease
Type I Anaphylactic	Antigen reacts with IgE (reaginic) antibody bound to mast cells	Release of vasoactive substances* Vasodilation and chemotaxis	Anaphylactic shock, e.g. bee and wasp venom Atopic diseases, e.g. asthma, hay fever and rhinitis Drug allergies **Useful test: specific IgE test and skin prick testing (with caution)** **(see Box below table)**
Type II Cell-bound†	Circulating antibody (IgG or IgM) reacts with antigen on cell surface	Complement activation Phagocytosis Promotion of killer cell cytotoxicity Cell lysis	Transfusion reactions and Rhesus incompatibility Autoimmune haemolytic anaemia Myasthenia gravis Poststreptococcal glomerulonephritis Myxoedema and thyrotoxicosis Idiopathic thrombocytopenic purpura Goodpasture's syndrome Drug-induced disease (mainly haematological effects)
	Some IgG antibodies stimulate the cells against which they are directed	TSH receptor antibody results in prolonged hypersecretion of thyroid hormone	Graves' disease **Useful test: Coombs' test**
Type III Immune complex†	Free antigen and antibody (IgG or IgM) combine in the presence of complement, and precipitate as immune complexes	Platelet aggregation Complement activation Activation of clotting factor XII, leading to fibrin and plasmin formation Damage to small blood vessels	Immune complex diseases:‡ *1. Exogenous antigens* Serum sickness with monoclonal antibodies Drug-induced haemolytic anaemia and thrombocytopenia, e.g. quinine, quinidine and phenacetin Hypersensitivity pneumonitis, e.g. farmer's lung *2. Microbial antigens* Poststreptococcal glomerulonephritis Glomerulonephritis associated with endocarditis Syphilis Quartan malaria Schistosomiasis *3. Autologous antigens* SLE, rheumatoid arthritis, mixed cryoglobulinaemia **Useful test: Antibody levels**

Table 3.13 (Cont'd)

Type	Mechanism	Result	Disease
Type IV Cell-mediated or delayed hypersensitivity	Sensitized T lymphocytes are stimulated by an appropiate antigen	Lymphokine release	Tuberculin skin reaction and tuberculosis (systemic reaction = Koch phenomenon) Tuberculoid leprosy Contact dermatitis Graft rejection (late) and GVHD Tumour immunity
Type V			**Useful test: Patch testing**

* Histamine, kinins, platelet-activating factor (PAF), leucotriene C4 (LTC4) and leucotriene D4 (LTD4), prostaglandins, thromboxanes and chemotactic factors (eosinophil chemotactic factor of anaphylaxis (ECF-A), neutrophil chemotactic factor (NCF)).
†Complement dependent.
‡Immune complex diseases successfully treated by plasma exchange include: SLE, rapidly progressive glomerulonephritis, Wegener's granulomatosis, polyarteritis nodosa, mixed essential cryoglobulinaemia, cutaneous vasculitis.

Skin testing

- *Type I* (prick test) An urticarial weal and flare develops within 20 minutes and resolves within 2 hours.
- *Type II* (intradermal injection) An ill-defined weal develops over several hours, is maximal at 5–7 hours and resolves within 24 hours.
- *Type IV* (intradermal or patch test; delayed hypersensitivity) An indurated area develops within 2–4 days and resolves over several days.

Different types of hypersensitivity reactions in skin conditions

Skin disease	Hypersensitivity type	Mechanisms involved
Urticaria	I	IgE, mast cells, histamine
Bullous diseases	II	Autoantibody to skin components, complement
Vasculitis	III	Immune complexes, PMN, complement
Allergic contact dermatitis	IV	T cells, cytokines

PRIMARY IMMUNODEFICIENCY

- Rare: in about half the children affected no defect is ever found, and then it is usually in the phagocytic cells.
- Primary B-cell deficiency is very rare, and of T cells even more so.
- Respiratory system is the most common site of infection. The pattern of infection depends on the type of defect (Tables 3.14 and 3.15).

B-CELL DISORDERS

- Decreased production of some or all antibody isotypes due to B-cell defects or impaired T-cell helper function.
- Pathogens are pyogenic bacteria (e.g. staphylococci, streptococci, *H. influenzae* and pneumococci), yeasts, giardia and campylobacter.
- Treated with gammaglobulin.

1. Bruton's congenital agammaglobulinaemia

- Rare, X-linked recessive inheritance. Defective gene is *Btk* (Bruton's tyrosine kinase).
- Presents in male infants at about 6 months with recurrent pyogenic and gastrointestinal infections.
- Increased incidence of autoimmune disorders and lymphoreticular malignancies.
- No circulating B cells: very reduced IgG and no IgM, A, D, E.
- Normal T-cell function, i.e. normal delayed hypersensitivity.

2. Common variable immunodeficiency (CVID)

- Incidence of 10 per million. Acquired at any age and in either sex.
- Heterogeneous collection of conditions.
- Presents in late childhood or adult life with recurrent pulmonary infections and chronic diarrhoea. Characterized by high incidence of autoimmune disorders.
- Low serum immunoglobulin levels: cell-mediated immunity normal in 60%.

3. Dysgammaglobulinaemia

- Selective IgA deficiency is the commonest primary defect in the UK with 1:700 individuals affected.
- Usually asymptomatic but may present with recurrent respiratory tract or gastrointestinal infections, particularly if IgG2 is reduced.
- Increased frequency of allergic respiratory and autoimmune diseases.

4. Acquired hypogammaglobulinaemia

- Presents in infancy/adulthood.
- Associated conditions include autoimmune diseases, haemolytic anaemia and thymoma. IgG <250 mg/dl:IgM may be spared. Often normal B-cell count. Variable abnormalities in cell-mediated immunity.

5. Transient hypogammaglobulinaemia of infancy

- Usually presents between 3 and 6 months of age.
- Occurs when the onset of immunoglobulin synthesis (especially IgG) is delayed beyond the norm.

Table 3.14 Examples of infections related to cellular and humoral deficiency	
Defensive defect	*Opportunistic organism*
T cell	Viral pneumonias Varicella zoster virus Tuberculosis *Candida* *Toxoplasma gondii*
B cell	Bacterial pneumonias esp. *Pseudomonas* and *Klebsiella*
Neutropenia/phagocyte defects	Bacterial and fungal infections Cryptococcus Tuberculosis Strongyloides *Staphylococcus aureus*

T-CELL DISORDERS

- Compromised T_C-mediated cytotoxicity and DTH response.
- Opportunistic infections (e.g. *Pneumocystis carinii,* fungi) (see Table 2.28), severe viral and chronic bacterial infections, e.g. TB.
- Treatment by:
  1. Thymus grafts
  2. Bone marrow transplantation.

1. Congenital thymic aplasia (DiGeorge's syndrome)
- Rare, non-familial.
- Absence of the thymus is due to a defect in the development of the 3rd and 4th branchial pouches and arches.
- Presents in infancy/adulthood with cardiovascular defects, hypoparathyroidism, convulsions and opportunistic infections.
- Variable reduction in T-cell number and function. B-cell function often normal, i.e. normal Ab levels.

2. Chronic mucocutaneous candidiasis
- Some cases are familial.
- Severe candida infection of mucous membranes, nails and skin with associated endocrine abnormalities, e.g. hypoparathyroidism.
- Negative skin testing to candida.

3. Hyper-IgM syndrome
- X-linked. Defective gene is CD40L.
- Decreased B-cell activation due to T-cell defect: ↑ IgM, ↓ IgG and IgA.
- Recurrent infections, especially with *Pneumocystis carinii*. Often associated with autoimmune blood disorders.

COMBINED B- AND T-CELL DISORDERS

- Pathogens are pyogenic bacteria, viruses, fungi, TB and *Pneumocystis carinii*.
- Treatment by bone marrow transplantation.

1. Severe combined immunodeficiency (SCID)
- Mostly autosomal recessive inheritance: 50% are deficient in enzyme adenosine deaminase (ADA). Several defective genes have been identified.
- Presents in first few months of life with failure to thrive, chronic diarrhoea, recurrent pneumonia and widespread candidiasis.
- Complete absence of B- and T-cell immunity.

2. Ataxic telangiectasia syndrome

- Autosomal recessive inheritance.
- Presents in infancy with cerebellar ataxia, oculocutaneous telangiectasia and recurrent sinopulmonary infections.
- Increased incidence of malignancy, especially lymphomas.
- Low IgA and IgE levels. T-cell deficiency is variable.

3. Wiskott–Aldrich syndrome

- Incidence of four per million male births: X-linked recessive inheritance.
- Presents with severe eczema, thrombocytopenia and recurrent pyogenic infections, e.g. *Strep. pneumoniae, N. meningitidis, H. influenzae.*
- Increased incidence of tumours of lymphoreticular system.
- Low antibody levels, especially IgM, but increased IgE levels.

NEUTROPHIL DISORDERS

- Pathogens are Gram –ve (e.g. *E. coli* and *Klebsiella*) and Gram +ve (e.g. *Staph. aureus*) bacteria, some viruses and fungi (e.g. aspergillus).
- Treatment is with antibiotics.

1. Chronic granulomatous diseases (CGD)

- Rare, X-linked defect in the NADPH oxidase system (occasionally autosomal recessive). Results in reduced production of H_2O_2 and superoxide anion.
- Presents in first 2 years of life with recurrent bacterial (catalase-producing, e.g. staphylococcal species) infections, lymphadenopathy, hepatomegaly, pneumonia, osteomyelitis and abcesses. High susceptibility to aspergillus infections.
- Impaired opsonization and bactericidal activity (nitroblue tetrazolium test).
- Hypergammaglobulinaemia.
- May respond to IFN-γ treatment.

2. Chediak–Higashi syndrome

- Very rare deficiency of NADH or NADPH oxidase in the polymorphonuclear cells resulting in a reduced ability of phagocytes to store materials in lysosymes and release their contents.
- Presents with recurrent bacterial infections (especially Neisseria, staphylococcal and streptococcal), hepatosplenomegaly, lymphadenopathy and pancytopenia. Partial oculocutaneous albinism.
- Defective neutrophil function.

3. Leucocyte adhesion deficiency (LAD)

- Rare autosomal recessive defect in the biosynthesis of the β chain (CD18) common to three glycoproteins (three integrin receptors) on the surface of leucocytes.
- Usually presents with infections of skin, mouth, respiratory tract and around rectum.
- Characterized by failure of neutrophils to migrate to sites of tissue infection.

4. Job's syndrome

- Reduced chemotactic response by neutrophils and high IgE levels.
- Presents with recurrent cold staphylococcal abscesses and eczema. Often associated with red hair and fair skin.

5. Lazy leucocyte syndrome

- Severe impairment of neutrophil chemotaxis and migration.
- Presents with recurrent low-grade infections.

6. Myeloperoxidase deficiency

- Decreased production of hypochlorous acid and other reactive intermediates.
- Clinical features are of delayed killing of staphylococci and *Candida albicans.*

SECONDARY IMMUNODEFICIENCY

- Most immunodeficiency in adults is secondary to other conditions.
- Infection is usually with opportunistic pathogens, such as pneumocystis, CMV or yeasts.

HYPOGAMMAGLOBULINAEMIA

Causes

1. Artefactual, e.g. haemodilution during IV therapy.
2. Decreased production:
   (i) Severe malnutrition
   (ii) Lymphoproliferative diseases, e.g. chronic lymphatic leukaemia and myeloma
   (iii) Infection, e.g. malaria, septicaemia, trypanosomiasis
   (iv) Drugs, e.g. cytotoxic agents, gold, phenytoin, penicillamine and irradiation
   (v) Splenectomy.
3. Increased loss or catabolism:
   (i) Protein-losing enteropathy and intestinal lymphangiectasia.
   (ii) Malabsorption
   (iii) Nephrotic syndrome
   (iv) Exfoliative dermatitis
   (v) Burns.

T-CELL DEFICIENCY

Causes

1. Drugs, e.g. high-dose steroids, cyclophosphamide, ciclosporin.
2. Lymphoproliferative disorders, e.g. Hodgkin's disease and advanced malignancy.
3. Infections, e.g. measles, rubella, infectious mononucleosis, TB, brucellosis, leprosy; HIV-1 and -2 and secondary syphilis.
4. Protein-calorie malnutrition.
5. Other diseases, e.g. pyoderma gangrenosum, advanced rheumatoid arthritis, sarcoidosis, diabetes and alcoholism.

HIV-1 infection and acquired immune deficiency syndrome (AIDS)

(See also p. 65.)

- Syndrome first reported in 1981.
- Clinical spectrum of HIV-1 infection includes an acute mononucleosis-like seroconversion illness, asymptomatic infection, AIDS-related complex (ARC), and overt AIDS.
- AIDS is characterized by the development of severe, disseminated opportunistic infections, especially *Pneumocystis carinii* pneumonia, Kaposi's sarcoma and, less commonly, other neoplasms.
- Destruction of CD4 cells is the primary immune abnormality.

Laboratory findings
- (i) Detection of anti-HIV-I antibodies using ELISA (sensitivity approximately 100% specificity 99%). Western blot analysis is used to confirm positive ELISA test. HIV proteins are electrophoresed and the putative serum antibody of the patient is then reacted and read by antihuman antibody conjugated with enzyme or radioactive label.
- (ii) Reduction in absolute blood CD4$^+$ T cell counts (used in monitoring progression of disease and inversion of CD4/CD8 ratio to <0.5 (normal >1.5)).
- (iii) Many factors affect CD4 cell counts, e.g. endogenous and exogenous corticosteroids, race, gender, age and exercise.
- (iv) Reduced delayed hypersensitivity responses.
- (v) Decreased proliferation to soluble antigens.
- (vi) Decreased synthesis of IL-2 in vitro following stimulation with antigens.
- (vii) Decreased mitogen response in vitro.
- (viii) Increased serum β2 microglobulin levels.
- (ix) Hypergammaglobulinaemia especially of IgA, IgG1, IgG3 and IgM.
- (x) Moderate decrease in natural killer cell numbers and function.
- (xi) Increased cytokine levels.

Possible mechanisms of HIV-related T-cell depletion
- Virus-induced lysis
- Syncytia formation
- Immune lysis (by antibody or cellular mechanisms)
- Induction of apoptosis.

Senescence of the immune response
Depressed humoral and cellular immune response. Also characterized by a loss in some T-cell functions, especially release of interleukin 2 and suppressor cells. Occurrence of autoimmune disease is increased.

HYPERGAMMAGLOBULINAEMIA

Causes of polyclonal hypergammaglobulinaemia:
1. Artefactual, e.g. prolonged venous stasis before venepuncture
2. Haemoconcentration secondary to dehydration
3. Chronic infection, e.g. TB, infective endocarditis, leishmaniasis
4. Autoimmune disease, e.g. SLE, rheumatoid arthritis
5. Ulcerative colitis and Crohn's disease
6. Sarcoidosis
7. Hepatic disease.

Commonly recognized immunoglobulin changes in liver disease
(usually accompanied by a decrease in albumin) are:

IgG ↑ in: chronic active hepatitis, cryptogenic cirrhosis
IgM ↑ in: 1° biliary cirrhosis, alcoholic cirrhosis
IgA ↑ in: alcoholic cirrhosis.

Table 3.15 Monoclonal hypergammaglobulinaemia

Disorder	Class of protein	Light chain
Multiple myeloma	IgG, IgA, IgD, or IgE	κ or λ
Macroglobulinaemia	IgM	κ or λ
Heavy chain disease	IgG, IgA, or IgM	None

Causes of monoclonal hypergammaglobulinaemia

1. Multiple myeloma, Waldenström's macroglobulinaemia and heavy chain disease (Table 3.15)
2. Leukaemia, lymphoma or carcinoma
3. Bence Jones proteinuria
4. 'Benign' paraproteinaemia
5. Amyloidosis.

AUTOIMMUNE DISEASE (Table 3.16)

Table 3.16 Autoimmune diseases

Disease	Autoantibody present against
Organ specific	
Hashimoto's thyroiditis	Thyroglobulin, thyroid peroxidase
Graves' disease	TSH receptor
Myasthenia gravis	Acetylcholine receptor
Pernicious anaemia	Gastric parietal cells, intrinsic factor
Goodpasture's syndrome	Antiglomerular and lung basement membrane
Autoimmune thrombocytopenia	Platelets
Autoimmune haemolytic anaemia (AIHA)*	Red blood cells (see Table 3.17)
Primary antiphospholipid antibody syndrome	Anticardiolipin (antiphospholipid)
Premature ovarian failure	Corpus luteum, interstitial cells
Pemphigus†	Intercellular substance of epidermis
Pemphigoid†	Basement membrane
Non-organ-specific	
Vasculitis	ANCA
Drug-induced lupus	Histone
Primary biliary cirrhosis	Mitochondria
Rheumatoid arthritis	IgG (rheumatoid factor)
Sceloderma (CREST variant)	Centromere
Mixed connective tissue disorder	Extractable nuclear antigens
SLE	Nuclear antigens, e.g. ANA, anti-double stranded (ds) DNA, smooth muscle antigen and IgG. Lupus anticoagulation (up to 40% of patients)

*AIHA: autoimmune haemolytic anaemia (primary: idiopathic > 50% secondary: to SLE/RA, chronic lymphatic leukaemia, non-Hodgkin's lymphoma, infection, e.g. mycoplasma, EBV and drug treatment).
†Immunofluorescent staining pattern: pemphigus (IgG, C3); pemphigoid (IgG, C3), herpes gestationis (IgG, C3); dermatitis herpetiformis (IgA, C3 on dermal papillae).

Table 3.17 Red blood cell conditions

Type of anaemia	%	Damage due to
Warm antibody	70	Mainly IgG; opsonization and phagocytosis
Cold antibody	18	Mainly IgM, except paroxysmal cold haemoglobinuria
Drug-induced, e.g.	12	Antibodies to adsorbed drug
penicillin, α-methyldopa		Attachment of immune complexes (drug/IgG)
		Autoantibodies to RBC (Rhesus neg.)

EXPLANATORY THEORIES FOR BREAKDOWN IN SELF TOLERANCE

1. **Cross-reactive antigens:** Microbial antigens cross-reacting with host tissues induce an immune response against self.
2. **Aberrant antigen presentation:** Usually only certain cells present antigen to CD4+ T cells because they have MHC class II molecules. Other cells may be able to express these molecules and present self antigens e.g. via cytokines induced by infectious agents.
3. **Attachment of foreign hapten to self molecule** forming a hapten–carrier complex.
4. **Regulatory abnormalities:** Deficiency of suppressor T cells e.g. SLE.
5. **Polyclonal activation:** Some microorganisms, e.g. EBV, stimulate B lymphocytes to secrete antibodies irrespective of their antigen specificities. Some B cells are also capable of mounting an immune response against self.
6. **Release of sequestered antigen:** Lens and sperm proteins do not pass through the primary lymphoid organs so that autoreactive cells are not eliminated, e.g. mumps-induced orchitis, sympathetic uveitis.

AUTOANTIBODIES

Rheumatoid factor (Table 3.18)
* Circulating immunoglobulin, usually IgM (also IgG or IgA), which is directed against the Fc fragment of the patient's own IgG.
* Detected by latex agglutination tests and sheep red cell agglutination test (SCAT) or Rose–Waaler test (see p. 129).

Positive in 80% of cases with rheumatoid arthritis. A high titre of seropositivity is associated with systemic complications (i.e. nodules, vasculitis and neuropathy).

False positives occur in:
1. General population, rising with age (4%).
2. Collagen vascular disease, e.g. Sjögren's syndrome (25–30%), essential mixed cryoglobulinaemia, systemic sclerosis, SLE, dermatomyositis
3. Juvenile rheumatoid arthritis (15%).
4. Bacterial and viral infections (especially HIV, viral hepatitis, rubella, infectious mononucleosis and chronic infections, e.g. TB, syphilis and leprosy).
5. Infective endocarditis (<50%).
6. Chronic fibrosing lung disease.
7. Chronic liver disease.
8. Others: Waldenström's macroglobulinaemia, glomerulonephritis, renal transplant, advanced age, blood transfusion, myocardial infarction.

Anti-smooth muscle antibody

Positive in:
1. Chronic active hepatitis (40–90%)
2. Primary biliary cirrhosis (30–70%)
3. Idiopathic cirrhosis (25–30%)
4. Viral infections (80%)

Anti-mitochondrial antibody

Positive in:
1. Primary biliary cirrhosis (60–94%)
2. Chronic active hepatitis (25–60%)
3. Idiopathic cirrhosis (25–30%)

Gastric parietal cell antibody

Positive in:
1. Pernicious anaemia (>90%)
2. Atrophic gastritis (♀ 60%, ♂ 15–20%)
3. Autoimmune thyroid disease (33%)

Thyroid autoantibodies (microsomal and thyroglobulin)

Positive in:
1. Hashimoto's thyroiditis (70–90% microsomal: 75–95% thyroglobulin)
2. Graves' disease (50–80% microsomal; 33–75% thyroglobulin)
3. Hypothyroidism (40–65% microsomal; 50–80% thyroglobulin)
4. Pernicious anaemia (55% microsomal)

Antireticulin antibody

Positive in:
1. Coeliac disease (37%)
2. Crohn's disease (24%)
3. Dermatitis herpetiformis (17–22%)

ANTINUCLEAR ANTIBODIES (ANA) (Table 3.18)

- IgG or IgM antibody directed against a variety of nuclear constituents, e.g. DNA, RNA or nucleolar material.

High positive titres occur in:
1. SLE.
2. Other connective tissue disorders, e.g. Sjögren's syndrome, systemic sclerosis, rheumatoid arthritis.
3. Others: Hashimoto's thyroiditis, myasthenia gravis, pernicious anaemia, TB, leprosy, pulmonary fibrosis, lymphoma, malignancy, ulcerative colitis, advanced age.
4. Other autoimmune disease, e.g. chronic active hepatitis, myasthenia gravis.
5. Use of certain drugs.

- Antiribonucleoprotein (anti-RNP) antibody is seen in high titres with mixed connective tissue disorders and in lower titres with SLE and other connective tissue disorders.
- Anticentromere antibody is present in 70% of patients with CREST and 15% of patients with diffuse scleroderma.
- CREST syndrome: calcinosis, Raynaud's phenomenon, oesophageal dysfunction, sclerodactyly and telangiectasia.
- Antihistone antibody is seen in SLE and drug-induced lupus.
- Antibodies that bind *single-stranded* denatured DNA (ss-DNA) are present in 90% of patients with SLE, but also in drug-induced lupus and other connective tissue disorders.
- Antibodies to native *double-stranded* DNA (ds-DNA) are highly specific for SLE.

Table 3.18 Summary of frequency of antinuclear antibodies (ANA) and rheumatoid factor (RF) in various diseases

Disease	ANA (%)	RF (%)
SLE	90	20
Rheumatoid arthritis	20	70
Sjögren's syndrome	70	90

Antineutrophil cytoplasmic antibodies (ANCAs) (Table 3.19)

Table 3.19 Different types of antineutrophil cytoplasmic antibody (ANCA)-associated diseases and their epitopes

Type of ANCA	Epitope	Disease association
cANCA	Proteinase 3	Wegener's granulomatosis Microscopic polyangiitis (rarely)
pANCA	Myeloperoxidase	Idiopathic crescentic glomerulonephritis Microscopic polyangiitis Churg–Strauss syndrome Wegener's granulomatosis (rarely)
False-positive ANCA		Infection, HIV, bacterial endocarditis, cystic fibrosis Bronchial carcinoma, atrial myxoma Sweet's syndrome, eosinophilia–myalgia syndrome

BLOOD GROUP IMMUNOLOGY

ABO GROUP

- Complex oligosaccharides, A, B and H, are located on the surface of red blood cells. Present in the tissue fluids and secretions of approximately 75% of people.
- An individual inherits one of three ABO antigen groups (*agglutinogen*) from each parent—A, B or neither.
- Individuals also inherit antibodies (*agglutinins*) which react against red cells of groups other than their own, i.e. anti-A or anti-B (Table 3.20).

Table 3.20 ABO group characteristics

Genotype	Phenotype	Agglutinogen on cell	Agglutinins in plasma	% Frequency in population
OO	O	Nil or H substance	Anti-A, Anti-B	46
AA/AO	A	A	Anti-B	42
BB/BO	B	B	Anti-A	9
AB	AB	AB	None	3

> Agglutinogen A + agglutinin anti-A → agglutination
> Agglutinogen B + agglutinin anti-B → agglutination

- Significant associations between ABO blood groups, secretor status and disease include peptic ulcer disease (O), duodenal ulcer (non-secretor status), gastric carcinoma (A), and pernicious anaemia (A).

Summary of principles of blood transfusion

- Blood group O is the universal donor group because there are no A or B antigens on the red cell membrane.

Therefore blood transfusion may be given thus (Fig. 3.11):

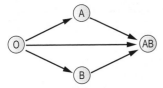

Fig. 3.11 ABO groups in blood transfusion.

RHESUS (CDE) GROUP

- Three further agglutinogens, C, D and E, occur in association with red cells, of which Group D is the most important agglutinogen.
- 84% of caucasians are Rhesus-positive, i.e. Rhesus (D) antigen is present on the surface of red blood cells. Africans and Japanese are generally Rhesus-negative.

RHESUS INCOMPATIBILITY

- There is no preformed Rhesus agglutinin (anti-D). A Rhesus-negative person can make anti-D only after sensitization with Rhesus-positive blood, i.e. a Rhesus-*negative* mother and a Rhesus-positive father may produce a Rhesus-*positive* fetus. If fetal red blood cells escape into the blood of the mother she produces anti-D antibodies. If these IgG antibodies cross the placenta in subsequent pregnancies, they destroy the fetal red blood cells, resulting in haemolytic disease of the newborn.
- Sensitization can be prevented by administering a single dose of anti-Rh D antibodies in the form of Rh immune globulin during the postpartum period to Rhesus-negative women after the birth of a Rhesus-positive child or following a miscarriage. This will destroy the Rhesus-positive fetal red blood cells, preventing maternal sensitization and the production of her own anti-D, which can affect the next pregnancy.

MINOR BLOOD GROUP SYSTEM

Proteins expressed on erythrocytes which display allelic variation can also act as blood antigens, e.g. Kell antigen, a zinc endopeptidase, the Duffy antigen receptor for chemokines (DARC).

TRANSPLANTATION IMMUNOLOGY

TERMINOLOGY (Table 3.21)

Table 3.21 Summary of terms used in tissue transplantation

	Genetic term	Transplantation
Relationship between donor and host		
Same individual	Syngeneic (autologous)	Autograft
Identical twin	Syngeneic (isologous)	Isograft e.g. kidney transplant between monozygotic identical twins
Different individuals (same species)	Allogeneic (homologous)	Allograft e.g. cadaveric renal transplant
Different species	Xenogeneic (heterologous)	Xenograft e.g. baboon kidney transplanted into a human
Location of graft		
In a different type of tissue		Heterotopic
In the tissue from which the graft came		Isotopic e.g. corneal grafts
In same type of tissue as graft origin, but a different anatomical position		Orthotopic e.g. skin grafted from the thigh to the arm

> **Tissue typing techniques** ✓
>
> These are used to identify donor/recipient pairs with the lowest risk of complications:
>
> 1. HLA typing with anti-HLA antibodies for the presence of specific HLA antigens on host and potential donor cells.
> 2. HLA cross-matching (mixed lymphocyte reaction (MLR)) determines the extent to which potential donor cells stimulate activation and proliferation of donor T cells. This in vitro test provides a quantitative assessment of tissue compatibility when a perfect HLA match is not available.

GRAFT REJECTION AND SURVIVAL

Three types of rejection reaction (Table 3.22) can take place following transplantation:

1. **Hyperacute rejection** where the recipient has preformed antibodies, occurs within hours or days. There is rapid vascular spasm, occlusion and failure of organ perfusion.
2. **Acute accelerated rejection** due to sensitized T lymphocytes and a cell-mediated immune response, occurs 10–30 days after transplantation. There is infiltration of small lymphocytes and mononuclear cells which destroy the graft.
3. **Chronic rejection** is characterized by the slow loss of tissue function over a period of months or years. May be a cellular immune response, an antibody response or a combination of the two.

Table 3.22 Rejection reactions

Type	Time	Cause
Hyperacute	Hours	Preformed donor circulating antibodies activate complement
Acute	Days–weeks	Occurs when there is HLA incompatibility. Starts when allogenic dendritic cells or autologous cells present to T cells in local lymphocytes. Alloreactive T cells become stimulated, secrete IL-2 and proliferate. CD4$^+$ cells then migrate to the organ and initiate a delayed hypersensitivity reaction
Chronic	Months–years	Causes are unclear. There is some inflammation and T cells are present. Advancing vascular disease represents the main problem.

Table 3.23 Graft survival

Organ	Characteristics	Graft survival (%)
Cornea	No immunosuppression required because cornea does not become vascularized	Over 90
Kidney	Live related kidney donation often used; graft survival optimized by HLA match; immunosuppression required	Over 80
Pancreas	Usually transplanted along with kidneys in diabetics with renal failure; separated islet cells have also been infused into the vena cava	About 50

Table 3.23 (Cont'd)

Organ	Characteristics	Graft survival (%)
Heart	Used for coronary artery disease, cardiomyopathy and some congenital heart disease; immunosuppression required	Over 80
Liver	Used for alcoholic liver disease, primary biliary cirrhosis and virus-induced cirrhosis	Over 60: outcome not affected by degree of HLA matching
Stem cells	Used in malignancy, haematological conditions and some primary immunodeficiency; best results when there is a match of HLA *A, B, C* and *DR*	Up to 80

STEM CELL TRANSPLANTATION

- Used to restore myeloid and lymphoid cells in haematological malignancy; when myeloid cell production is reduced or abnormal, e.g. aplastic anaemia; and in primary immunodeficiencies, e.g. SCID (Table 3.24).
- Following transplantation, myeloid cells are regenerated from pluripotent stem cells, which can be obtained from several sources: e.g. bone marrow, peripheral blood stem cells and cord blood. An advantage of cord blood is that the immature lymphocytes are less likely to cause GVHD.

Table 3.24 Indications for stem cell transplantation

Indication	Specific disease
Anaemia	Aplastic (severe forms) Fanconi's anaemia
Leukaemia	Acute lymphoblastic Acute myeloid Chronic myeloid
Immunodeficiency	Reticular dysgenesis Severe combined immunodeficiency (SCID) Chronic granulomatous disease Wiskott–Aldrich syndrome
Inborn errors in metabolism	Gaucher's disease Hurler's disease Thalassaemia Osteopetrosis

GRAFT VERSUS HOST DISEASE (GVHD)

- A condition resulting from an attack by the donor's immunologically reactive T lymphocytes against the foreign allogenic antigens of the recipient, i.e. where there is an antigen difference between the donor and recipient; occurs up to 4 weeks after SCT.
- When severe, acute GVHD carries a 70% mortality. Chronic GVHD occurs later and affects skin and liver.
- The skin, gastrointestinal tract, liver and lungs are most commonly affected.
- It is a major factor limiting allogeneic bone marrow on stem cell transplantation in humans, but does not occur with heart or kidney transplantation.
- All patients receiving BMT or SCT are given immunosuppressive drugs to prevent GVHD, even if donor and recipients are HLA identical. Removing mature T cells from the source of the stem cells reduces the risk of GVHD. T-cell depletion increases the risk of graft rejection.

XENOTRANSPLANTATION

There are several key problems that need to be overcome before xenotransplantation from other species becomes an option:

1. Primates assemble sugar side-chains differently from other species. All humans possess natural antibodies against a sugar (gal-α1,3-gal) on cells. These antibodies bind onto xenotransplanted organs and trigger complement activation and hyperacute rejection.
2. Complement inhibitors from other species do not inhibit human complement. As a result of this molecular incompatibility, xenotransplanted organs activate complement.
3. With pig donor organs there may be acute rejection, as pig proteins elicit a T-cell response.
4. Pigs are infected with endogenous retroviruses which may infect humans following transplantation and use of immunosuppressive drugs.

TUMOUR IMMUNOLOGY

- Tumour cells are cells transformed by virus or by physical or chemical means. They are usually not well differentiated, proliferate uncontrollably, lack contact inhibition and have *tumour-associated antigen* (TAA) expression on their surface.

TUMOUR-ASSOCIATED ANTIGEN (TAA) (Table 3.25)

- TAAs are molecules produced by tumour cells that may elicit both humoral and cell-mediated responses.

Table 3.25 Examples of tumour-associates antigens

Type	Antigen	Distribution
Developmental proteins	Carcinoembryonic antigen (CEA)	Fetal gut cells: very small amounts on adult colonic cells but much higher on colonic tumour cells; antigen shed into serum aids early diagnosis and detection of progression
	Alpha-fetoprotein	Secreted by fetal liver/yolk sac cells; serum of patients with liver or germinal cell tumours
	Cell antigen (CD10)	Present on common acute lymphoblastic leukaemic cells; also on B-lymphoid precursor cells in regenerating bone marrow or in fetal bone marrow
Lineage specific proteins	Tyrosine	Normal melanocytes and melanoma cells both express the enzyme tyrosine, which is not expressed in other cells, normal or abnormal
Viral proteins	EBV and human papillomavirus	EBV immortalizes cells by producing cells that drive B-cell proliferation and inhibit apoptosis. The marked polyclonal B-cell proliferation increases the risk of translocation involving lung myc, leading to the growth of a malignant population
Proteins produced through translocations	bcr-abl fusion protein	Product of the bcr/abl translocation

127

B-cell involvement is characterized by:
1. Attachment of antibody to Fc receptors on macrophages and polymorphonuclear cells with phagocytosis.
2. Attachment of antibody to Fc receptors on killer cells with subsequent lysis by antibody-dependent cell cytotoxicity.
3. Activation of the classical complement cascade, causing tumour lysis.

T-cell involvement is characterized by:
1. Production of lymphokines such as macrophage-activating factor (MAF) and macrophage chemotactic factor.
2. Production of tumour necrosis factor (TNF) by activated macrophages.
3. Killing of tumour cells without prior sensitization by natural killer (NK) cells.

- Tumours in immunodeficient and immunosuppressed patients (Table 3.26): most of these tumours are caused by multiple factors, including virally induced pathological changes.

Table 3.26 Tumours associated with immunodeficiency and immunosuppression

Disease	Tumour type
Immunodeficiency	
DiGeorge syndrome	
Wiskott–Aldrich syndrome	
Ataxia telangiectasia	All lymphoreticular
Severe combined immunodeficiency (SCID)	
Chediak–Higashi syndrome	
Immunosuppression	
Organ transplants	
Azathioprine/steroids	Non-Hodgkin's lymphoma (NHL), liver cancer, Kaposi's sarcoma, cervical cancer
Ciclosporin A	Lymphoma, skin cancer, Kaposi's sarcoma
Inflammatory disease	
Rheumatoid arthritis	NHL
Malaria	Burkitt's lymphoma
HIV infection	NHL, Kaposi's sarcoma

TUMOURS OF THE IMMUNE SYSTEM

1. **Lymphomas:** T- and B-cell lymphomas can be distinguished in tissue sections using specific anti-T-cell (e.g. CD3) and anti-B-cell (e.g. CD20) antibodies, or enzymes. Anti κ and λ light chain antibodies are used to analyse the monoclonal nature of B-cell malignancies such as lymphomas, leukaemias and myelomas.
2. **Lymphoid and myeloid leukaemias:** These derive from different cell types and antibodies of the lymphohaematopoietic system, and are distinguished by enzyme staining, e.g. CD13/CD33 for myeloid cells, CD3/CD5 for T cells and CD19/CD20 for B cells. CD10 antigen is expressed on common acute lymphoblastic leukaemic cells.
3. **Myelomas and other plasma cell tumours:** Electrophoresis of serum and urine detect a variety of paraproteins, e.g. IgG (myeloma), IgM (Waldenström's macroglobulinaemia, and heavy or light chain diseases).

IMMUNOLOGICAL ASSAYS

Relative sensitivity of serological procedures to detect antibody		✓
MOST SENSITIVE	RIA	
	ELISA	
	Agglutination	
	Flocculation	
LEAST SENSITIVE	↓ Precipitation	

1. AGGLUTINATION ASSAYS

- Red cells or inert particles, e.g. latex, are clumped by antiserum that cross-links antigens on the surface particles.
- *Examples:* Coombs' antiglobulin test, Widal test, ABO blood grouping and the Rose–Waaler test for the detection of rheumatoid factor.

COOMBS' ANTIGLOBULIN TEST

- Two-stage reaction (Fig. 3.12). The direct Coombs' test is used to detect cell-bound antibody. It involves adding an antibody directed against an antiglobulin reagent, thus providing a bridge between two antibody-coated cells or particles.
- The direct test detects cells coated with IgG in vivo; the indirect test detects antibodies that bind cells.

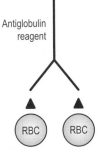

Fig. 3.12 Coombs' test.

Causes of a positive Coombs' test

1. Idiopathic acquired haemolytic anaemia and autoimmune haemolytic anaemia.
2. Haemolytic transfusion reactions.
3. Alloantibodies, e.g. haemolytic disease of the newborn (i.e. detects maternal anti-Rh antibody bound to fetal red blood cells with rhesus incompatibility).
4. SLE, lymphoma, leukaemia and carcinoma.
5. Drugs, e.g. methyldopa.

2. COMPLEMENT FIXATION TESTS

- An antigen–antibody reaction may fix complement, and the presence of a complement-fixing antibody may be detected using an indicator system.
- In the *presence* of complement-fixing antibody, complement is unavailable to lyse indicator red cells with anti-red cell antibody. In the *absence* of antibody, complement will remain unfixed and available for lysis of the indicator system.

- There are two stages to the test:
  1. Test system: patient's serum + known antigen + complement
  2. Indicator system: sheep red blood cells ± haemolysis.
- *Examples:* tests for viral antibodies, HBsAg, anti-DNA, anti-platelet antibodies and the Wassermann reaction for syphilis.

3. IMMUNOFLUORESCENCE TESTS (Fig. 3.13)

- Antigen fixed to a solid phase combines with antibody in a test serum.
- Anti-human antibody (IgG or IgM) labelled with fluorescein (F) is added, and the Ag–Ab complexes visualized with ultraviolet light.
- *Examples:* detection of organ-specific auto-antibodies (thyroid) and non-organ-specific autoantibodies (ANA in SLE) using indirect IF; identification of T and B cells in blood, rapid identification of microorganisms in tissues or cultures (e.g. rabies virus, herpes simplex virus in biopsy) using direct IF, and localization of hormones and enzymes.

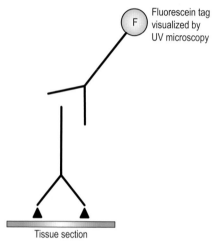

Fluorescein tag visualized by UV microscopy

Tissue section

Fig. 3.13 Immunofluorescence test.

FLOW CYTOMETRY

- Measures cell properties, e.g. cell viability, proliferation, surface antigen expression and intracellular enzyme activity.
- Relies on labelling with fluorescent markers.
- Main applications:
  1. Cell surface antigen detection, e.g. CD4 cell count in HIV infection, and cell markers in haematological malignancies
  2. Measurement of cellular DNA, e.g. study of cell cycle and cell viability in evaluation of cytotoxic drugs.

4. IMMUNOENZYME ASSAYS

Example: enzyme-linked immunoabsorbent assay (ELISA) (see Note).
- Similar to immunofluorescent assays, except label used is an enzyme, such as horse radish peroxidase, instead of fluorescein, and purified antigen is required. Enzyme will cause a colour change on the addition of a specific

substrate. The intensity of the colour change is proportional to the amount of patient antibody that has bound to fixed antigen.
- Can be used to assay both antigen and antibody.
- *Examples:* HIV-1 antibody and hepatitis B antigen.
- Used routinely to supplement indirect IF tests, e.g. gliadin antibodies.

Note: Antibody capture tests: both ELISA and RIA can be made more sensitive and specific by 'capturing' patients' IgM reacting with the virus, then adding labelled monoclonal antiviral antibody.

5. RADIOIMMUNOASSAY (RIA)

- Generally the most sensitive assay for antigen.
- Similar to above, except label used is a radioactive isotope, e.g. ^{125}I. Increasing known amounts of unlabelled antigen are reacted with a constant amount of antibody, followed by labelled antigen. The bound antigen–antibody versus the free antigen ratio is determined and the amount of antigen in the unknown sample is calculated by reference to a standard curve. The partitioning of the activity indicates the concentration of the antibody in the test solution.
- *Examples:* assay of polypeptide hormones, anti-DNA-Ab, hepatitis B surface antigen, drugs (e.g. digoxin).

6. IMMUNODIFFUSION

- Technique for estimating antigen concentration.
- Radial immunodiffusion: antigen diffuses out of a well cut into an agar plate which has a specific antibody incorporated. The distance of the line of precipitation from the well is proportional to the concentration of antigen in the well.
- Double diffusion: solutions of antigen and antibody are placed in two adjacent wells, with antibody in the central well. The further the line of precipitation is from the latter well, the greater the concentration of antigen.
- *Examples:* cryptococcal antigen in CSF, carcinoembryonic antigen and alpha-fetoprotein.

4

ANATOMY

PERIPHERAL NERVOUS SYSTEM   134
Dermatomes   134
Spinal nerves   138
  Cervical plexus   138
  Brachial plexus   138
  Lumbosacral plexus   140

AUTONOMIC NERVOUS SYSTEM   141
Sympathetic system   142
Parasympathetic system   144

CENTRAL NERVOUS SYSTEM   147
Basal ganglia   147
Midbrain   147
Pons   147
Medulla   147
Spinal cord   148
Cerebral cortex   148
Ventricles of the brain and cerebrospinal
   fluid system   151
Skull foramina   152
Cranial nerves   152

PRINCIPAL VESSELS   163
Principal arteries   163
Principal veins   165

HEAD AND NECK   167
Thyroid gland   167
Larynx   167

THORAX   169
Surface markings   169
Trachea and bronchi   169
Lung   171
Heart   171
Fetal circulation   174

ABDOMEN   175
Surface markings   175
Diaphragm   175
Thoracic duct   176
Oesophagus   176
Stomach   176
Duodenum   177
Liver   177

PERIPHERAL NERVOUS SYSTEM

DERMATOMES (Table 4.1)

Table 4.1 Summary of dermatomal supply

Root value	Area innervated
C5–T1	Upper limb
T4	Nipple
T7	Lower ribs
T10	Umbilical area
T12	'Lowest' nerve of the anterior abdominal wall
L1	Inguinal region
L2,3	Anteromedial and lateral thigh
L4,5*	Medial border of the foot and sole, front and back of the calf up to the knee
S1*	Lateral side of the foot (fifth toe) and sole
S2	Posterior surface of the leg and thigh
S3,4	Buttocks and perianal region

* L5 supplies the first toe; S1 supplies the fifth toe.

Dermatomes of the head and neck (Fig. 4.1)

Anterior to the auricle, the scalp is supplied by the three branches of the trigeminal nerve.
Posterior to the auricle, the scalp is supplied by the spinal cutaneous nerves from the neck.

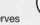

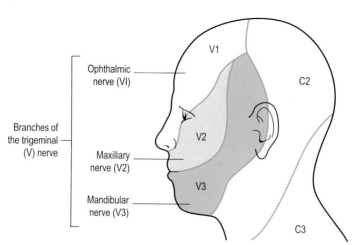

Fig. 4.1 Dermatomes: head and neck.

Dermatomes in the thorax and abdomen (Fig. 4.2)

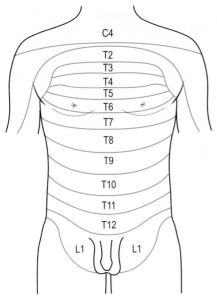

Fig. 4.2 Dermatomes: thorax and abdomen.

Dermatomes in the upper limb (Fig. 4.3)

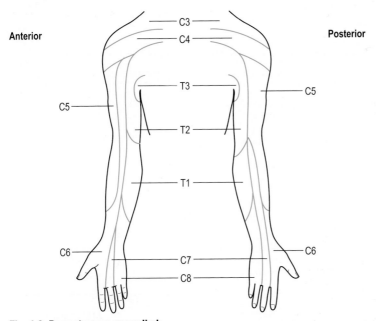

Fig. 4.3 Dermatomes: upper limb.

Dermatomes in the lower limb (Fig. 4.4)

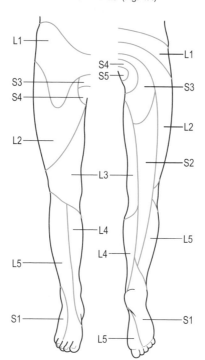

Anterior   Posterior

Fig. 4.4 Dermatomes: lower limb.

Table 4.2 Motor root values and peripheral nerve supply of important muscle groups			
Joint movement	*Muscle*	*Root value*	*Peripheral nerve*
Shoulder			
• abduction	Deltoid	C4, 5	Axillary
• external rotation	Infraspinatus	C4, 5	Suprascapular
• adduction	Pectoralis/	C6–8	Medial and
	Latissimus dorsi		lateral pectoral
Elbow			
• flexion	Biceps	C5, 6	Musculocutaneous
• extension	Triceps	C7, 8	Radial
• pronation		C6, 7	
• supination	Biceps/	C5, 6	Musculocutaneous
	brachioradialis	C6	Radial
Wrist			
• flexion	Flexor muscles	C7, 8	Median and ulnar
	of forearm		
• dorsiflexion	Extensor muscles	C7	Radial
	of forearm		
Finger			
• flexion	Long finger flexors	C8	Median and ulnar
• extension	Long finger extensors	C7	Radial
• opposition of	Small hand muscles	T1	Ulnar
thumb or splaying			
of fingers			

Table 4.2 (Cont'd)

Joint movement	Muscle	Root value	Peripheral nerve
Hips			
• flexion	Iliopsoas	L1–3	—
• extension	Glutei	L5 and S1	Sciatic
• adduction	Adductors	L2, 3	Obturator
• abduction	Glutei and tensor fasciae latae	L4, 5 and S1	Sciatic
Knee			
• flexion	Hamstrings	L5 and S1,2	Sciatic
• extension	Quadriceps	L3, 4	Femoral
Ankle			
• dorsiflexion	Anterior tibial	L4, 5	Sciatic (peroneal)
• plantar flexion	Calf (gastrocnemius and soleus)	S1, 2	Sciatic (tibial)
• eversion	Peronei	L5 and S1	Sciatic (peroneal)
• inversion	Anterior tibial and posterior tibial	L4 / L4, 5	Sciatic (peroneal) / Sciatic (tibial)
Toes			
• flexion		S2, 3	
• extension	Extensor hallucis longus	L5 and S1	Sciatic (peroneal)

Note: All muscles on back of upper limb (triceps, wrist and finger extensors) are innervated by C7.

Table 4.3 Quick screening tests for muscle power

Shoulder	Abduction	C5	Hip	Flexion	L1–L2
	Adduction	C5–C7		Extension	L5–S1
Elbow	Flexion	C5–C6	Knee	Flexion	S1
	Extension	C7		Extension	L3–L4
Wrist	Flexion	C7–C8	Ankle	Dorsiflexion	L4
	Extension	C7		Plantar flexion	S1–S2
Fingers	Flexion	C7–C8			
	Extension	C7			
	Abduction	T1			

Table 4.4 Tendon jerks and abdominal reflexes

Tendon jerk	Muscle	Root value	Peripheral nerve
Biceps	Biceps	C5, 6	Musculocutaneous
Triceps	Triceps	C7	Radial
Supinator	Brachioradialis	C6	Radial
Finger	Long finger flexors	C8	Median and ulnar
Knee	Quadriceps	L3,4	Femoral
Ankle	Gastrocnemius	S1	Sciatic (tibial branch)
Abdominal		T8–12	
Cremasteric		L1, 2	
Anal		S3, 4	

Table 4.5 Effects of nerve root compression

C4–C5	Elbow sensation, supraspinatus muscle
C5–C6	Thumb sensation, biceps muscle
C6–C7	Middle finger sensation, latissimus dorsi muscle, triceps reflex
C7–C8, T1	Little finger sensation, flexor carpi ulnaris muscle

SPINAL NERVES

> 31 pairs of spinal nerves:
> - 8 cervical
> - 12 thoracic
> - 5 lumbar
> - 5 sacral
> - 1 coccygeal.

CERVICAL PLEXUS (C1–4)

Phrenic nerve (C3–5)
The most important branch of the cervical plexus.
- Descends beneath sternocleidomastoid muscle, and passes in front of the subclavian artery. Right phrenic passes lateral to the superior vena cava. Left phrenic crosses the lateral aspect of the aortic arch. Both right and left nerves then descend vertically in front of the root of the lung and pass between pericardium and mediastinal pleura to the diaphragm.
- Motor fibres supply the diaphragm. Sensory fibres supply the pericardium, pleura and diaphragmatic pleura.

BRACHIAL PLEXUS

- Formed by the union of the ventral rami of the 5th to 8th cervical nerves and most of the ventral ramus of the 1st thoracic nerve.
- The three posterior divisions unite to form the posterior cord: the superior and two anterior divisions unite to form the lateral cord, and the inferior and anterior divisions form the medial cord.

Brachial plexus injuries
1. **Erb-Duchenne paralysis:** damage to C5, 6 roots.
   (i) Paralysis of the deltoid, biceps and brachialis: 'winged scapula', i.e. arm internally rotated at the shoulder and elbow extended.
   (ii) Sensory loss on the lateral aspect of shoulder and upper arm, and radial border of the forearm.
   Causes: breech presentation (with traction on the head).

2. **Klumpke's paralysis:** damage to T1 root.
   (i) Paralysis of intrinsic hand muscles: 'claw hand'.
   (ii) Sensory loss on the medial border of forearm and hand, and over medial two fingers.
   (iii) Horner's syndrome due to traction on the sympathetic chain.
   Causes: birth injury (traction with the arm extended).

Radial nerve (C5–8)
Main branch of the posterior cord of the brachial plexus (see Note).
Motor to: extensor muscles of the forearm, wrist, finger and thumb.
Sensation: see Fig. 4.5.

Radial nerve damage in the arm
1. Wrist drop.
2. Atrophy of triceps (if trauma occurred in the axilla), i.e. unable to extend elbow, wrist or digits.
3. Small area of anaesthesia on the dorsum of the hand between 1st and 2nd metacarpals (see Fig. 4.5)

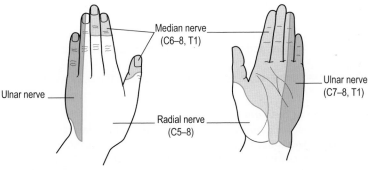

Fig. 4.5 Sensory supply to the hand.

Causes: fractures of neck of humerus, pressure palsy, badly placed injections, lead poisoning, and polyarteritis.
Note: The axillary nerve (C5, 6) is the smaller terminal branch, and supplies both the deltoid and teres major muscle.

Median nerve (C6–8, T1)
Arises from the lateral and medial cords of the brachial plexus.
Motor to:
1. Lateral 2 lumbricals (**L**),
2. Opponens policis (**O**), abductor pollicis brevis (**A**) and flexor pollicis brevis (**F**), i.e. the thenar eminence muscles.
3. All muscles on the flexor aspect of the forearm, apart from flexor carpi ulnaris and the ulnar half of the flexor digitorum profundus.
Note: As with the ulnar nerve, it supplies no muscles in the upper arm.

> Mnemonic: **LOAF** and forearm flexors.

Sensation: see Fig. 4.5.

Median nerve damage at the elbow
1. Pronation of forearm lost. 2. Wrist flexion weak: ulnar deviation.

Median nerve damage at the wrist
1. Paralysis and wasting of thenar muscles.
2. Paralysis of opponens pollicis.
3. Loss of sensation as shown (Fig. 4.5).
Causes: trauma, amyotrophic lateral sclerosis, heavy metal poisoning, carpal tunnel syndrome, polyarteritis nodosa, and diabetes.

Ulnar nerve (C7–8, T1)
Main continuation of the medial cord of the brachial plexus.
Motor to:
1. Medial and lateral interossei and lumbricals (**M**).
2. Adductor pollicis (**A**).
3. 1st dorsal interosseus (**F**).
4. Interossei (**I**).
5. Abductor digiti minimi and flexor digiti minimi: hypothenar muscles (**A**) and

> Mnemonic: **MAFIA**

ANATOMY

6. Flexor carpi ulnaris and medial half of flexor digitorum profundus in the forearm.

i.e. it supplies all the intrinsic muscles of the hand apart from those of the thenar eminence and the 1st and 2nd lumbricals which are innervated by the median nerve.

Note: As with the median nerve, it supplies no muscles in the upper arm.
Sensation: see Fig. 4.5.

Ulnar nerve damage at the wrist

1. Wasting and paralysis of intrinsic hand muscles (apart from lateral 2 lumbricals), i.e. fingers cannot be abducted or adducted, the thumb cannot be adducted due to paralysis of adductor pollicis: 'claw hand' (see Note).
2. Wasting and paralysis of hypothenar muscles.
3. Loss of sensation as shown (Fig. 4.5)

Note: Distinguish from Volkmann's contracture – another claw hand deformity where ischaemia causes muscle contraction throughout the forearm.

Ulnar nerve damage at the elbow

1. Clawing less marked in the 3rd and 4th fingers due to additional paralysis of flexor digitorum profundus.
2. Radial deviation of the wrist (paralysis of flexor carpi ulnaris).

Causes: laceration at the wrist, fractures/dislocation at the elbow, pressure palsy, carpal tunnel syndrome, machine vibrating tools, polyarteritis, leprosy and lead poisoning.

LUMBOSACRAL PLEXUS

Sciatic nerve (L4, 5, S1–3)

Most important branch of lumbosacral plexus and largest nerve in the body. Terminates by dividing into medial and lateral popliteal nerves (tibial and common peroneal nerves respectively) in the proximal part of the popliteal fossa.

Motor to:

1. The hamstring muscles (biceps femoris, semimembranous and semitendinous).
2. Adductor magnus.

Sensation: back of thigh and distal to knee.

Sciatic nerve damage

1. Paralysis of flexion of the knee and all movement below the knee, resulting in a foot drop.
2. Sensory loss is complete below the knee, except for a small area on the medial side of the leg.
3. Ankle jerk and plantar response is lost, but knee jerk is retained.

Causes: penetrating injuries, badly placed injections, fractures of pelvis or femur, and posterior dislocation of the hip.

Branches of sciatic nerve

- Medial popliteal (tibial) nerve.
- Lateral popliteal (common peroneal) nerve.

1. Medial popliteal (tibial) nerve

- Anterior divisions L4, 5 and S1–3.
- Larger of the two terminal branches of the sciatic nerve.
- Divides into medial and lateral planter nerves.

Motor to:
1. Calf muscles (gastrocnemius, soleus, and popliteus).
2. Flexor hallucis longus and tibialis posterior.
3. Terminal plantar branches supply the intrinsic muscles and the sole of the foot.
4. Mediates the ankle and plantar reflexes.

Sensation: lateral aspect of the foot and 5th toe (sural nerve branch) and sensation to the sole.

Tibial nerve damage
1. Unable to plantarflex, invert the foot, or flex the toes.
2. Claw-like deformity of the toes.
3. Sensation lost to the sole of the foot.

2. Lateral popliteal (common personeal) nerve
- Posterior divisions of L4, 5 and S1, 2.
- Passes through the popliteal fossa, winding around the head of the fibula close to biceps femoris.
- Divides into terminal branches: deep peroneal (anterior tibial) and superficial nerves.

Motor to: anterior compartment of the leg (extensor digitorum longus, extensor hallucis longus, tibialis anterior, peroneus tertius and extensor digitorum brevis); turns the foot upwards and outwards.

Sensation: anterolateral aspect of the lower half of the leg, including the ankle and dorsum of the foot.

Common peroneal nerve lesions
More susceptible to injury than the tibial nerve.
1. Foot drop with paralysis of dorsiflexion.
2. Paralysis of eversion and weak inversion (only with the foot in plantar flexion) and of toe extension.
3. Sensory loss to anterolateral aspect of lower half of leg.

Causes: pressure palsy, Charcot–Marie–Tooth neuropathy, fractures of tibia and fibula.

AUTONOMIC NERVOUS SYSTEM (ANS) (Fig. 4.6)

- Controls visceral functions, e.g. circulation, digestion and excretion, without voluntary control and modulates endocrine gland function which regulates metabolism.
- Sensory and motor components, and divided into sympathetic and parasympathetic systems.
- The axons of the ANS leave their cell body located in the CNS as preganglionic fibres, synapse in the appropriate ganglion and leave as postganglionic fibres.
- The neurotransmitter released by preganglionic fibres at the ganglia is acetylcholine (ACh), regardless of whether sympathetic or parasympathetic.
- The ACh receptors on postganglionic fibres are of nicotinic type.
- In general the sympathetic and parasympathetic systems mediate opposite effects.

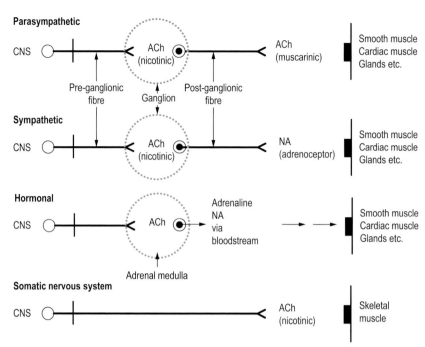

Fig. 4.6 Anatomy and neurotransmitters of the autonomic nervous system.

SYMPATHETIC SYSTEM

- The sympathetic system is controlled by centres in the hypothalamus and brainstem.
- The sympathetic outflow from the brain is in the descending reticular system of synapsing neurons.
- Nerve fibres leave the spinal cord with the nerve roots between T1 and L2, and pass into the sympathetic trunk where most synapse (Table 4.6).
- The 'first order' neurons are referred to as preganglionic.
- Postganglionic fibres then pursue a lengthy course finally reaching the heart, blood vessels, bronchi, papillary muscles and gut (Table 4.7).

Table 4.6 Sympathetic outflow (T1–L2)		
Spinal segments	*Sympathetic innervation*	*Destination*
T1–T2	Via internal carotid and vertebral arteries	Head and neck Ciliary muscle and iris Blood vessels Sweat glands
T1–T4	Via cardiac and pulmonary plexuses	Heart and bronchi
T2–T7		Upper limb
T4–L2	Via coeliac, mesenteric, hypogastric and pelvic plexuses	Adrenal medulla Alimentary tract Colon and rectum Bladder and genitalia
T11–L2		Lower limb
T1–T4: relay in sympathetic ganglion. T4–L2: do not relay in sympathetic ganglion.		

Table 4.7 Adrenergic receptors* (adrenoceptors): effects of sympathetic nervous system

System affected	ADRENERGIC RECEPTORS			
	α_1 • Postsynaptic, found esp. on smooth muscle	α_2 • Postsynaptic (outside CNS) • Postsynaptic (inside CNS)	β_1 • Mainly located in heart	β_2 • Widely distributed (esp. smooth muscle of blood vessels, bronchi and uterus)
Heart	↓ Rate ↓ Atrial contractility ↓ AVN conduction		↑ Rate and contractility ↑ AVN conduction ↑ Renin secretion	
Vessels	Little effect	Vasoconstriction of arterioles (esp. skin, abdominal viscera and coronary circulation) Constriction of systemic veins		Vasodilatation of coronary arterioles and in skeletal muscle
Bronchus	Bronchoconstriction			Bronchial muscle relaxation
Gut	↑ Motility; relaxation of sphincters	↓ Motility		↓ Motility
Urogenital	Contraction of detrusor muscles of bladder; relaxation of sphincters	Relaxation of detrusor muscles; contraction of sphincters and pregnant uterus		Relaxation of pregnant uterus
Pancreas	↑ Exocrine secretion No effect on β-cells of islets	↓ Exocrine secretion		↑ Endocrine secretion by β-cells; lipolysis, glycogenolysis, gluconeogenesis
Eye (see Fig. 4.18)	Miosis: sphincter pupillae contracts			Mydriasis: dilator pupillae contracts
Glands		↑ Secretion (lacrimal, salivary, alimentary)		↑ Secretion by sweat glands

AVN = atrioventricular node.
* Also dopamine receptors. Most numerous within the CNS, but they are also important in control of renal blood flow. Stimulation produces renal vasodilatation.

Sympathetic trunk

- Extends for the whole length of the spinal cord.
- Ganglia are associated with each spinal segment, except in the cervical region where there are only three ganglia:
  1. Superior cervical ganglion (C2–4)
  2. Middle cervical ganglion (C5,6)
  3. Inferior cervical ganglion, which fuses with 1st thoracic ganglion to form the stellate ganglion (C7, 8 and T1).

Consequences of sympathectomy
1. Division of the stellate ganglion (T1) results in Horner's syndrome due to interruption of the sympathetic fibres to the eyelid and pupil.
2. 'Cervicothoracic' sympathectomy (T2–4) results in a warm, dry hand, due to interruption of sudomotor and vasoconstrictor pathways to head and upper limb.
3. 'Lumbar' sympathectomy (L2–4) results in a warm, dry and pink lower limb.

PARASYMPATHETIC SYSTEM

- Also controlled by the hypothalamus and brainstem by a series of specific nuclei.
- Preganglionic fibres leave the CNS with the cranial nerves (especially the vagus nerve) and sacral nerve roots.
- Ganglia of the parasympathetic system are close to their destination, and postganglionic fibres are short (in contrast to sympathetic ganglia).

Parasympathetic (craniosacral) outflow

- Cranial outflow supplies the visceral structures in the head via the oculomotor, facial and glossopharyngeal nerves and those in the thorax and upper abdomen via the vagus nerves.
- Sacral outflow supplies the pelvic viscera via the pelvic branches of the 2nd to 4th sacral spinal nerves.

Neurological control of bladder function (Fig 4.7)

- The afferent branch of the micturition reflex runs in the spinal cord via parasympathetic nerves to the pontine micturition centre, which is under voluntary control.
- The efferent branch runs from the pontine micturition centre to the sacral micturition centre (S2, 3, 4), from which preganglionic parasympathetic nerves run to the pelvic plexus and then to the bladder to cause contraction.
- At the same time, the efferent branch inhibits the hypogastric and pudendal nerves, leading to relaxation of the outflow region and the pelvic floor.

Summary of bladder function
- An **automatic** bladder (partial emptying when bladder volume is approx. 250 ml) occurs with cord section above S2, 3, 4.
- An **autonomous** bladder (weak uncoordinated bladder contractions without desire to micturate occurs with lower motor neuron cord lesions at S2, 3, 4 level.
- An **atonic** bladder (distended bladder with overflow) occurs with sensory neuropathies (e.g. diabetes).

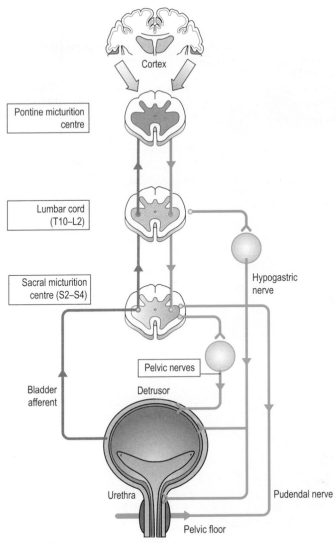

Cortex

Pontine micturition centre

Lumbar cord (T10–L2)

Sacral micturition centre (S2–S4)

Hypogastric nerve

Pelvic nerves

Bladder afferent

Detrusor

Urethra

Pudendal nerve

Pelvic floor

Fig. 4.7 Neurological control of bladder function.

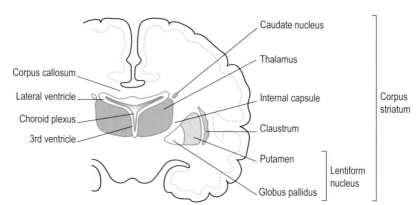

Fig. 4.8 Basal ganglia.

Caudate nucleus
Thalamus
Internal capsule
Claustrum
Putamen
Globus pallidus

Corpus striatum

Lentiform nucleus

Corpus callosum
Lateral ventricle
Choroid plexus
3rd ventricle

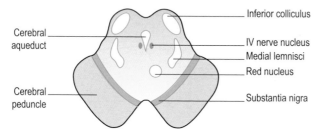

Fig. 4.9 Midbrain.

Inferior colliculus
IV nerve nucleus
Medial lemnisci
Red nucleus
Substantia nigra

Cerebral aqueduct
Cerebral peduncle

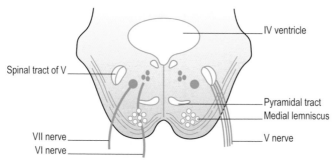

Fig. 4.10 Pons.

IV ventricle
Pyramidal tract
Medial lemniscus
V nerve

Spinal tract of V
VII nerve
VI nerve

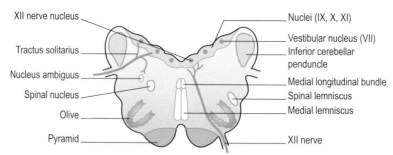

Fig. 4.11 Medulla.

XII nerve nucleus
Tractus solitarius
Nucleus ambiguus
Spinal nucleus
Olive
Pyramid

Nuclei (IX, X, XI)
Vestibular nucleus (VII)
Inferior cerebellar penduncle
Medial longitudinal bundle
Spinal lemniscus
Medial lemniscus
XII nerve

BASAL GANGLIA

- Consists of the corpus striatum (caudate nucleus, putamen, globus pallidus), claustrum, amygdala and the thalamus.
- Has afferent and efferent connections with the cerebral cortex, thalamus, subthalamus and brainstem.
- Controls motor function by an effect on the cerebral hemispheres.

MIDBRAIN

- Connects the pons and cerebellum to the diencephalon (hypothalamus and thalamus). Contains the cerebral peduncles (corticobulbar, corticospinal tracts), red nucleus, substantia nigra and the cranial nerve nuclei of III and IV and a portion of the large sensory nucleus of V.
- Ascending sensory fibres travel in the lateral and medial lemnisci.
- Descending motor fibres pass en route to pons and spinal cord.

PONS

- Lies between the medulla and midbrain and is connected to the cerebellum by the middle cerebellar peduncle.
- Upper pons: most prominent features are the pontine nuclei and the pontocerebellar fibres anteriorly.
- Lower pons: dorsal surface forms the upper part of the floor of the fourth ventricle. Contains the nuclei of the VI, VII and VIII cranial nerves. (The sensory nucleus of V is extensive, extending from the midbrain to the upper cervical level, with the most important part in the pons and the medulla. The motor nucleus of V is in the pons. The corticospinal tracts cross in the lower pons.)

MEDULLA

- Continuous through the foramen magnum with the spinal cord, and above with the pons.
- Connected to the cerebellum by the inferior cerebellar peduncle.
- Contains the nucleus ambiguus (motor to IX and X) and the solitary nucleus (sensory VIII, IX and X).
- Most prominent cranial nerve nuclei are IX, X, XI and XII.
- The dorsal column nuclei cross to form the medial lemniscus.
- Sensory decussation contains some uncrossed fibres.

Limbic system

- Collection of connected structures in the cerebrum, including deep structures, e.g. amygdala, hippocampus, certain areas of cerebral cortex, e.g. the cingulated, and segments of other structures, e.g. hypothalamus.
- Limbic system circuit transmits information from the hippocampus, via hypothalamus, thalamus and internal capsules back to hippocampus.
- Precise function unclear, but lesions in specific parts may lead to amnesia, e.g. in temporal lobes or mamillary bodies (Korsakoff's syndrome).

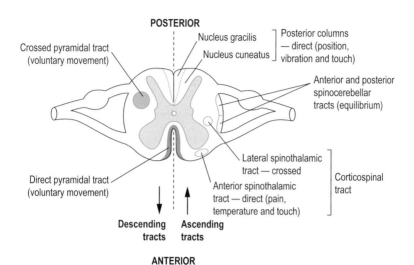

Fig. 4.12 Spinal tracts.

SPINAL CORD (Fig. 4.12)

- Average length is 45 cm. Extends from the foramen magnum and ends in the filum terminale at the level of L2, 3. Below this the nerve roots form the cauda equina.
- A total of 31 pairs of spinal nerves originate from the cord (see p. 138).
- Expansion of spinal cord at the lower end is called the *conus medullaris,* from which a fibrous band runs to the back of the coccyx. The dura fuses with this band at S2, 3 and obliterates the subarachnoid space.
- Blood supply: two anterior spinal arteries supply the anterior two-thirds of the cord (branches of the vertebral arteries) and two posterior arteries (branches of the vertebral or posterior cerebellar arteries) supply the remainder.

CEREBRAL CORTEX

Arterial supply and effects of occlusion (Fig. 4.13)

Anterior cerebral artery
- Supplies the medial aspect of the hemisphere.
- Occlusion may cause a weak, numb, contralateral leg +/– similar milder arm signs. The face is spared. Bilateral infarction is associated with an akinetic mute state due to damage to the cingulate gyri.

Middle cerebral artery
- Supplies the lateral (external) aspect of each hemisphere.
- Occlusion may cause contralateral hemiplegia, sensory loss mainly of face and arm, dysphasia and dyspraxia (dominant hemisphere), contralateral neglect (non-dominant hemisphere) and sometimes contralateral homonymous hemianopia.

Posterior cerebral artery
- Supplies the occipital lobe.
- Occlusion may cause many effects including contralateral homonymous hemianopia.

Circle of Willis arterial supply and effects of occlusion (Fig. 4.14)
Located at the base of the brain, mainly in the interpeduncular fossa.

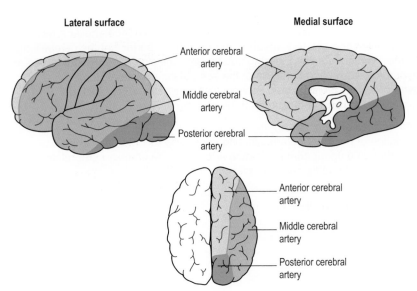

Fig. 4.13 Arterial supply to the cerebral cortex.

Vertebrobasilar circulation
- Supplies the brainstem, cerebellum and posterior cerebral artery.
- Occlusion may cause hemianopia, cortical blindness, diplopia, vertigo, nystagmus, hemi- or quadriplegia, unilateral or bilateral sensory symptoms, cerebellar symptoms and drop attacks.

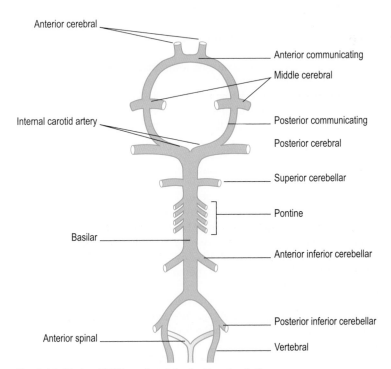

Fig. 4.14 Circle of Willis and vertebrobasilar circulation.

Lateral medullary
- Occlusion of one vertebral artery or the posterior inferior cerebellar artery.
- Due to infarction of lateral medulla and the inferior surface of the cerebellum.
- Causes vertigo, vomiting, nystagmus towards the side of the lesion, ipsilateral hypotonia, ataxia and paralysis of the soft palate, ipsilateral Horner's syndrome, and a dissociated sensory loss (analgesia to pin-prick on ipsilateral face and contralateral trunk and limbs).

Common sites of berry aneurysm
1. Junction of posterior communicating artery with the internal carotid.
2. Junction of anterior communicating artery with the anterior cerebral artery.
3. Bifurcation of middle cerebral artery.
15% are multiple.

Localization of function (Fig. 4.15)

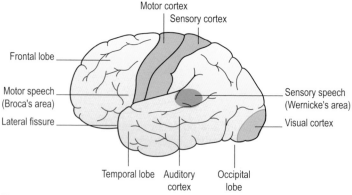

Fig. 4.15 Cerebral cortex: function.

- **Lateral (Sylvian) fissure:** lies between the temporal, frontal and parietal lobes.
- **Central sulcus:** runs obliquely downwards from the superior margin of the brain almost to the lateral fissure.
- **The primary voluntary motor cortex:** lies along the posterior part of the precentral gyrus adjoining the central sulcus.
- **The primary sensory cortex:** lies in the postcentral gyrus.
- **The primary auditory area:** lies on the cephalic border of the superior temporal gyrus in the depths of the lateral fissure.
- **The primary visual cortex:** lies in the calcarine fissure area of the occipital pole.
- **Broca's area:** lies in the posterior part of the inferior frontal gyrus.
- **Wernicke's area:** lies in the posterior part of the superior temporal lobe.
- **Frontal lobes:** involved in the formation of personality, higher reasoning and intellectual functioning. Part of the dominant frontal lobe has a primary role in the production of speech.
- **Temporal lobes**: provide a large part of memory function and integration as well as the auditory centres.
- **Parietal lobes:** complex integrating function for sensory, motor and to a lesser extent emotional functioning. Allows planning of complex actions and crucial role in object and word recognition and association with emotion.

Classification of dysphasias

1. *Broca's expressive dysphasia*
   Lesion: inferolateral frontal lobe.
   Non-fluent speech with malformed words. Reading and writing are impaired, but comprehension is intact. Understands questions and attempts to convey meaningful answers.
2. *Wernicke's receptive dysphasia*
   Lesion: posterior superior temporal lobe.
   Fluent speech but many errors, e.g. neologisms such as comb for brush, of which patient is unaware. Reading, writing and comprehension are impaired and so replies are inappropriate.
3. *Conduction aphasia*
   Lesion: communication between Broca's and Wernicke's areas interrupted.
   Repetition is impaired, and to a lesser extent, comprehension and fluency.
4. *Transcortical dysphasias*
   Lesion: areas of cortex surrounding classical language areas.
   Repetition is affected.
5. *Anomic aphasias*
   Naming is affected in all dysphasias, but especially with left temperoparietal lesions.

Classification of dyspraxias

1. *Dressing dyspraxia*
   Mostly non-dominant hemisphere lesions.
2. *Construction apraxia*
   Non-dominant hemisphere lesions. Occurs with hepatic encephalopathy.
3. *Gait dyspraxia*
   Bilateral function lesions, lesions in the posterior temporal region, hydrocephalus.

VENTRICLES OF THE BRAIN AND CEREBROSPINAL FLUID (CSF) SYSTEM

- 500–750 ml of cerebrospinal fluid (CSF) is produced per day by a process of ultrafiltration and active secretion (Fig. 4.16). The total volume of CSF is 100–150 ml.

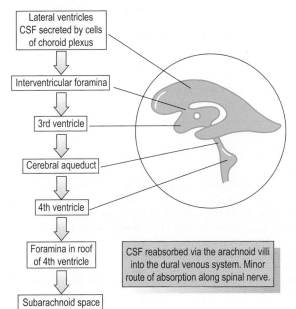

Lateral ventricles CSF secreted by cells of choroid plexus

⬇

Interventricular foramina

⬇

3rd ventricle

⬇

Cerebral aqueduct

⬇

4th ventricle

⬇

Foramina in roof of 4th ventricle

⬇

Subarachnoid space

CSF reabsorbed via the arachnoid villi into the dural venous system. Minor route of absorption along spinal nerve.

Fig. 4.16 Ventricles and CSF secretion.

Composition of CSF
See page 301.

SKULL FORAMINA (Table 4.8)

Base of the skull forms three fossae that contain the brain and meninges.
- Anterior fossa contains the frontal lobes.
- Middle fossa contains the hypothalamus and temporal lobes.
- Posterior fossa contains the brainstem and cerebellum.

Table 4.8 Skull foramina and contents

Foramen	Contents
Optic canal	Optic (II) nerve and ophthalmic artery
Superior orbital fissure*	III, IV, VI and ophthalmic division of V cranial nerves, sympathetic nerve and ophthalmic veins
Stylomastoid foramen	VII cranial nerve
Foramen rotundum	Maxillary division of V
Foramen ovale†	Mandibular division of V and accessory meningeal artery
Foramen spinosum	Middle meningeal artery, meningeal branch of the mandibular nerve
Foramen magnum	Spinal cord, accessory (XI) nerve, vertebral and spinal arteries
Foramen lacerum	Internal carotid artery, lesser petrosal nerve (branch of IX), greater petrosal nerve (branch of VII), deep petrosal nerves (autonomic)
Jugular foramen‡	Internal jugular vein and IX, X, XI cranial nerves
Hypoglossal foramen	XII cranial nerve, meningeal branch of ascending pharyngeal artery
Internal auditory meatus	VII and VIII cranial nerves, labyrinthine (internal auditory) artery

* Forms a communication between the middle cranial fossa and the orbit.
† Communication from middle cranial fossa to the infratemporal fossa.
‡ Lies lateral to the foramen magnum.

CRANIAL NERVES (Table 4.9)

Olfactory (I) nerve
Course: Olfactory cells reside in the mucosa of the superior nasal conchae and the upper part of the nasal septum. The axons pass through the cribriform plate of the ethmoid bone to reach the overlying olfactory bulb in the anterior cranial fossa. The olfactory tracts pass from the olfactory bulb to the medial surface of the cerebral hemisphere and the temporal lobes.

Optic (II) nerve
Course: Axons of ganglion cells from the retina make up the optic nerve. The optic disc is the central collecting point for these axons. The orbital portion of

---

Pupillary reflexes (Fig. 4.17)
Balance between parasympathetic (constrictor) and sympathetic (dilator) tone controls pupil size.
1. **Light reflex:** relayed via the optic nerve, optic tract, lateral geniculate nuclei, the Edinger–Westphal nucleus of the III nerve and ciliary ganglion. The cortex is not involved. Lesions of the brain stem may result in an Argyll Robertson pupil with loss of direct light reflex, but preservation of convergence reflex ('light-near dissociation'), e.g. neurosyphilis, diabetes and some hereditary neuropathies.
2. **Accommodation reflex:** convergence originates within the cortex and is relayed to the pupil via the III nerve nuclei. The optic nerve and tract and the lateral geniculate nucleus are not involved. Lesions of the cerebral cortex may result in absence of the convergence reflex, with preservation of the light reflex, e.g. cortical blindness.

Table 4.9 Summary of cranial nerves and their functions

Nerve	Origin	Cranial exit	Type	Chief functions
I. **Olfactory**	Nasal mucosa	Cribriform plate	Sensory	Smell
II. **Optic**	Retina	Optic canal	Sensory	Vision and light reflexes (direct and consensual)
III. **Oculomotor**	Midbrain a. III nerve nucleus b. Edinger–Westphal nucleus	Superior orbital fissure	a. Motor b. Parasympathetic	a. Motor to four extrinsic eye muscles and levator palpebrae superioris b. Motor to ciliary and sphincter pupillae muscles for light and accommodation reflexes
IV. **Trochlear**	Midbrain (below inferior colliculus)	Superior orbital fissure	Motor	Motor to superior oblique muscle
V. **Trigeminal** a. Ophthalmic b. Maxillary c. Mandibular	Pons Trigeminal ganglion and motor V nucleus	a. Superior orbital fissure b. Foramen rotundum c. Foramen ovale	a. Sensory b. Sensory } a,b,c c. Mixed	Motor to muscles of mastication and for jaw jerk Sensation from skin of face, scalp, nasal cavity, mouth and palate: corneal reflex
VI. **Abducent**	Pons	Superior orbital fissure	Motor	Motor to lateral rectus muscle
VII. **Facial**	Pons	Stylomastoid foramen	Motor, sensory (taste) and parasympathetic	Motor to muscles of facial expression, corneal reflex efferent part Secretomotor to lacrimal and salivary glands Sensation and taste from anterior two-thirds of tongue and soft palate

Table 4.9 (Cont'd)

Nerve	Origin	Cranial exit	Type	Chief functions
VIII. Vestibulocochlear a. Vestibular b. Cochlear	Pons (organ of Corti; the cochlear and spiral ganglion)	Does not leave skull Final common pathway: superior temporal gyrus	Sensory	Hearing; balance and position of head
IX. Glossopharyngeal	Medulla	Jugular foramen	Motor, sensory (taste) and parasympathetic	Motor to pharyngeal muscles (gag reflex) Secretomotor to parotid salivary gland Sensation and taste from posterior one-third of tongue, tonsil and pharynx
X. Vagus	Medulla	Jugular foramen	Motor, sensory and parasympathetic	Motor to heart, lungs and alimentary tract Motor to the muscles of the larynx, pharynx and palate Sensation from pharynx, larynx, heart, lungs and abdominal viscera
XI. Accessory (two parts: cranial and spinal)	Medulla (nucleus ambiguus) and spinal cord (cervical)	Jugular foramen	Motor	Motor to sternocleidomastoid and trapezius muscles Motor to muscles of pharynx, larynx and soft palate
XII. Hypoglossal	Medulla	Hypoglossal canal	Motor	Motor to strap muscles of neck Motor to muscles of tongue

the nerve extends from where the optic nerve pierces the sclera to the optic foramen in the skull. It leaves the orbit through the optic foramen and then unites with the other optic nerve to form the optic chiasma.

Posterior to the optic chiasma, the nerves continue as the optic tract and synapse with the neurons in the lateral geniculate body in the thalamus. From the lateral geniculate body, the optic radiation curves backward to the occipital visual cortex. A small number of fibres concerned with pupillary and ocular reflexes bypass the lateral geniculate body and go to the pretectal nucleus and superior colliculus in the midbrain.

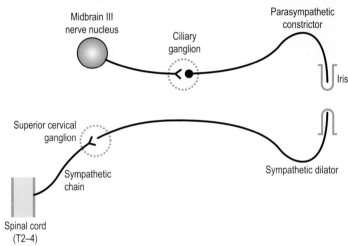

Fig. 4.17 Anatomy of pupillary reflexes.

Lesions of the optic nerve

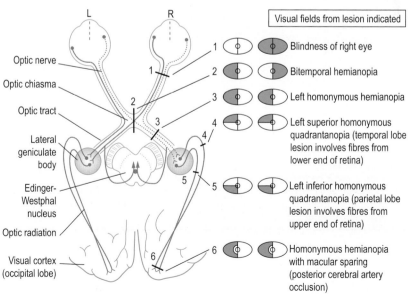

Fig. 4.18 Optic nerve and tract.

Horner's syndrome (Fig. 4.19)

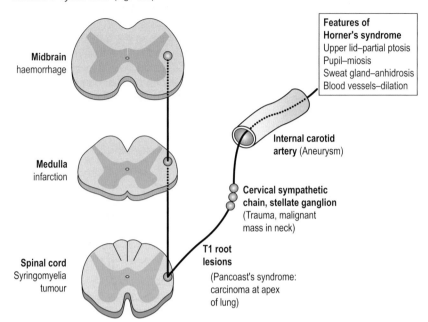

Midbrain
haemorrhage

Medulla
infarction

Spinal cord
Syringomyelia
tumour

> **Features of
> Horner's syndrome**
> Upper lid–partial ptosis
> Pupil–miosis
> Sweat gland–anhidrosis
> Blood vessels–dilation

**Internal carotid
artery** (Aneurysm)

**Cervical sympathetic
chain, stellate ganglion**
(Trauma, malignant
mass in neck)

**T1 root
lesions**
(Pancoast's syndrome:
carcinoma at apex
of lung)

Fig. 4.19 Causes of Horner's syndrome.

Eye movements and disturbance of gaze

Vertical
- The centres governing vertical eye movements lie in the midbrain.
- Lesions of the upper midbrain cause paresis of conjugate upward gaze, often with loss of pupillary light and accommodation reflexes (Parinaud's syndrome); e.g. encephalitis, tumours around the IIIrd ventricle, midbrain or pineal body, Wernicke's encephalopathy or infarction.
- Disturbances of vertical gaze also seen with progressive supranuclear palsy, Huntington's chorea, hydrocephalus and vascular syndromes.

Horizontal
- Centre is located in prepontine reticular formation in the pons.

Lesions
- Internuclear ophthalmoplegia: ipsilateral adduction weakness, contralateral abduction nystagmus, caused by a medial longitudinal fasiculus lesion.
- Wernicke's encephalopathy: weakness of abduction, gaze-evoked nystagmus, internuclear ophthalmoplegia, horizontal and vertical gaze palsies.

Frontal eye fields
- Responsible for contralateral horizontal saccades.
  1. Unilateral obliteration will lead to gaze deviation toward the affected side.
  2. A seizure causing hyperactivity in that area will cause gaze deviation away from the affected side.

Interpretation of eye signs in the comatosed patient (Fig. 4.20)

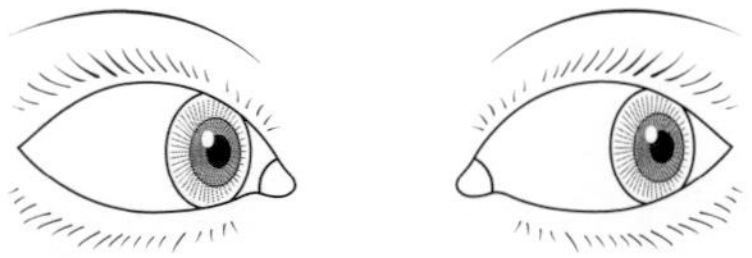

1. Conjugate lateral deviation. Looking away from hemiplegic side is caused by ipsilateral cerebral haemorrhage or infarction. Looking towards hemiplegic side is caused by a contralateral pontine infarction.

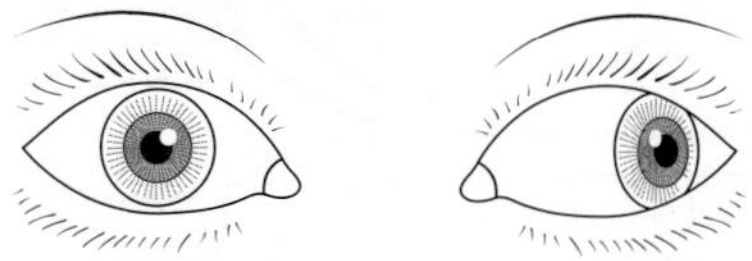

2. Dysconjugate (vertical or horizontal) deviation. Brainstem lesion, e.g. haemorrhage, infarction or space-occupying lesion.

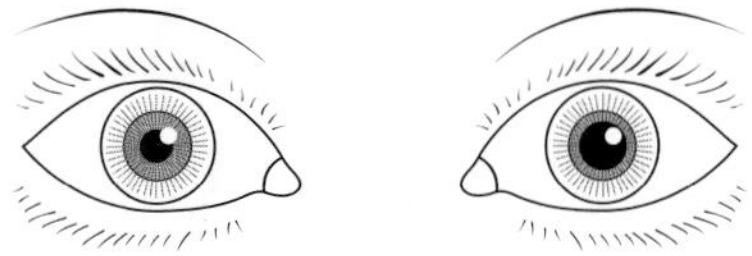

3. Unilateral dilated pupil. Supratentorial mass lesion, e.g. haemorrhage or infarction with cerebral oedema, uncal herniation and IIIrd nerve compression.

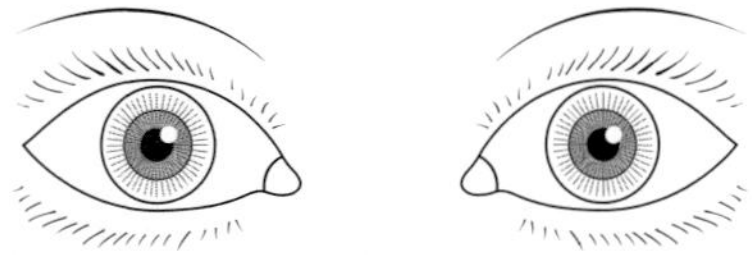

4. Bilateral mid-position, fixed pupils. Mid-brain lesion, e.g. haemorrhage, infarction, space-occupying lesion.

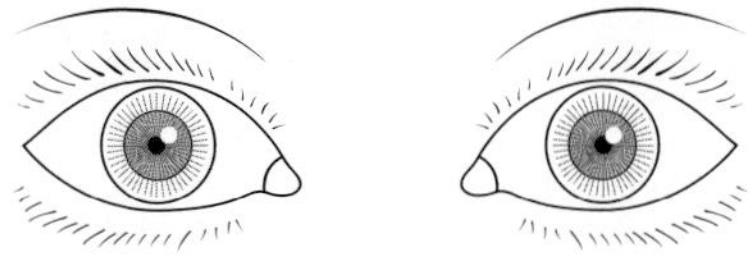

5. Pinpoint pupils. Narcotic overdose (oculocephalic reflex intact). Pontine haemorrhage (oculocephalic reflex absent). Barbiturate, phenytoin and tricyclic overdose can abolish the reflex; the pupils are normal size.

Fig. 4.20 Interpretation of eye signs.

Oculomotor (III) nerve (Figs 4.21, 4.22)

Course: The nerve emerges from the anterior aspect of the midbrain medial to the cerebral peduncle. It passes forward in the subarachnoid space to pierce the dura mater, and lies in the lateral wall of the cavernous sinus, close to the IV and VI nerves and the ophthalmic branch of the trigeminal nerve. The nerve enters the orbit through the superior orbital fissure.

Complete IIIrd nerve lesion

1. Ptosis: paralysis of levator palpebrae superioris.
2. Mydriasis: dilator action of sympathetic fibres unopposed.
3. Deviation of eye laterally and downwards: unopposed action of superior oblique and lateral rectus.
4. Loss of accommodation-convergence and light reflexes due to paralysis of constrictor pupillae.

Causes: vascular lesions *(Weber's syndrome),* and aneurysm of the posterior communicating artery. An isolated IIIrd nerve lesion is associated with diabetes, encephalitis and meningitis (especially due to TB, sarcoid and syphilis).

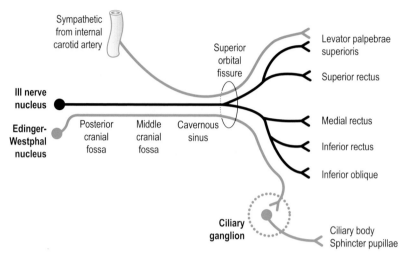

Fig. 4.21 Oculomotor nerve.

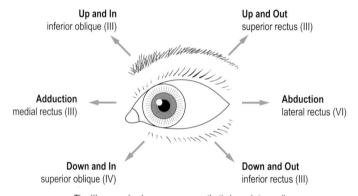

The III nerve also has a parasympathetic branch to pupil ciliary muscle and levator palpebrae superioris

Fig. 4.22 Muscles of the eye.

Trochlear (IV) nerve (Fig. 4.23)
Course: The nerve emerges from the posterior aspect of the midbrain, just below the inferior colliculi. It passes forward in the subarachnoid space to pierce the

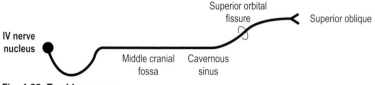

Fig. 4.23 Trochlear nerve.

dura mater and then lies in the wall of the cavernous sinus, just below the oculomotor nerve. The nerve enters the orbit through the superior orbital fissure.

IVth nerve lesions
1. Rare, but most commonly seen after trauma.
2. Two images appear at an angle when the affected eye is abducted, and one above the other when the other eye is adducted. Diplopia typically occurs when looking downward and medially, e.g. descending stairs.

Trigeminal (V) nerve
Course: This is the largest of the cranial nerves. The trigeminal nerve emerges from the pons by a large sensory and a small motor root. The nerve passes forward out of the posterior cranial fossa, and on reaching the petrous part of the temporal bone in the middle cranial fossa the large sensory root expands to form the trigeminal ganglion. Impulses reach the ganglion via its three divisions; the ophthalmic, maxillary and mandibular nerves. The ophthalmic nerve passes through the superior orbital fissure. The maxillary nerve leaves the middle cranial fossa through the foramen rotundum, passes through the pterygopalatine fossa and the inferior orbital fissure, and crosses the floor of the orbit to emerge through the infraorbital foramen. The mandibular nerve leaves the skull via the foramen ovale.

The motor root is situated below the sensory ganglion and is completely separate from it. It passes independently out of the cranial cavity to join the mandibular division and supplies eight muscles; the muscles of mastication, the tensor tympani, the tensor veli palatini, the myelohyoid and the anterior belly of digastric.

Vth nerve lesions
1. Damage to the central organization of sensory innervation results in sensory loss, of an 'onion' skin distribution, with loss or dissociation starting over the angle of the jaw and cheek and spreading across the face.
2. Unilateral paralysis of the muscles of mastication: jaw deviates to the affected side.

Causes: brainstem vascular lesion, intrinsic brainstem tumours, syringomyelia, herpes zoster, trigeminal neuralgia, acoustic neuroma, cavernous sinus lesions, multiple sclerosis.

Abducent (VI) nerve (Fig. 4.24)
Course: Emerges from the anterior surface of the brain, in the groove between the lower border of the pons and the medulla oblongata. It runs upwards, forwards and laterally in the subarachnoid space, and traverses the cavernous sinus, lying at first lateral and then inferolateral to the internal carotid artery. The nerve enters the orbital cavity through the medial part of the superior orbital fissure.

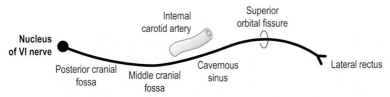

Fig. 4.24 Abducent nerve.

VIth nerve lesions

1. Convergent squint with failure of abduction.
2. Diplopia is maximal on looking to the affected side.

Causes: osteitis *(Gradenigo's syndrome),* acoustic neuroma, aneurysm, meningitis, raised intracranial pressure (as a false localizing sign).

Facial (VII) nerve (Fig. 4.25)

Course: Consists of three roots, a large motor root and a small mixed sensory and parasympathetic root *(nervus intermedius)* which arise from the lateral surface of the brainstem close to the lower border of the pons. Leaving the brainstem, it accompanies the VIII nerve through the internal acoustic meatus. It then traverses the facial canal within the temporal bone, to emerge from the skull at the stylomastoid foramen, where it divides into terminal muscular branches in the substance of the parotid gland.

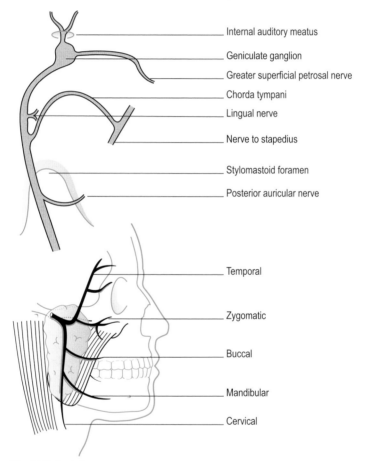

Internal auditory meatus
Geniculate ganglion
Greater superficial petrosal nerve
Chorda tympani
Lingual nerve
Nerve to stapedius
Stylomastoid foramen
Posterior auricular nerve
Temporal
Zygomatic
Buccal
Mandibular
Cervical

Fig. 4.25 Facial nerve.

Branches

1. Greater petrosal nerve: mixed nerve with parasympathetic fibres to the lacrimal gland and sensory fibres to the geniculate ganglion.
2. Nerve to stapedius muscle.
3. Chorda tympani nerve: taste fibres to the anterior two-thirds of the tongue. Parasympathetic fibres are secretomotor to the submandibular and sublingual glands.

4. Muscular branches to all muscles of facial expression: temporal, zygomatic, buccal, mandibular and cervical.

VIIth nerve lesions

1. Supranuclear (i.e. upper motor neuron lesions): e.g. cerebrovascular accident. Sparing of forehead muscles which receive bilateral cortical fibres.
2. Nuclear: bulbar paralysis e.g. polio.
3. Infranuclear: e.g. Bell's palsy, acoustic neuroma, fractures of the temporal bone, and invasion by a malignant parotid tumour.

Lower motor neuron lesion. Complete facial paralysis (i.e. affects all the muscles of one side of face).

If the intracranial part of the nerve is involved, there is:
  (i) Loss of taste over the anterior two-thirds of the tongue, due to chorda tympani nerve involvement (Table 4.10).
  (ii) Hyperacusis due to paralysis of the stapedius muscle.
  (iii) Decreased secretion from the lacrimal, submandibular and sublingual glands.

Vestibulocochlear (VIII) nerve (Fig. 4.26)

Course: Consists of two sets of sensory fibres. Cochlear nerve consists of the central processes of the bipolar neurons which have their cell bodies in the petrous temporal bone. The peripheral processes of the vestibular nerve are distributed to the semicircular canals, the utricle and the saccule. The vestibular and cochlear components enter the internal auditory meatus with the facial nerve and run in the petrous temporal bone to the inner ear.

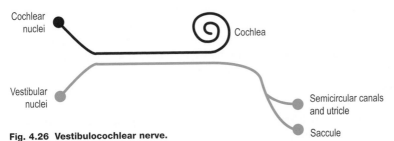

Fig. 4.26 Vestibulocochlear nerve.

Glossopharyngeal (IX) nerve

Course: Arises from the lateral aspect of the medulla just caudal to the pons. The nerve runs laterally and separates from the vagus nerve as it pierces the dura to enter the anterior compartment of the jugular foramen. Outside the foramen, it passes forward between the internal jugular vein and the internal carotid artery.

IXth nerve lesions

Rare in isolation. Interruption of all fibres results in:
1. Loss of sensation, including taste, on the posterior third of the tongue (Table 4.10)
2. Unilateral loss of the gag reflex
3. Difficulty with swallowing.

Table 4.10 Summary of sensory innervation of the tongue

Region	Sensation	Taste
Posterior one-third	IX, X	IX, X
Anterior two-thirds	Chorda tympani (VII)	Chorda tympani (VII)

Vagus (X) nerve

Course: Emerges from the anterior surface of the upper part of the medulla oblongata by 8–10 rootlets. Leaves the skull via the jugular foremen with the IX and XI cranial nerves. Passes vertically downwards to the root of the neck, lying in the posterior part of the carotid sheath between the internal jugular vein and first the internal and then the common carotid artery.

Branches

1. In the neck: *pharyngeal, superior laryngeal* and *cardiac nerves.* Below the level of the subclavian artery, the nerve has a different course on each side:
   - *Right vagus:* The recurrent laryngeal nerve is given off as it crosses the subclavian artery. Below this the nerve descends through the superior mediastinum posterior to the right brachiocephalic and superior vena cava and passes posterior to the lung root.
   - *Left vagus:* Enters the thorax between the left common carotid and left subclavian arteries, posterior to the left brachiocephalic vein and passes posterior to the lung root. The left recurrent laryngeal nerve is given off as the vagus crosses the arch of the aorta.
2. In the thorax: *pulmonary* and *oesophageal plexuses.*
   - The two vagi enter the abdomen through the oesophageal opening. The *left* vagus passes onto the anterior surface and the *right* onto the posterior surface of the stomach.
3. In the abdomen: *coeliac, hepatic* and *renal plexuses.*

Xth nerve lesions

See page 168.

Accessory (XI) nerve

Course: Consists of a spinal and cranial nerve. The spinal root passes upwards along the side of the spinal cord and joins the cranial root from the brainstem. Fibres of the cranial root travel with the nerve for a short distance and then branch to join and be distributed with the vagus nerve. The spinal root descends as a separate nerve to supply the trapezius and sternocleidomastoid muscles.

XIth nerve lesions

Paralysis of the sternocleidomastoid muscle causes weakness on turning the head away from the paralysed muscle, e.g. trauma to the base of the skull. Usually associated with other cranial nerve lesions: IX, X and XII cranial nerves.

Hypoglossal (XII) nerve

Course: Arises from the medulla between the olive and pyramid as 10–15 rootlets. The fibres pass anterolaterally and leave the posterior cranial fossa via the hypoglossal canal just in front of the foramen magnum. Descends between the internal carotid artery and the internal jugular vein and hooks around the occipital branch of the external carotid, to lie on the hypoglossus muscle before entering the tongue.

Unilateral XIIth nerve lesions

1. Ipsilateral paralysis and wasting of the tongue muscles on the affected side.
2. Deviation of the tongue to the side of the lesion on protrusion, e.g. tumours and penetrating injuries in the neck.

Bilateral XIIth nerve lesions

1. Generalized atrophy of the tongue (with or without fasiculation).
2. Protrusion impossible and articulation disturbed, e.g. motor neuron disease.

PRINCIPAL ARTERIES

See Fig. 4.27.

Ascending aorta
Extends from base of left ventricle at level of lower border of 3rd costal cartilage, upwards and to the right of 2nd right costal cartilage

Arch of aorta
Commences at sternal angle and crosses to left side of 4th thoracic vertebra (superior mediastinum)

Thoracic aorta
Runs from the 4th–12th thoracic vertebra (superior mediastinum)

Abdominal aorta
Begins in the median plane at the lower border of T12, continues downwards and slightly to the left of the midline. Bifurcates into the common iliac arteries in front of L4

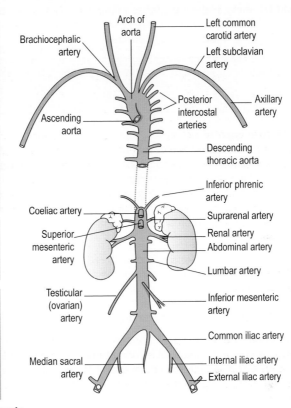

Fig. 4.27 Branches of the aorta.

Common carotid artery

Surface marking: On a line from the upper border of the sternal end of the clavicle to a point midway between the apex of the mastoid and the angle of the mandible.
Course: Right common carotid and subclavian arteries originate from the brachiocephalic artery at the level of the upper part of the right sternoclavicular joint.

Left common carotid and subclavian arteries arise directly from the arch of the aorta. The former has a short intrathoracic course between the trachea and the left lung, and enters the neck opposite the left sternoclavicular joint.

Both common carotid arteries ascend in the neck under cover of the anterior border of the sternocleidomastoid muscle. Each divides at the upper margin of the thyroid cartilage, opposite the lower border of the 3rd cervical vertebra into internal and external carotid arteries.

The carotid sinus (baroreceptor) is located at the bifurcation of the common carotid artery, and the carotid body (chemoreceptor) in the posterior wall of the sinus. Both sinus and body are innervated by the glossopharyngeal (IX) nerve.

Internal carotid artery

Supplies the major part of the cerebral hemisphere on its own side, and communicates via the circle of Willis with the opposite internal carotid artery and usually both vertebral arteries. Also supplies eye, forehead and nose.
Course: Lies within the carotid sheath posterior and then medial to the external carotid artery. Has no branches in the neck, but enters the base of the skull via the carotid canal, where it gives rise to the ophthalmic artery and bifurcates into anterior and middle cerebral arteries.

> Occlusion may cause total infarction of the anterior two-thirds of the ipsilateral hemisphere and basal ganglia (striate arteries). Usually clinical features are similar to a middle cerebral artery occlusion.

External carotid artery

Supplies the thyroid gland, tongue, throat, face, ear, scalp and dura mater. Plays no part in the arterial supply to the cerebral hemisphere.
Course: Lies anteromedial to the internal carotid artery. Ascends lateral to the carotid sheath, glossopharyngeal nerve and pharyngeal branch of the vagus. Terminates by dividing into the superficial temporal and maxillary arteries just lateral to the temporomandibular joint.

Carotid sheath

Formed by the condensation of all three layers of deep cervical fascia.
Course: Extends from the base of the skull to the root of the neck. Lies deep to the sternocleidomastoid muscle. Contains common and internal carotid arteries, the internal jugular vein and the vagus nerves. The sympathetic trunk lies posterior to the sheath, embedded in the prevertebral layer of fascia.

Subclavian artery

Surface marking: Indicated by an arch between the medial end of the sternoclavicular joint and lateral end at the middle of the clavicle.
Course: Originates on the right from the brachiocephalic trunk and on the left from the arch of the aorta. Passes deep to the lower end of the anterior scalene muscle and becomes the axillary artery at the lateral border of the 1st rib.
Branches: Vertebral, internal thoracic, deep cervical and highest intercostal arteries and thyrocervical trunk.

> **Subclavian steal syndrome:**
> - Stenosis of the subclavian artery proximal to the ipsilateral vertebral artery may cause blood to be 'stolen' by retrograde flow from this vertebral artery down into the arm. Results in brainstem ischaemia after arm exertion.
> - Diagnosis is by demonstrating a > 20 mmHg difference in blood pressure between the arms.

Femoral artery

Surface marking: Upper two-thirds of a line connecting the mid-inguinal point with the adductor tubercle.
Course: Distal continuation of external iliac artery beyond inguinal ligament. Accompanied by femoral vein throughout its course which lies first on medial side of artery and then passes posteriorly to it at apex of the femoral triangle.
Branches: Superficial circumflex, superficial inferior epigastric and superficial external pudendal arteries. Divides into profunda femoris and superficial femoral artery (Fig. 4.28).

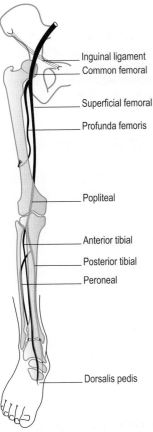

Fig. 4.28 Arteries of the lower limb.

- Inguinal ligament
- Common femoral
- Superficial femoral
- Profunda femoris
- Popliteal
- Anterior tibial
- Posterior tibial
- Peroneal
- Dorsalis pedis

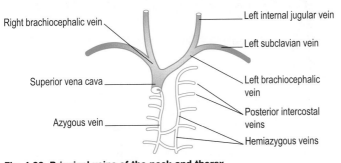

PRINCIPAL VEINS (Fig. 4.29)

- Right brachiocephalic vein
- Superior vena cava
- Azygous vein
- Left internal jugular vein
- Left subclavian vein
- Left brachiocephalic vein
- Posterior intercostal veins
- Hemiazygous veins

Fig. 4.29 Principal veins of the neck and thorax.

Superior vena cava
- Formed by the right and left brachiocephalic veins at the lower border of the 1st costal cartilage.
- Drains veins of head, neck, upper extremities, thorax and azygous veins.

Course: Runs downwards behind the right border of the sternum and enters upper border of right atrium at 3rd costal cartilage.

Internal jugular vein
- Drains the cranial cavity and a few of the superficial veins of the head and neck.
- Contains valves in dilated segments at the superior and inferior ends (bulbs).

Course: Originates at the jugular foramen, descending forwards and medially within the carotid sheath to the root of the neck. Passes behind the clavicle where it joins the subclavian vein to form the brachiocephalic trunk and thence into the superior vena cava. Lies lateral first to the internal and then to the common carotid artery within the sheath.

Subclavian vein
Continuation of the axillary vein in the neck, beginning at the lateral border of the 1st rib.

Course: Passes medial, anterior and slightly inferior to the subclavian artery. Joins internal jugular vein to form the brachiocephalic vein just lateral to the sternoclavicular joint.

Inferior vena cava
- Largest vein of the body. Formed by the union of right and left common iliac veins at the level of the 5th lumbar verterbra.
- Drains veins of the abdomen, pelvis, lower extremities and azygous veins. Also receives the lumbar veins, the renal veins and the right inferior phrenic veins. The left suprarenal and testicular veins drain into the left renal vein. (**Note:** Hence increased risk of varicocoele on left.)

Course: Runs to the right of the aorta, and lies anterior to the bodies of the lumbar vertebrae on the right sympathetic trunk. It extends to the central tendon of the diaphragm, and thereafter behind the bare area of the liver, before opening into the right atrium.

Principal veins of the lower limb
- Deep veins which accompany the major arteries.
- Superficial veins: long and short saphenous veins and their tributaries (Fig. 4.30).

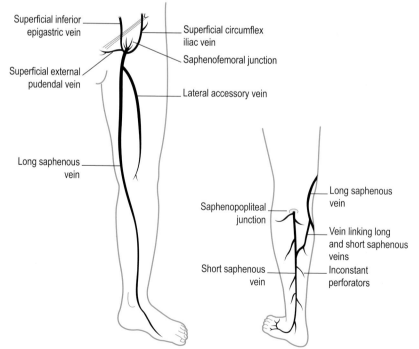

Fig. 4.30 Principal veins of the lower limb.

THYROID GLAND

Upper border marks the site of the cricothyroid membrane. Inferior border marks the beginning of trachea and oesophagus, and the level at which the common carotid may be compressed against the transverse process of the 6th vertebra.

Cricoid cartilage surface markings:

Structure
1. The isthmus overlies the 2nd to 4th rings of the trachea.
2. The two lateral lobes extend from the side of the thyroid cartilage downwards to the 6th tracheal ring.
3. An inconstant pyramidal lobe projects up from the isthmus.
4. Parathyroid glands lie in close relation to the posterior border of the gland.

Important relations include: Trachea and oesophagus posteriorly, and carotid sheath posteriorly and laterally.

Embryology
The thyroid develops from a thyroglossal diverticulum which pushes out from the tongue at the foramen caecum. It descends to a definitive position in the neck, and loses all connections with its origin. This development accounts for the occasional occurrence of a lingual thyroid, thyroglossal cyst or sinus and retrosternal thyroid along the path of descent.

LARYNX

Structure
1. Extends from the level of the 3rd cervical vertebra to the lower border of the 6th where it is continuous with the trachea.
2. There are nine cartilages in the laryngeal skeleton: three are single (thyroid, cricoid and epiglottis) and three are paired (arytenoid, corniculate and cuneiform).

Nerve supply
1. All intrinsic muscles of the larynx, except the cricothyroid, are innervated by the recurrent laryngeal nerve.
2. Cricothyroid muscle is supplied by the superior laryngeal nerve.

Recurrent laryngeal nerve (RLN)
This is a branch of the vagus and has a different course on each side, because of embryonic development.
Course: Right RLN arises from the vagus in the neck and passes behind the right subclavian artery.
Course: Left RLN arises from the vagus on the arch of the aorta and winds behind it.
- Both nerves then ascend between the trachea and the oesophagus and enter the larynx below the lower border of inferior constrictor.
- The recurrent nerves supply all the intrinsic laryngeal muscles, apart from the cricothyroid, and the mucosa below the vocal cords.

ANATOMY

Recurrent laryngeal nerve lesions
1. Unilateral paralysis causes the affected cord to lie close to the midline and during phonation the unaffected cord moves across the midline to compensate. Results in dysphonia and a bovine cough.
2. Bilateral paralysis: the unopposed cricothyroids cause the cords to lie closely apposed. Results in a weak voice and stridor, especially after exertion.
Causes: damage during thyroidectomy, thyroid carcinoma, malignant lymph nodes, broncho-oesophageal carcinoma*, aortic aneurysm* and enlarged left atrium (mitral stenosis)*. * = left RLN lesion.

Superior laryngeal nerve
Course: This branch of vagus passes deep to the internal and external carotid arteries where it divides.

Superior laryngeal nerve lesions
Cause weakness of phonation.
With combined lesions of both the superior and recurrent laryngeal nerves the cords assume an intermediate or cadaveric position.

Muscles of the larynx (Table 4.11)

Table 4.11 Action of the muscles of the larynx

Muscle	Action
Cricothyroid	Lengthens, tenses and adducts
Posterior cricoarytenoid	Abducts
Lateral cricoarytenoid	Adducts
Transverse arytenoid	Adducts
Oblique arytenoid	Adducts
Thyroarytenoid	Relaxes

SURFACE MARKINGS

Sternal angle
Surface marking: 5 cm inferior to the floor of the jugular notch at the level of T5.

Lines of pleural reflection
Surface markings: Apex of pleura is 2.5 cm above the clavicle: medial border descends from the level of the sternal angle to the 6th rib in the midline, 8th rib in the midclavicular line, 10th in the midaxillary line and 12th rib adjacent to vertebral column posteriorly (mnemonic: 6, 8, 10, 12).

Lower borders of the lungs
Surface marking: Run two rib levels higher than the pleural reflections (i.e. 4, 6, 8).

Fissures
- The right lung has three lobes and two fissures: oblique and horizontal.
- The left lung has two lobes: superior (upper) and inferior (lower).
- The lingula is the lower part of the superior lobe between the cardiac notch and the oblique fissure.

Main (oblique) fissure
- Divides the lung into upper and lower lobes.
- Extends from the 2nd thoracic spine posteriorly to 6th rib, 5 cm from the midline.

Horizontal (transverse) fissure
- Divides the upper and middle lobes of the right lung.
- Horizontal line along the 4th rib from the midline to the oblique fissure.

TRACHEA AND BRONCHI

Surface marking: Commences at the lower border of the cricoid cartilage (C6); bifurcates at sternal angle (T4, 5) just to the right of the midline to form right and left bronchi. At full inspiration, bifurcation is at T6, 11 cm long and 2.5 cm in diameter.

Right main bronchus
Course: Wider, shorter (2.5 cm) and more vertical than the left (i.e. foreign objects more likely to enter), and passes directly to the root of the lung at the level of T5. Right main bronchus divides into upper, middle and lower bronchus in hilar region. Left main bronchus divides into an upper (lingular) and lower lobe bronchus.

Left main bronchus
Course: 5 cm long and passes downwards and outwards below the arch of the aorta and in front of the oesophagus and descending aorta. Undivided bronchus reaches the hilum of the lung at level of T6. The structures of the root of the left lung pass in front of the descending aorta where the recurrent laryngeal nerve hooks around the aortic arch.

Divisions of right main bronchus (Fig. 4.31)
Division of lobar bronchi into 10 segmental bronchi within the lung – one for each bronchopulmonary segment. Azygous vein arches over right main bronchus from behind to reach the superior vena cava, and the pulmonary artery lies first below and then anterior to it. The structures of the root of the right lung pass behind the ascending aorta.

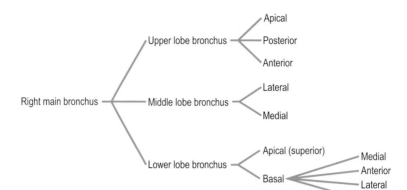

Fig. 4.31 Divisions of the right main bronchus.

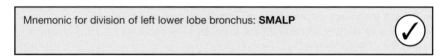

Mnemonic for division of left lower lobe bronchus: **SMALP**

Divisions of left main bronchus (Fig. 4.32)

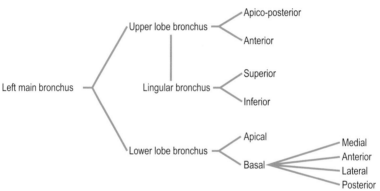

Fig. 4.32 Divisions of the left main bronchus.

Respiratory segments supplied by the segmental bronchus (Fig. 4.33)

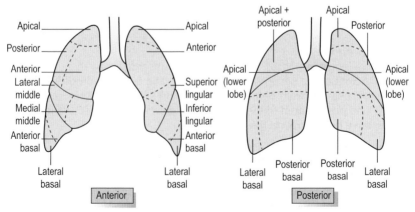

Fig. 4.33 Respiratory segments supplied by the segmented bronchus.

LUNG

Root of lung

Contents
1. Main bronchus
2. Pulmonary artery
3. Two pulmonary veins
4. Bronchial arteries and veins
5. Autonomic nerves
6. Lymphatics.

HEART

Arterial supply

Myocardium supplied by right and left coronary arteries (Fig. 4.34). Angiographic views illustrated in Figure 4.35.

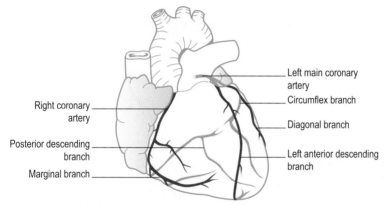

Fig. 4.34 Arterial supply to the myocardium.

Coronary dominance	
Right:	60%
Left:	20%
Equally balanced:	20%

Right coronary artery

Supplies: The right atrium, sinoatrial node, atrioventricular node, right ventricle and posterior part of interventricular septum. Arises from the anterior aortic sinus.
Course: Runs in the atrioventricular groove, then downwards to the inferior border and around the posterior aspect in the coronary sulcus. Two main branches: *posterior descending* branch runs in the posterior interventricular groove to the apex, *marginal* branch runs along the inferior border.

Left coronary artery

Supplies: Anterior part of the left and right ventricle, anterior part of the interventricular septum, atrioventricular groove and lateral wall of the left ventricle.
Course: arises from the *posterior* aortic cusp. Two main branches: *left anterior descending* (LAD) runs in the anterior interventricular groove to the apex, and

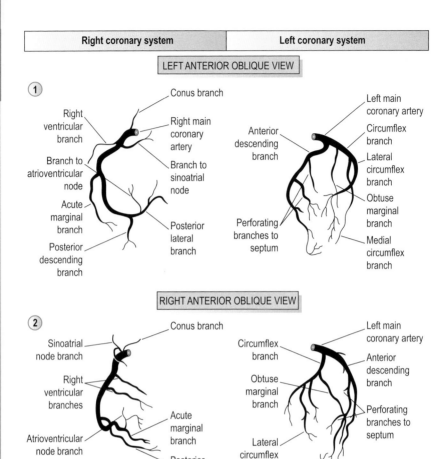

Right coronary system	Left coronary system

LEFT ANTERIOR OBLIQUE VIEW

1

Right ventricular branch

Conus branch

Right main coronary artery

Branch to atrioventricular node

Branch to sinoatrial node

Acute marginal branch

Posterior descending branch

Posterior lateral branch

Left main coronary artery

Anterior descending branch

Circumflex branch

Lateral circumflex branch

Obtuse marginal branch

Perforating branches to septum

Medial circumflex branch

RIGHT ANTERIOR OBLIQUE VIEW

2

Sinoatrial node branch

Conus branch

Right ventricular branches

Atrioventricular node branch

Acute marginal branch

Posterior descending branch

Circumflex branch

Obtuse marginal branch

Lateral circumflex branch

Left main coronary artery

Anterior descending branch

Perforating branches to septum

Fig. 4.35 Arterial supply to the myocardium: angiographic views.

around the inferior margin to the posterior interventricular groove. The *circumflex artery* passes to the left between atria and ventricles in the coronary sulcus.

Posterior descending branch of the right coronary artery anastomoses with the anterior descending branch of the left coronary artery at apex of heart and interventricular septum.

Venous drainage
1. 90% drains into right atrium through coronary sinus via the great, middle and small cardiac veins.
2. 10% drains into other chambers via the venae cordis minimae.

Nerve supply
1. Parasympathetic: right vagus innervates sinoatrial node and atria; left vagus innervates atrioventricular node and conducting tissue.
2. Sympathetic: cervical and upper thoracic sympathetic ganglia, via superficial and deep cardiac plexuses supplying all parts of the heart.

Valves

1. Atrioventricular:
   (i) Tricuspid (anterior, posterior and septal or medial cusps)
   (ii) Mitral (anterior and posterior cusps).
   Both have chordae tendinae and papillary muscles.

Table 4.12		
	Surface marking	*Auscultation point*
Tricuspid	Right half of the sternum at the level of the fourth intercostal space	Right half of the body of the sternum just above the junction with the xiphoid process
Mitral	Left half of the sternum at the level of the fourth intercostal space	Apex of the heart: left fifth intercostal space 7–8 cm lateral to the midline

2. Semilunar:
   (i) Pulmonary (anterior, right and left cusps)
   (ii) Aortic (right, left and posterior cusps).
   Each has a free border with a central nodule and lateral lunules.

Table 4.13		
	Surface marking	*Auscultation point*
Pulmonary	Upper edge of the left third costal cartilage at the lateral margin of sternum	Second left intercostal space just lateral to the sternum
Aortic	Lower edge of the left third costal cartilage at the lateral margin of the sternum	Second right intercostal space just lateral to the sternum

Nodes

1. The *sinoatrial node* is supplied by the right or left coronary artery and the right vagus nerve.
2. The *atrioventricular node* is supplied by the right coronary artery and by the left vagus nerve.

Embryology

1. Formation of paired endocardial tubes in splanchnic mesoderm.
2. Differentiation of heart tube into bulbis cordis, ventricle, atrium and sinus venosus (from arterial to venous end).
3. Septation:
   (i) Interatrial from septum primum and septum secundum.
   (ii) Interventricular: muscular and membranous parts.
   (iii) Spiral aorticopulmonary: fused bulbar ridges.

The aortic arches and their derivatives

Common arterial trunk	→	Truncus arteriosus → six pairs of aortic arches (1st, 2nd and 5th arches disappear)	✓
3rd arches	→	Carotid arteries	
Right 4th arch	→	Brachiocephalic and **right** subclavian artery	
Left 4th arch	→	Aortic arch → **left** subclavian artery	
6th arch	→	Right and left pulmonary arteries and ductus arteriosus	

FETAL CIRCULATION (Fig. 4.36)

Sequence of events at birth

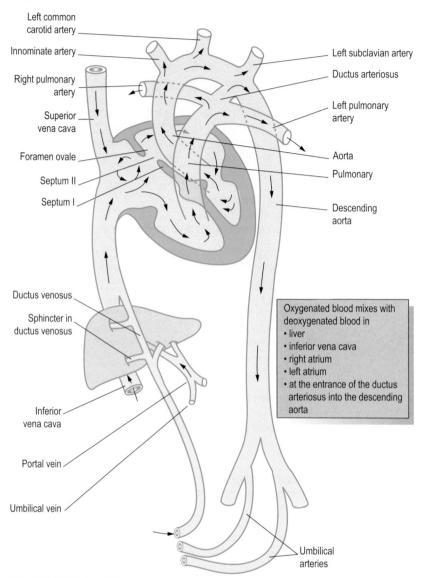

Left common carotid artery

Innominate artery

Right pulmonary artery

Superior vena cava

Foramen ovale

Septum II

Septum I

Left subclavian artery

Ductus arteriosus

Left pulmonary artery

Aorta

Pulmonary

Descending aorta

Ductus venosus

Sphincter in ductus venosus

Oxygenated blood mixes with deoxygenated blood in
• liver
• inferior vena cava
• right atrium
• left atrium
• at the entrance of the ductus arteriosus into the descending aorta

Inferior vena cava

Portal vein

Umbilical vein

Umbilical arteries

Fig. 4.36 Fetal circulation.

1. Expansion of lungs, causing a decrease in pulmonary vascular resistance. ✓

   ↓

2. Increased blood flow in pulmonary arteries.

   ↓

3. Closure of umbilical artery.

   ↓

4. Reversal of flow through ductus arteriosus and closure.

   ↓

5. Increased pressure in left atrium. Closure of foramen ovale (complete in one week).

   ↓

6. Interruption of placental flow.

   ↓

7. Ductus venosus collapses.

ABDOMEN

SURFACE MARKINGS

Costal margin
Surface marking: 7th costal cartilage to the tip of the 12th rib.

Transpyloric plane
Surface marking: Level is at disc between L1 and 2.

Transumbilical plane
Surface marking: Level is at disc between L3 and 4.

Liver
Surface marking: Upper border: right 4th rib in midline to 5th space in the anterior axillary line. Lower border: tip of right 10th rib and just below left; palpable in normal subjects. Moves down on inspiration.

Spleen
Surface marking: Underlies 9th, 10th and 11th ribs posteriorly on the left side; distinct notch on inferomedial border; enlarges diagonally downwards.

Gall bladder
Surface marking: Fundus is at the tip of the 9th costal cartilage, where the lateral border of rectus abdominis cuts the costal margin.

Kidneys
Surface marking: Upper pole lies deep to the 12th rib; lower pole lies at the upper part of L3; right kidney normally 2.5 cm lower than the left, and its lower pole is normally palpable; moves slightly downwards on inspiration.

DIAPHRAGM

Openings in the diaphragm
1. Aortic opening (T12) lies just to the left of the midline. Transmits the abdominal aorta, the thoracic duct and the azygous vein.
2. Oesophageal opening (T10) transmits the oesophagus, branches of the left gastric artery and vein and the two vagi.
3. Inferior vena cava opening (T8) lies to the right of the midline in the central tendon. Transmits the inferior vena cava and the right phrenic nerve.

Nerve supply

Innervated by the phrenic nerve (C3, 4, 5) and peripherally by the lower seven intercostal nerves.

Embryology

It is formed by the fusion of the septum transversum (forming the central tendon), dorsal oesophageal mesentery, the pleuroperitoneal membranes and the body wall.

THORACIC DUCT

Drains: Whole lymphatic field below the diaphragm and the left half of the lymphatics above it.

Course: Begins at and passes superiorly from the cisterna chyli to enter the thorax through the aortic opening on the right side of the aorta, to become the thoracic duct. It ascends first behind and then to the left of the oesophagus. The duct empties into the venous system of the neck at the union of the internal jugular and subclavian veins.

OESOPHAGUS

Surface markings: Continuous with the lower end of the pharynx and extends from the lower border of the cricoid cartilage (C6) to the cardiac orifice of the stomach at the level of the 10th thoracic vertebra to the left of the midline.

Arterial supply

Inferior thyroid branch of the thyrocervical trunk, branches of the thoracic aorta, bronchial arteries and ascending branches from the left gastric and inferior phrenic artery.

Venous drainage

Lower third: Drained by the portal venous system via the gastric veins.
Middle third: Drained by the azygous system.
Upper third: Drained by the superior vena cava.

STOMACH

Blood supply

All arteries are derived directly or indirectly from the coeliac trunk. Venous drainage via the portal system.

Nerve supply

1. Parasympathetic via the vagus (motor and secretory nerve supply to the stomach):
    (i) *Anterior* vagus branches to the cardia, lesser curvature and pylorus.
    (ii) *Posterior* vagus branches to the body of the stomach, and distribution of coeliac branch to the intestine as far as the mid-transverse colon and the pancreas.

    With vagotomy, neurogenic gastrin secretion is abolished, but the stomach is also rendered atonic, so vagotomy must always be accompanied by a drainage procedure, e.g. pyloroplasty.
2. Sympathetic via intrinsic nerve plexuses:
    (i) *Auerbach's* plexus lies between the circular and longitudinal muscle layers.
    (ii) *Meissner's* plexus lies in the submucosa.

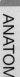

DUODENUM

Course: 30 cm in length and divided into four parts.
1. The first part is intraperitoneal; the bile duct and inferior vena cava pass behind.
2. The remainder is retroperitoneal. The 2nd part of the duodenum runs round the head of the pancreas. The ampulla of Vater is situated in this part.
3. The 3rd part crosses over the inferior vena cava, the aorta and origin of the inferior mesenteric artery. The superior mesenteric artery passes anteriorly.

Arterial supply of the intestine

The gastrointestinal tract develops from the foregut, mid and hindgut. Each has its own discrete arterial supply, but with extensive anastomoses.
Foregut: The stomach and duodenum are supplied by branches of the coeliac axis arising from the aorta at T12.
Midgut: Mid-duodenum to the distal transverse colon is supplied by the superior mesenteric artery, arising from the aorta at L1.
Hindgut: Distal transverse colon to the rectum is supplied by the inferior mesenteric artery, arising from the aorta at L3.

LIVER

Blood supply (Fig. 4.37)

Two blood supplies:
1. The common hepatic duct lies anteriorly.
2. The hepatic artery in the middle.
3. The portal vein posteriorly.

These structures lie in the free edge of the lesser omentum. The cystic artery commonly arises from the right hepatic artery in the angle between the common hepatic duct and the cystic duct.

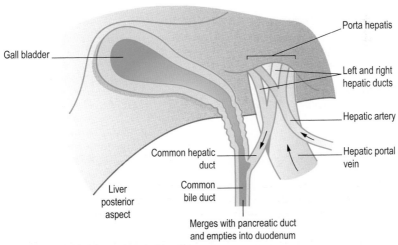

Gall bladder

Porta hepatis

Left and right hepatic ducts

Hepatic artery

Hepatic portal vein

Common hepatic duct

Liver posterior aspect

Common bile duct

Merges with pancreatic duct and empties into duodenum

Fig. 4.37 Gall bladder and porta hepatis.

Portal vein

Carries: Venous blood from the digestive tracts and spleen to the liver.
Accompanies hepatic artery and bile duct in the free edge of the lesser omentum.

Course: Formed by the union of the superior mesenteric and splenic veins behind the neck of the pancreas. During its course it lies behind the duodenum, gastroduodenal artery and bile duct. It passes up to the porta hepatis where it divides into right and left branches, before entering the liver with and posterior to the corresponding branches of the hepatic artery and the common hepatic ducts.

Hepatic venous portal system

Main connections between portal and systemic venous systems

1. Oesophageal branch of the left gastric veins and the oesophageal veins of the azygous system.
2. Inferior mesenteric vein of the portal system and the inferior haemorrhoidal veins draining into the internal iliac veins.
3. Portal tributaries in the mesentery and mesocolon and the retroperitoneal veins communicating with the renal, lumbar and phrenic veins.
4. Portal branches in the liver and the veins of the anterior abdominal wall via veins passing along the falciform ligament to the umbilicus.
5. Portal branches in the liver and the veins of the diaphragm across the bare area of the liver.

5
PHYSIOLOGY

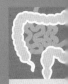

FLUID BALANCE   180
Distribution and measurement of body
   fluids   180
Control of fluid flow between plasma and
   interstitial compartments   181
Osmolality   182

ACID–BASE BALANCE   183
Glossary   183
Buffer systems   184
   Important buffer mechanisms in the
     body   185
Acid–base disturbances   187
   Respiratory acidosis   187
   Respiratory alkalosis   188
   Metabolic acidosis   188
   Metabolic alkalosis   188
   Mixed disorders   189
   Hyperchloraemic acidosis   189
   Hypochloraemic acidosis   189
   Metabolic effects of prolonged vomiting
     189
   Lactic acidosis   189

RENAL PHYSIOLOGY   190
Functions of the kidney   190
   Glomerular filtration   190
   Proximal tubule function   192
   Loop of Henle function   192
   Distal tubule/collecting duct function
     193
   Endocrine function   193
Renal transport of sodium   193
   Regulation of sodium balance and
     blood pressure   193
   Aldosterone   193
   The renin–angiotensin system   194
   Atrial natriuretic peptide   196
   Endothelins and nitric oxide   196
Salt and water balance abnormalities
   196
   Salt depletion   196

Water depletion   197
Water excess   197
Sodium excess   197
Renal transport of other solutes   198
   Potassium secretion   198
   Hydrogen secretion and bicarbonate
     reabsorption   198
   Chloride transport   199
   Sugars and amino acids   199
   Urea   199
Renal transport of water   199
   Antidiuretic hormone   199

RESPIRATORY PHYSIOLOGY   201
Lung volumes and capacities   201
   Volumes   202
   Capacities   202
   Spirometric measures   203
Pulmonary dynamics   204
   Work of breathing   204
   Compliance   205
   Airways resistance   205
   Intrapleural pressure   205
   Respiratory cycle   206
Pulmonary gas exchange and blood gas
     transport   206
   Partial pressures of gases in respiration
     206
   Blood–gas barrier   206
   Diffusing capacity of the lung or transfer
     factor   206
   The alveolar – arteriolar oxygen
     difference   207
Pulmonary circulation   207
   Ventilation/perfusion ratio   208
Control of breathing   208
Response to chronic hypoxia   209

CARDIAC PHYSIOLOGY   209
Conducting system of the heart   209
   Ventricular muscle   209
   Pacemaker cells   210

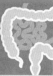

Cardiac cycle   210
   Phases of the cardiac cycle   210
   Intracardiac pressures   211
   Heart sounds   212
   Venous pressure changes   213
Cardiac performance   213
   Ventricular end-diastolic volume   213
   Central venous pressure   213
   Ventricular end-systolic volume   213
   Stroke volume   214
   Ejection fraction   214
   Cardiac output   214
   Blood pressure   216
   Peripheral resistance   216
The circulation   217
   Circulation through special areas   217
   Circulatory adaptations   218

GASTROINTESTINAL PHYSIOLOGY
   219
   Gastrointestinal polypeptide hormones
   219
Stomach   219
   Gastric secretion   219
Pancreas   220
   Pancreatic secretion   220
Biliary system   221
   Haem and bilirubin catabolism   221
Small intestine   222
   Intestinal secretion   222
   Small intestine motility   223
   Digestion and absorption in the small
      intestine   223

Colon   223
   Large intestine motility   224

ENDOCRINE PHYSIOLOGY   224
Classification of hormones   224
Mechanisms of hormone action   224
Hypothalamic regulatory hormones   224
Anterior pituitary hormones   225
   Adrenocorticotrophic hormone   226
   Thyroid-stimulating hormone   226
   Luteinizing hormone and
      follicle-stimulating hormone   227
   Melanocyte-stimulating hormone   228
   Growth hormone   228
   Prolactin   229
Posterior pituitary hormones   229
   Antidiuretic hormone   229
   Oxytocin   230
Adrenal cortex   230
   Glucocorticoids   232
   Mineralocorticoids   232
   Sex hormones   232
Adrenal medulla   233
   Catecholamines   233
Thyroid   233
   Thyroid hormone   234
Pancreas   235
   Insulin   235
   Glucagon   237
   Somatostatin   238

**PHYSIOLOGICAL RESPONSE OF
   MOTHER TO PREGNANCY**   238

FLUID BALANCE

DISTRIBUTION AND MEASUREMENT OF BODY FLUIDS

The volumes of the various fluid compartments are measured indirectly by an *indicator dilution method*. This approach requires that the introduced substance be evenly distributed in the body fluid compartment being measured.

$$\text{Volume of compartment} = \frac{\text{amount of substance introduced} - \text{amount of substance removed}}{\text{final concentration of substance in the compartment}}$$

- *Total body water* (TBW) constitutes approximately 50–60% of the body weight and is measured using tritiated water (^3H_2O), or deuterium oxide (^2H_2O).
- *Extracellular fluid* (ECF) volume is measured using saccharides, e.g. inulin, mannitol or ions like thiocyanate.
- *Plasma volume* is measured using Evans Blue dye, radioiodinated serum albumin or red blood cells labelled with ^{32}P or ^{51}Cr.

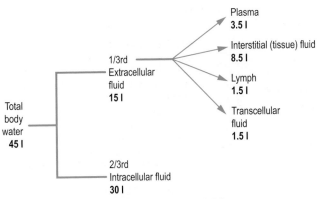

Fig. 5.1 Distribution of water in an average 70 kg man.
Transcellular fluid includes digestive secretions, gut luminal fluids, bile sweat, CSF, pleural pericardial, synovial and intraocular fluid.

- *Intracellular fluid* (ICF) volume cannot be measured directly from dilution: it is calculated from the difference between total body water and ECF volume. Similarly the interstitial fluid volume cannot be measured directly, and is calculated from the difference between the ECF volume and the plasma volume.

Table 5.1 Ion composition of body fluids		
Ion	ECF* (plasma) concentration (mmol/l)	ICF concentration (mmol/l)
Cations		
Sodium	142	10
Potassium	4.0	145
Calcium	2.5	0.001
Magnesium	1.0	40
Anions		
Chloride	104	5
Bicarbonate	25	10
Phosphate	1.1	100
Sulphate	0.5	20
Organic anions	3.0	0
Protein[†]	1.1	8

* ECF: sodium and potassium are the major cations; chloride and bicarbonate are the major anions.
† The plasma has a similar ion composition to that of the interstitial fluid except that it contains a much higher concentration of dissolved proteins.

CONTROL OF FLUID FLOW BETWEEN PLASMA AND INTERSTITIAL COMPARTMENTS (Fig. 5.2)

- A hydrostatic pressure difference across the capillary endothelium results in fluid flow from vascular to tissue space, but the retention of proteins within the vasculature is a retarding force (plasma oncotic pressure).
- The *Starling equation* describes the relationship between hydrostatic pressure, oncotic pressure and fluid flow across a capillary membrane.

PHYSIOLOGY

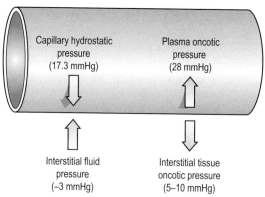

Fig. 5.2 Fluid flow between vascular and tissue compartments.

Capillary hydrostatic pressure
+ tissue oncotic pressure
(OUTWARD PRESSURES)
=
Interstitial fluid pressure +
plasma oncotic pressure
(INWARD PRESSURES)

Note: Tissue oncotic pressure: proteins in the interstitial space produce a force (generally 5–10 mmHg) causing outward filtration of fluid from the vascular space.

Interstitial pressure increases as the interstitial volume increases (oedema), which impedes further fluid filtration from the capillaries.

1. At the arterial end, the net intracapillary hydrostatic pressure (32 mmHg) exceeds the net interstitial oncotic pressure (18 mmHg), driving fluid out of the capillaries (32 − 18 = 14 mmHg).
2. At some point, the net hydrostatic pressure equals the net oncotic pressure with no net fluid movement.
3. The effective hydrostatic pressure falls to 12 mmHg on the venous side and is exceeded by the net plasma oncotic pressure (18 mmHg) and so reabsorption begins (12 − 18 = 6 mmHg). Any fluid not reabsorbed at this point is returned to the circulation by the lymphatic system. Thus filtration is favoured on the arterial side and absorption on the venous side.

Oedema

- A collection of excess interstitial fluid, i.e. interstitial fluid pressures become positive.

Causes

1. Increased capillary hydrostatic pressure, e.g. venous obstruction, excess blood volume, cardiac failure.
2. Decreased plasma oncotic pressure, e.g. causes of hypoproteinaemia (nephrotic syndrome, cirrhosis).
3. Increased capillary permeability, e.g. allergic, bacterial diseases and sepsis.
4. Increased tissue oncotic pressure, e.g. lymphatic blockage.

OSMOLALITY

- *Osmolality* is the number of particles (osmoles) of solute dissolved in one *kg* of solution (i.e. mosmol/kg) or mosmol/l. Osmolality is usually measured directly in the laboratory or using an osmometer.

- *Osmolarity* is the number of particles dissolved in a litre of solution (i.e. mosmol/l).

> - *Calculated plasma osmolarity* $\approx 2[Na^+ + K^+] + [glucose] + [urea]$
>   Plasma osmolality = 280–295 mosmol/l; (Normal urine osmolality = 300–1400 mosmol/l).
> - In most cases, plasma osmolarity calculated in this way is numerically very similar to the measured osmolality.
> - Main determinant of ECF osmolality is plasma $[Na^+]$, $[Cl^-]$ and $[HCO_3^-]$; main determinant of ICF osmolality is intracellular $[K^+]$.

- *Osmotic equilibration* between the ECF and ICF is achieved by water movement between the two compartments.
- *Osmolar gap* is the disparity between the measured osmolality and the calculated osmolality. Other osmotically active substances increase measured serum osmolality without altering serum $[Na^+]$, and therefore the measured serum osmolality exceeds the calculated value.

ACID–BASE BALANCE

GLOSSARY

Acid
A proton or hydrogen ion donor. It can dissociate to yield H^+ ions and the corresponding base. A strong acid completely or almost completely dissociates in aqueous solution, e.g. hydrochloric acid. A weak acid only partially dissociates in aqueous solution, e.g. acetic acid.

Anion gap
Routine serum electrolyte determination measures most of the cations but only a few of the anions. This apparent disparity between the total cation and the total anion concentration is called the anion gap.

> Anion gap $\approx [Na^+ + K^+] - [Cl^- + HCO_3^-]$.
> It is normally about 10–16 mmol/l and reflects the concentration of those anions actually present but not routinely measured, such as plasma proteins, phosphates, sulphates and organic acids.
> *Causes of an **increased** anion gap:* Marked renal failure, diabetic and alcoholic ketoacidosis, lactic acidosis, ingestion of salicylate, methanol, ethylene glycol or paraldehyde.
> Mild: dehydration, exogenous anions, e.g. penicillin and carbenicillin.
> *Causes of a **decreased** anion gap:* Increased unmeasured cation, e.g. potassium, magnesium and calcium. Decreased unmeasured anion, e.g. hypoalbuminaemia.

Arterial blood gases
Normal ranges:
$[H^+]$ = 36–44 mmol/l
pH = 7.35–7.45
Po_2 = 10.6–14.0 kPa
Pco_2 = 4.7–6.0 kPa
Bicarbonate (actual) = 23–33 mmol/l.

Base
A proton or hydrogen ion acceptor, e.g. HCO_3^- can accept H^+, thereby forming the corresponding undissociated acid, carbonic acid (H_2CO_3).

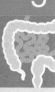

Base excess

This measures the change in the concentration of a buffer base (sum of the buffer anions of blood or plasma) from its normal value, i.e. base excess equals the observed buffer base minus the normal buffer base of whole blood. The normal range for base excess is ± 2.3 mmol/l in arterial whole blood. Metabolic acidosis is associated with a base excess below –5 mmol/l and metabolic alkalosis with a base excess above +5 mmol/l.

Henderson–Hasselbach equation

This describes the relationship of arterial pH to Pa_{CO_2}, bicarbonate and two constants.

$$pH = 6.1 + \log \frac{[HCO_3^-]}{0.235 \times [Pa_{CO_2}]}$$

where Pa_{CO_2} is the arterial partial pressure of CO_2.

Partial pressure

The pressure of a gas in a mixture of gases which is proportional to its concentration in the mixture. The sum of the partial pressures of the constituent gases is equal to the total pressure of the mixture. The partial pressure of any gas can therefore be calculated by multiplying its percentage composition by the ambient barometric pressure.

pH

The logarithm (to the base 10) of the reciprocal of the hydrogen ion concentration.
$pH = \log (1/[H^+])$ or $pH = -\log [H^+]$.
Note: A decrease in pH of 0.3 represents a twofold increase in $[H^+]$ and a decrease in pH of 1.0 represents a 10-fold increase in $[H^+]$.
Regulation of pH is achieved through control of:
(i) excretion of H^+ and reabsorption of HCO_3^- by the kidneys
(ii) excretion of CO_2 by the lungs through regulation of alveolar ventilation
(iii) buffering of H^+ by the body's buffering system.

pKa

The pH of a buffer at which half the acid molecules are undissociated and half are associated. The extent to which weak acids (or bases) dissociate in aqueous solution depends on the *dissociation constant* (pKa) for that acid or base.
$pH = pKa$ when equimolar concentrations of weak acid and base exist.

BUFFER SYSTEMS

- The *main source of H*+ in the body is the CO_2 produced as an end-product of the oxidation of carbon compounds, e.g. glucose and fatty acids during aerobic metabolism. Control of $[H^+]$ is achieved by buffering.
- Buffers consist of a weak acid (H^+ donor) in the presence of its base (H^+ acceptor). A buffer system minimizes changes in $[H^+]$ in response to the addition of acid or base, either by binding part of the additional hydrogen ion, or by dissociating further to release hydrogen ion, e.g.:

$$H^+ + Cl^- \quad + \quad NaHCO_3 \quad \rightarrow \quad H_2CO_3 \quad + \quad NaCl$$
$$\text{strong acid} \qquad \text{buffer} \qquad \qquad \text{weak acid} \qquad \text{neutral salt}$$

A buffer is most effective when the pH of the solution equals the pKa of the buffer.

IMPORTANT BUFFER MECHANISMS IN THE BODY (Table 5.2)

Table 5.2 Buffering according to body compartments

Compartment and major buffers	% of total body buffering
Plasma Bicarbonate Inorganic phosphate Plasma proteins	13
Erythrocytes Haemoglobin Bicarbonate Inorganic and organic phosphate	6
ICF (excluding erythrocytes) Bicarbonate Tissue protein Organic phosphate in skeletal muscle	51
Kidneys Bicarbonate Inorganic phosphate Ammonium	30

Buffer mechanism in the erythrocytes (Fig. 5.3)
- CO_2^- is produced in the tissues, and diffuses into the erythrocytes. Carbonic acid is formed, and catalysed by carbonic anhydrase dissociates to HCO_3^- and H^+.
- Most of the HCO_3^- diffuses into the plasma in exchange for chloride (chloride shift) to maintain electrical neutrality, and is converted to CO_2 which is blown off in the lungs.
- The hydrogen ion is buffered by reduced haemoglobin (the carbamate reaction). This minimizes the rise in pH that usually accompanies the deoxygenation of haemoglobin.

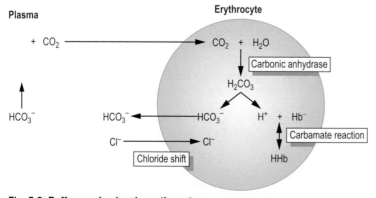

Fig. 5.3 Buffer mechanism in erythrocytes.

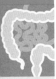

PHYSIOLOGY

Buffer mechanisms in the kidney

The kidneys play an important role in both the regeneration of bicarbonate buffer and in excretion of acids produced in cells during metabolism.

1. Renal bicarbonate reabsorption (Fig. 5.4)

- **H^+ secretion** into the tubular lumen occurs by active transport and is coupled to sodium reabsorption. For each H^+ secreted, one Na^+ and one HCO_3^- are reabsorbed.
- **HCO_3^- reabsorption**. Most of the H^+ secreted into the tubular fluid reacts with HCO_3^- to form carbonic acid which breaks down to form CO_2 and water. The CO_2 diffuses back into the proximal tubular cells, where it is rehydrated to H_2CO_3, which then dissociates into HCO_3^- and H^+. The buffering of secreted H^+ by filtered HCO_3^- is not a mechanism for H^+ excretion, since the CO_2 formed in the lumen from secreted H^+ returns to the tubular cell to form another H^+ and no net secretion of H^+ occurs.

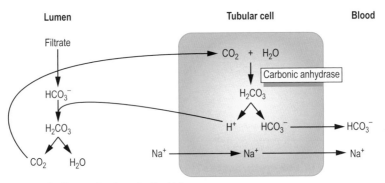

Fig. 5.4 Buffer mechanisms in the kidneys.

2. Ammonium secretion (NH_4^+)

- Ammonia (NH_3) is produced by the deamination of amino acids, mainly glutamine, to form glutamic acid, and the oxidative deamination of other amino acids to form keto-acids in the renal tubule cells. NH_3 diffuses into the tubular lumen, where it accepts H^+ to become ammonium (NH_4^+), which is then excreted. NH_3 secretion is an important mechanism in the renal response to chronic respiratory or metabolic acidosis.

3. Excretion of H^+ as dihydrogen phosphate

- The major titratable acid in the tubular fluid is phosphate. The titratable acidity measures that fraction of the acid excreted that did not combine with HCO_3^- or with NH_3.
- The exchange of H^+ for Na^+ converts monohydrogen phosphate into dihydrogen phosphate in the glomerular filtrate, which is excreted in the urine as titratable acid.
- Approximately 2/3rds of excess H^+ is excreted in the form of ammonium; the remaining 1/3rd of the excess acid is excreted as dihydrogen phosphate.

ACID–BASE DISTURBANCES (Table 5.3 and Fig. 5.5)

Table 5.3 Acid–base disturbances

Acid–base abnormality	Primary disturbance	Effect		Base excess	Compensatory response
		pH	P_{O_2}		
Respiratory acidosis	$\uparrow P_{CO_2}$	$\downarrow$	$\downarrow$		$\uparrow [HCO_3^-]$
Metabolic acidosis	$\downarrow [HCO_3^-]$	$\downarrow$	N or $\uparrow$	−ve	$\downarrow P_{CO_2}$
Respiratory alkalosis	$\downarrow P_{CO_2}$	$\uparrow$	N or $\uparrow$		$\downarrow [HCO_3^-]$
Metabolic alkalosis	$\uparrow [HCO_3^-]$	$\uparrow$	N or $\uparrow$	+ve	$\uparrow P_{CO_2}$

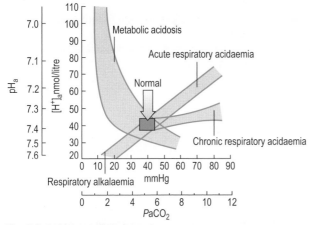

Fig. 5.5 Acid–base disturbances.

In general:
- Metabolic disturbances are compensated acutely by changes in ventilation, and chronically by appropriate renal responses.
- Respiratory disturbances are compensated by renal tubular secretion of H^+.
- A reduction in plasma $[HCO_3^-]$ may be due to metabolic acidosis or can indicate renal compensation for respiratory alkalosis.
- An elevated plasma $[HCO_3^-]$ can result from metabolic alkalosis or the secondary response to respiratory acidosis.

RESPIRATORY ACIDOSIS ($\downarrow$pH, $\uparrow CO_2$)

This is often mixed.

Causes
Any cause of *hypoventilation*:
1. Obstructive airways disease (acute or chronic)
2. CNS depression, e.g. sedative drugs, head injury, encephalitis, Pickwickian syndrome
3. Neuromuscular disease, e.g. myasthenia gravis, Guillain–Barré syndrome
4. Skeletal disease, e.g. flail chest, kyphoscoliosis, ankylosing spondylitis
5. Artificial ventilation.

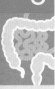
Compensatory mechanisms
In acute respiratory failure (e.g. asthmatic attack or bronchopneumonia), rapid erythrocyte mechanisms are the major compensatory response. In chronic respiratory failure (e.g. emphysema) the renal tubular mechanism is the most important compensatory mechanism.

RESPIRATORY ALKALOSIS ($\uparrow$pH, $\downarrow$CO$_2$)

Causes
Any cause of *hyperventilation*:
1. Psychogenic, e.g. hysteria, pain and anxiety
2. Central, e.g. raised intracranial pressure, encephalitis, meningitis, cerebral haemorrhage
3. Pulmonary, hypoxia (high altitude), pulmonary embolism, pneumonia, pulmonary oedema and pneumothorax
4. Metabolic, e.g. hyperthyroidism, fever, metabolic acidosis, acute liver failure
5. Drugs, e.g. early salicylate poisoning
6. Artificial ventilation
7. Gram-negative septicaemia.

METABOLIC ACIDOSIS ($\downarrow$pH, $\downarrow$HCO$_3^-$)

Causes
Normal anion gap: (see p. 183)
1. Intestinal loss of base, e.g. diarrhoea, fistulae, ureterosigmoidostomy (transplantation of ureters)
2. Renal loss of base, e.g. renal tubular acidosis (types 1 and 2), pyelonephritis
3. Therapy with carbonic anhydrase inhibitors, e.g. acetozolamide, ammonium chloride and rarely with hyperalimentation.
Conditions that cause a metabolic acidosis without an increase in unmeasured anions are associated with a high serum chloride.

Increased anion gap due to an increased acid pool:
1. Overproduction of organic acid, e.g. diabetic and alcoholic ketoacidosis or lactic acidosis secondary to hypoxia
2. Decreased ability to conserve/generate HCO$_3^-$ and to excrete acid, e.g. acute or chronic renal failure
3. Advanced salicylate poisoning, ingestion of ethanol, methanol or paraldehyde
4. Inborn errors of metabolism, e.g. maple syrup urine disease.

METABOLIC ALKALOSIS ($\uparrow$pH, $\uparrow$HCO$_3^-$)

Causes
1. Excess oral intake of alkali or forced alkaline diuresis
2. Excess acid loss, e.g. gastric aspiration or persistent vomiting as in pyloric stenosis (hypochloraemic alkalosis, see below)
3. Diuretic therapy (thiazide/loop)
4. Renal tubular acidosis due to chloride deficiency, potassium deficiency, hyperaldosteronism, Cushing's syndrome, corticosteroid treatment, or Bartter's syndrome.

MIXED DISORDERS

Causes
1. Respiratory alkalosis and metabolic acidosis in: salicylate overdose, renal failure with sepsis and septicaemia
2. Respiratory acidosis and metabolic acidosis in: respiratory distress syndrome, cardiac failure, shock, hypothermia, cardiac arrest, severe CNS depression (e.g. drug overdose) and severe pulmonary oedema, or uncontrolled diabetes in patients with chronic lung disease
3. Respiratory acidosis and metabolic alkalosis in: chronic lung disease and diuretic therapy or treatment of acute or chronic lung disease with steroids
4. Respiratory and metabolic alkalosis in: overventilation of chronic respiratory acidosis.

HYPERCHLORAEMIC ACIDOSIS

Often associated with hypokalaemia. Occurs when HCO_3^- is lost in a one-to-one exchange for chloride.

Causes
1. Ureterosigmoidostomy (transplantation of ureters into upper sigmoid colon). Urine which contains chloride enters the intestinal lumen, where cells reabsorb some of this chloride in exchange for bicarbonate, causing bicarbonate depletion.
2. Renal tubular acidosis.
3. Acetazolamide treatment.
4. Hyperventilation.

HYPOCHLORAEMIC ACIDOSIS

Causes
1. Loss of gastrointestinal fluids, e.g. vomiting and diarrhoea
2. Overtreatment with diuretics
3. Chronic respiratory acidosis
4. Diabetic acidosis
5. Adrenal insufficiency, i.e. Addison's disease.

METABOLIC EFFECTS OF PROLONGED VOMITING

Prolonged vomiting may be caused by, e.g. pyloric stenosis.

Causes
1. Continued vomiting of acid gastric fluid with no loss of alkaline duodenal fluid
2. Hypovolaemia and metabolic alkalosis due to HCl and K^+ loss
3. Renal/HCO_3^- excretion inhibited by *hypochloraemic alkalosis*, hypokalaemia and reduced glomerular filtration rate
4. Paradoxical aciduria
5. Compensatory hypoventilation.

LACTIC ACIDOSIS

This is defined as a level >5 mmol/l. Normal plasma lactate (resting) = <1 mmol/l.

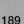

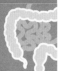

Causes
Increased generation of lactate:
1. Cardiac arrest due to decreased tissue perfusion
2. Large tumour masses (leukaemia, lymphoma)
3. Cyanide and carbon monoxide poisoning
4. Mitochondrial toxicity with antiretroviral drugs, especially nucleoside reverse transcriptase inhibitors, e.g. zidovudine, stavudine.

Decreased utilization of lactate:
1. Phenformin and metformin intoxication
2. Diabetes mellitus
3. Alcoholism
4. Hepatic failure due to decreased hepatic perfusion.

RENAL PHYSIOLOGY

FUNCTIONS OF THE KIDNEY

A. GLOMERULAR FILTRATION

Involves passage through three layers:
1. Capillary endothelium lining the glomerulus
2. Glomerular basement membrane
3. Epithelial layer of Bowman's capsule.

Depends on:
1. The balance of Starling forces where:
   Net filtration pressure across the glomerular membrane = (glomerular capillary hydrostatic pressure – hydrostatic pressure in Bowman's capsule) – colloid osmotic pressure of blood.
2. Permeability of glomerular capillary wall.
3. Total capillary area and number of glomeruli.
4. Glomerular capillary plasma flow.
   - The glomerular filtrate is an ultrafiltrate of plasma, with an identical composition except for a few proteins (0.03%).

Glomerular filtration rate (GFR)
- Total volume of plasma per unit time leaving the capillaries and entering the Bowman's capsule.
- GFR is approximately 180 l per day, or 120 ml/min.

Renal clearance
- Volume of plasma from which all of a given substance is removed per minute by the kidneys.

Measurement
- The measurement of clearance involves a comparison of the rate of urinary excretion (urine volume × urinary concentration) with the plasma concentration.
- Various substances can be used for measuring the GFR by determining its clearance. The properties of these include:
  1. Biologically inert, i.e. not metabolized.
  2. Freely filtered from the plasma at the glomerulus, i.e. not plasma protein bound.
  3. Neither reabsorbed nor secreted by the tubules.
  4. Concentration in plasma remains constant throughout the period of urine collection.

If the substance is neither excreted nor reabsorbed, i.e. all of the plasma filtered has been cleared of the substance, e.g. inulin, then Clearance = GFR.

Measurement of clearance

$$\text{Clearance} = \frac{\text{Amount excreted/min}}{\text{Plasma concentration of substance } x}$$

$$\text{GFR} = \frac{U_x V}{P_x}$$

where
U_x = urine concentration (mmol/l)
V = urine volume (ml/min)
P_x = plasma concentration (mmol/l)
GFR = ml/min

- If Clearance >GFR, then there must be net secretion, as with para-amino hippuric acid (PAH).
- If Clearance <GFR, then there must be net reabsorption, as with urea.

Creatinine clearance

The 24-hour renal clearance of endogenous creatinine is often used clinically as an estimate of GFR (small amount of creatinine excreted). It declines with age, due to a decline in renal function and reduction in muscle mass. The plasma creatinine remains constant throughout life. Normal value is >100 ml/min.

Measurement of creatinine clearance (24 hour urine collection)

$$\text{Creatinine clearance} = \frac{\text{Urine creatinine concentration } (\mu) \times 24\text{ h urine volume } (v)/1440}{\text{Plasma creatinine concentration } (p)/1000}$$

1440 converts urine rate volume from per 24 h to per min.
1000 is used to convert μmol to mmol:
1000/1440 mmol.

Therefore if:
μ = 8 mmol/l
p = 110 μmol/l
v = 2000 ml

$$\text{Clearance} = \frac{8 \times 2000}{120} \times 0.7$$

$$= 93 \text{ ml/min}$$

If 24 hour urine collection is unreliable, then Clearance calculated from:

$$\text{Creatinine clearance (ml/min)} = \frac{140 - \text{age (years)} \times \text{weight (kg)}}{72 \times \text{serum creatinine (mg/dl)}}$$

Unreliable with unstable renal function, gross obesity and oedema.

Renal blood flow (RBF)

- RBF = 1200 ml/min of whole blood (i.e. approximately 25% of the cardiac output).

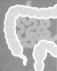

PHYSIOLOGY

- GFR and renal blood flow remain approximately constant, within a BP range of 80–180 mmHg, through the mechanism of autoregulation mediated by changes in the afferent arteriolar resistance.

Renal plasma flow (RPF)

- RPF is commonly measured using para-amino hippuric acid (PAH), by determining the amount of PAH in the urine per unit time, divided by the difference in its concentration in renal arterial or venous blood.
- RPF = 660 ml/min. Approximately 120 ml/min of the 660 ml/min is filtered at the glomerulus as ultrafiltrate, 65% is reabsorbed in the proximal tubule, 14% in the loops of Henlé, 15% in the distal tubules and 6% in the collecting ducts. Average urine output = 1.2 ml/min, i.e. only 1% of 120 ml/min of ultrafiltrate filtered at the glomerulus.

B. PROXIMAL TUBULE FUNCTION

1. *Iso-osmotic reabsorption* of 2/3rds of the glomerular filtrate.
2. *Active reabsorption* of sodium, potassium, glucose, galactose, fructose, amino acids, calcium, uric acid and vitamin C. Na^+ reabsorption can be coupled to the transport of other solutes by either co-transport with glucose, amino acids, bicarbonate and phosphate or exchange with, for example, H^+.
3. *Passive reabsorption* of urea and water due to the osmotic gradient generated by solute reabsorption.
4. *Active secretion* of organic acids, e.g. PAH, diuretics, salicylates, penicillins and probenicid.

Renal transport maximum (Tm) is the maximum amount of a given solute that can be transported (reabsorbed or secreted) per minute by the renal tubules. When the filtered load exceeds the transport maximum, the excess is not reabsorbed but excreted. Substances that have a Tm include phosphate, HPO_4^{2-}, SO_4^{2-}, glucose, many amino acids and uric acid.

C. LOOP OF HENLE FUNCTION

A counter current multiplier system exists between the ascending loop of Henle, the collecting ducts (counter current multipliers), the vasa recta, which represent the vasculature of the juxtaglomerular nephrons (counter current exchangers) and the interstitial tissues. This establishes an interstitial concentration gradient, whereby osmotic pressure of the interstitial tissue of the kidney increases from cortex to medulla. In the presence of a normally functioning antidiuretic hormone (ADH) feedback mechanism, this permits maximum reabsorption of water and concentration of urine. In the absence of ADH, the kidney forms a dilute urine.

Mechanism

- Blood entering the outer medulla in the vasa recta receives NaCl from the descending loop of Henle and so the interstitium becomes more concentrated.
- The tubular fluid in the descending limb loses water and so becomes more concentrated.
- The fluid in the ascending limb of the loop of Henle loses NaCl, and so is hypotonic as it enters the distal convoluted tubule.
- The filtrate in the distal tubule and collecting ducts loses both water and urea (ADH increases permeability to water), so tubular urine becomes more concentrated again.

Summary
Fluid entering loop – isotonic
Fluid at tip of loop – hypertonic
Fluid leaving loop – hypotonic

D. DISTAL TUBULE/COLLECTING DUCT FUNCTION

1. *Reabsorption* of approximately 5% of sodium and 3% of bicarbonate. Variable water reabsorption in the collecting ducts, depending on the presence of ADH. Reabsorption is not iso-osmotic.
2. *Tubular secretion* (active or passive) of ammonium and H^+, and K^+ is under the influence of aldosterone. Also important for eliminating unwanted metabolic products and drugs. Both the distal convoluted tubule and collecting ducts are subject to the actions of aldosterone.

E. ENDOCRINE FUNCTION

1. Synthesis of erythropoietin under stimulus of hypoxia and anaemia
2. 1,25-dihydroxycholecalciferol (vitamin D)
3. Renin
4. Prostaglandins A_2, E_2 and bradykinin.

RENAL TRANSPORT OF SODIUM

- 99% of filtered sodium load is reabsorbed (60% in proximal tubule, 25% in loop of Henle, 10% in distal tubule/collecting ducts where 2% is under the control of aldosterone).

Reabsorbed by three principal mechanisms:
1. In proximal tubule by Na^+/H^+ exchange. Intracellular H^+ is provided by HCO_3^- absorption and carbonic anhydrase action.
2. In the thick ascending limb, Na^+ is absorbed by $Na^+/Cl^-/2K^+$ co-transport. The transport protein is inhibited by furosemide, and so prevents urine concentration by the loop of Henle.
3. In the distal tubule, Na^+ is absorbed through an epithelial Na^+ channel which is electrically coupled to a K^+ channel. This dual channel mechanism results in net Na^+ absorption, coupled to net K^+ excretion. This mechanism is regulated by aldosterone.

REGULATION OF SODIUM BALANCE AND BLOOD PRESSURE

1. Glomerular filtration rate
2. Aldosterone via the renin–angiotensin system
3. Atrial natriuretic peptide (see p. 196)
4. Endothelins and nitric oxide.

ALDOSTERONE

- C-21 mineralocorticoid hormone secreted by the zona glomerulosa of the adrenal cortex.
- Normal plasma range = 0.9–3 μmol/l (on salt-restricted diet) and 0.1–0.4 μmol/l (on high-salt diet).

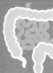

PHYSIOLOGY

Action

Promotion of sodium and chloride reabsorption in the distal tubules and collecting ducts, and excretion of K⁺ and H⁺. Similar exchange mechanism in the sweat glands, ileum and colon.

Control of secretion

1. Via the renin–angiotensin system (Fig. 5.6); cAMP-mediated and independent of ACTH.
2. ACTH enhances aldosterone production by stimulating steroidogenesis. Negligible role.
3. Plasma K⁺ and Na⁺ in the absence of changes in plasma volume: a 10% increase in plasma [K⁺] and a 10% decrease in plasma [Na⁺] (effect often overridden by changes in the circulating volume), can stimulate the synthesis and release of aldosterone by a direct action on the zona glomerulosa.
   (i) Changes in ECF volume are detected by pressure receptors in the afferent arteriole; a fall in [Na⁺] or rise in [K⁺] is detected by receptors at the macula densa.
   (ii) Renin is secreted into the bloodstream, where it combines with the substrate, angiotensinogen, synthesized by the liver, to form angiotensin I. This is converted in the lung by angiotensin-converting enzyme (ACE), produced by pulmonary epithelial cells, to the physiologically active octapeptide (angiotensin II). This exhibits a negative feedback on its own production by inhibiting renin secretion.

THE RENIN–ANGIOTENSIN SYSTEM

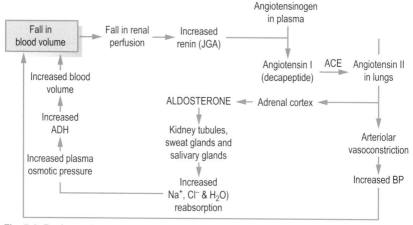

Fig. 5.6 Renin–angiotension system.
ACE = angiotensin-converting enzyme; JGA = juxtaglomerular apparatus.

Actions of angiotensin II

1. Potent arterial and venous vasoconstrictor.
2. Increases synthesis and release of aldosterone and ADH centrally.
3. Increases thirst by a central mechanism.
4. Increases level of prostaglandins.

Losartan is a non-competitive antagonist of the angiotensin II receptors AT1 and AT2. It is 30 000 times more selective for the AT1 than the AT2 receptor. It is now licensed for the treatment of essential hypertension.

Unlike angiotensin-converting enzyme (ACE) inhibitors, it has no action on bradykinins, or substance P, i.e. no dry cough as associated with ACE inhibitors.

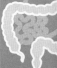

Causes of increased renin release
1. A decrease in the effective circulating blood volume and Na$^+$ depletion.
2. Catecholamines, oral contraceptives.
3. Chronic disorders associated with oedema (cirrhosis, congestive heart failure and nephrotic syndrome).
4. Standing.

Causes of decreased renin release
1. Angiotensin II, ADH, hypernatraemia and hyperkalaemia.
2. Indometacin and β-blockers reduce renin secretion.
3. Angiotensin-converting enzyme inhibitors (ACE-I) prevent conversion of angiotensin I to II.

Angiotensin-converting enzyme
1. Plays a key role in the renin–angiotensin and kallikrein-kinin systems by activating angiotensin I to angiotensin II. These two peptide hormones have opposite effects on vascular tone and on smooth muscle proliferation. It remains unclear whether ACE levels are a risk factor for ischaemic heart disease.
2. The ACE gene has been cloned and is located on chromosome 17. Polymorphism exists with three genotypes: II, ID and DD. A DD genotype may be associated with increased risk of myocardial infarction.

Causes of increased aldosterone secretion
1. Upright position and when ambulant.
2. High potassium/low sodium intake.
3. Loss of ECF, e.g. haemorrhage.
4. Surgery, anxiety.
5. Primary hyperaldosteronism (Conn's syndrome).
   Biochemical features of primary hyperaldosteronism:
   (i) elevated plasma (and urinary) aldosterone, with decreased levels of plasma renin and angiotensin
   (ii) hypertension due to Na$^+$ and water retention
   (iii) hypokalaemic alkalosis
   (iv) decreased haematocrit due to expansion of plasma volume
   (v) absence of peripheral oedema.
6. Secondary hyperaldosteronism, e.g. cardiac failure, cirrhosis.
   Biochemical features of secondary hyperaldosteronism:
   (i) elevated plasma (and urinary) aldosterone, with increased levels of plasma renin and angiotensin
   (ii) hypertension with oedema due to Na$^+$ and water retention in the interstitial space
   (iii) hypokalaemic alkalosis.
7. Renal artery stenosis.
8. Constriction of inferior vena cava in thorax.

Causes of decreased aldosterone secretion
1. Increase in dietary sodium intake or intravenous saline infusion.
2. Adrenalectomy.
   Main effects of adrenalectomy:
   (i) Na$^+$ lost in the urine and also Na$^+$ enters the cells, so plasma Na$^+$ falls: K$^+$ is retained, so plasma K$^+$ rises. Hypoglycaemia occurs through inhibition of gluconeogenesis.
   (ii) Plasma volume is reduced, resulting in hypotension and shock.

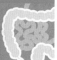

ATRIAL NATRIURETIC PEPTIDE (ANP)

Three peptides have been isolated: A, B and C
A: stored in right atrium and causes natriuresis and vasodilatation.
B: stored in cardiac ventricles and has similar effects to A.
C: stored in vascular endothelial cells and causes vasodilatation.
Receptors A and B are active in signal transduction, while receptor C binds the peptides and terminates their effect.
Endopeptidase breaks down peptides, and inhibitors have been developed that may have a role in treatment of hypertension, heart failure and myocardial ischaemia.

Actions
1. Marked natriuresis.
2. Lowers the blood pressure.
3. Decreases the responsiveness of vascular smooth muscle to many vasoconstrictor substances.
4. Inhibits the secretion of renin and vasopressin.
5. Decreases the responsiveness of the kidney to stimuli that would normally increase aldosterone secretion.
6. ↑ECF volume is associated with ↑ levels of ANP.

ENDOTHELINS (ET) AND NITRIC OXIDE (NO)

Endothelins

- Family of 21 amino acid peptides produced by a variety of tissues.
- All are potent vasoconstrictors.
- Modulate vasomotor tone, cell proliferation and hormone production.
- Three members of family: endothelin -1, -2, -3 interact with 2 receptor types (Type A and B). These bind to G-proteins which after activation cause an increase in intracellular calcium and stimulate protein kinase C.

Endothelin-1:
- Produced in endothelial and vascular smooth muscle cells.
- Most potent vasoconstrictor, and has mitogenic activation on vascular smooth muscle and myocardial cells.
- Involved in pathogenesis of heart failure, postischaemic renal failure, myocardial damage following infarction. Levels correlate with severity.

Nitric oxide

Previously called endothelial-derived relaxing factor. Production is regulated via the activity of NO synthase, a mainly cytosolic calcium-calmodulin-requiring enzyme, similar in structure to cytochrome P450 enzymes.

SALT AND WATER BALANCE ABNORMALITIES

SALT DEPLETION

Hypo-osmotic dehydration.
1. A net loss of salt in excess of water results in a decreased osmolality of the ECF, with a subsequent shift of fluid from the ECF to the ICF.
2. Resulting decreased ECF volume, with an increased ICF volume and a decrease in the osmolality of both.

Causes: Addison's disease (renal loss of salt).

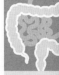
WATER DEPLETION

Hyperosmotic dehydration.
1. Main effect is a decreased ECF volume, with a fluid shift from the ICF to the ECF compartments.
2. Both the ECF and ICF volumes are decreased, and the osmolality of both is increased.
3. Resulting decreased GFR with associated release of aldosterone and ADH (i.e. renal tubular reabsorption of Na^+ and Cl^- increased).

Causes: decreased intake of water, diabetes insipidus, lithium.

WATER EXCESS

Hypo-osmotic overhydration.
1. Water enters the plasma, causing a decreased ECF osmolality, and hence a shift of fluid from the ECF to the ICF compartments.
2. Increase in the ECF and ICF volumes with a decrease in the osmolality of both compartments.

Causes: excessive intake of water, syndrome of inappropriate ADH secretion (SIADH).

SODIUM EXCESS

Hyperosmotic overhydration.
1. Sodium retention is usually accompanied by an equivalent retention of water and chloride.
2. The rise in plasma osmolality causes a shift of water from ICF to ECF. The ECF volume is increased and is borne by the interstitial fluid (oedema), whilst the ICF volume is decreased.
3. ADH release is inhibited, and the osmolality of both compartments is increased.

Causes: administration of large amounts of hypertonic fluid.

Causes of hypernatraemia

Normal extracellular sodium: water ratio is 140 mmol/l. Hypernatraemia occurs when the extracellular sodium:water ratio is greater than normal.
1. Sodium excess (i.e. increased total body sodium)
   - Excess IV saline, especially postoperatively
   - Primary hyperaldosteronism, e.g. steroid therapy, Cushing's or Conn's syndrome.
2. Water depletion (i.e. low total body sodium)
   - Reduced water intake, e.g. coma, heat stroke, confusion in the elderly
   - Extrarenal, e.g. fever, thyrotoxicosis, burns, diarrhoea and fistula
   - Renal, e.g. osmotic diuresis (some patients with hyperosmolar non-ketotic diabetic coma, postobstructive uropathy), diabetes insipidus (cranial/nephrogenic).

Causes of hyponatraemia

True hyponatraemia occurs when the extracellular sodium: water ratio is less than normal.
1. Water loading
   (i) *Hypertonic hyponatraemia* – with sodium retention (i.e. increased total body sodium and water)
   - Secondary hyperaldosteronism, e.g. congestive cardiac failure, nephrotic syndrome, liver cirrhosis
   - Reduced GFR, e.g. acute/chronic renal failure.

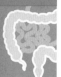

(ii) *Hypotonic hyponatraemia* – without sodium retention
- Acute water overload, e.g. excess IV fluids, esp. dextrose in postoperative period (spot urine [Na^+] <20 mmol/l)
- Psychogenic polydipsia
- Inappropriate ADH secretion, e.g. chlorpropamide, thiazide diuretics, carbamazepine, phenytoin, cytotoxic agents (cyclophosphamide, vincristine), TB, lung carcinoma, abscesses and other neoplasms.

2. Sodium depletion (i.e. decreased total body sodium)
   (i) Renal loss (spot urine [Na^+] >20 mmol/l), e.g. diuretics; osmotic diuresis due to diabetes, ketonuria, renal tubular damage (diuretic phase of acute renal failure), renal tubular acidosis, and Addison's disease
   (ii) Extrarenal loss (spot urine [Na^+] <20 mmol/l) e.g. sweating, extensive dermatitis, burns, vomiting, diarrhoea, fistulae, paralytic ileus and pancreatitis.

Other causes
Pseudohyponatraemia, e.g. hyperlipidaemia, sampling from IV infusion arm.

RENAL TRANSPORT OF OTHER SOLUTES

POTASSIUM SECRETION

- 7% of filtered potassium load is excreted. Almost all potassium is actively reabsorbed in the proximal tubule.
- Passive secretion of potassium occurs in the distal tubule in exchange for sodium, promoted by aldosterone. Hydrogen and potassium ions compete for this exchange.
- Metabolic acidosis is associated with cellular K^+ efflux, a decreased K^+ secretion and hyperkalaemia. The converse is true with metabolic alkalosis.

Causes of hypokalaemia (see p. 284)
1. Increased renal loss, e.g. diuretics, renal tubular acidosis, Fanconi syndrome, renal failure (diuretic phase of acute renal failure/chronic pyelonephritis), diabetic ketoacidosis, Cushing's syndrome and steroid excess, hyperaldosteronism (primary and secondary).
2. Increased gastrointestinal loss, e.g. diarrhoea and vomiting, laxative abuse, carbenoloxone ingestion, intestinal fistulae, chronic mucus-secreting neoplasms.
3. Other causes include insulin therapy, catabolic states, IV therapy with inadequate K^+ supplements, insulinoma, metabolic or respiratory alkalosis, familial periodic paralysis, drugs, e.g. carbenicillin, phenothiazines, amphotericin B and degraded tetracycline.

Causes of hyperkalaemia
1. Acute renal failure and advanced chronic renal failure.
2. Potassium-sparing diuretics.
3. Metabolic or respiratory acidosis.
4. Haemolysis (e.g. incompatible blood transfusion), tissue necrosis (e.g. major trauma and burns), severe starvation (e.g. anorexia nervosa), hypoaldosteronism.

HYDROGEN SECRETION AND BICARBONATE REABSORPTION

- Hydrogen ion secretion (acidification) takes place throughout the entire length of nephron, except the loop of Henlé (85% in the proximal tubule, 10% in the distal tubules and 5% in the collecting ducts), in exchange for sodium.
- Three major mechanisms of hydrogen ion excretion (see pH, p. 184).

CHLORIDE TRANSPORT

Cl⁻ moves passively in association with Na⁺ except in the ascending limb of the loop of Henlé, where it is actively transported. Plasma chloride level varies inversely with that of plasma bicarbonate because these anions exchange for each other across cell membranes. Depression of plasma chloride will result in an alkalosis caused by the increase in plasma bicarbonate following the release of HCO_3^- from cells.

SUGARS AND AMINO ACIDS

- Completely reabsorbed in proximal tubule via active, carrier-mediated mechanism. Sodium-dependent.
- Glucose reabsorption is saturatable: i.e. when blood glucose reaches 10 mmol/l, glycosuria occurs.

UREA

- 87% of filtered urea is reabsorbed; 50% is passively reabsorbed in the proximal tubule.
- Only one-fifth of the remaining urea entering the collecting duct leaves in the urine; the remainder is returned in the bloodstream.

Causes of changes in plasma urea and creatinine:
Normal ratio of urea to creatinine, 10:1
1. *Plasma urea and creatinine are raised in parallel*
   - Chronic renal failure, established acute renal failure
2. ↑*Urea* > ↑*creatinine*
   - Prerenal uraemia, e.g. sodium and water depletion, cardiac failure, gastrointestinal haemorrhage and trauma
   - High protein intake (oral or IV) in presence of renal disease.
   - Protein catabolism, e.g. starvation, postoperative states, corticosteroid therapy, tetracycline therapy in the presence of renal disease
   - Drugs via impairment of renal function, e.g. potent diuretics, indomethacin
3. ↑*Creatinine* > ↑*urea*
   - Rhabdomyolysis
4. ↓*Urea* > ↓*creatinine*
   - Pregnancy, low protein diet, acute liver failure, high fluid intake.

RENAL TRANSPORT OF WATER

Control of water excretion
- Water is reabsorbed passively along osmotic gradients set up by active transport of solutes, mainly Na⁺, Cl⁻ and urea. 80% of filtered water is reabsorbed isosmotically in the proximal tubule. 10–15% is reabsorbed in the loop of Henlé, distal tubule and partly in the collecting ducts, in the presence of ADH.
- Counter current exchange together with multiplication is essential for the concentration of urine, and can only occur in the presence of ADH.

ANTIDIURETIC HORMONE (ADH, OR VASOPRESSIN)

- Synthesized in the cell bodies of the supraoptic and paraventricular nuclei of the hypothalamus.
- Transported along nerve axons and released from posterior pituitary. The neurophysins are the physiological carrier proteins for the intraneuronal transport of ADH.
- Nonapeptide: the biologically active form is arginine vasopressin.

Control of secretion
- Release can occur in response to an increase in *osmolality* (via stimulation of osmoreceptors located in the anterior hypothalamus) and a decreased *fluid volume* (via a decrease in the tension or stretch of the volume receptors located in the left atrium, vena cavae, great pulmonary veins, carotid sinus and aortic arch).

Actions (Fig. 5.7)
- Acts via cyclic AMP on the distal tubules and collecting ducts.
- In absence of ADH, the distal tubule and collecting duct are fairly impermeable to water (8% is reabsorbed in distal convoluted tubules and collecting ducts, 12% is lost in the urine) and the urine is hypotonic.
- With maximal ADH effect, the walls of the collecting duct are permeable to water (19% is reabsorbed in distal convoluted tubule and collecting ducts, 1% is lost in the urine) and the urine is hypertonic.

Causes of ADH excess: syndrome of inappropriate ADH secretion (SIADH)
1. Increased pituitary ADH
   - Hypoadrenalism, stress
   - Drugs, e.g. nicotine, barbiturates, clofibrate, vincristine
   - Lung disease, e.g. pneumonia, TB, pleural effusion, positive pressure ventilation
   - Intracranial disease, e.g. head injury, stroke, cerebral tumours and encephalitis
   - Systemic disease, e.g. acute intermittent porphyria

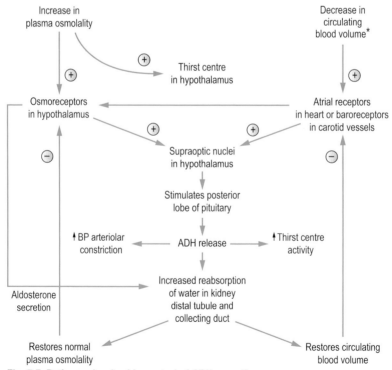

Fig. 5.7 Pathways involved in control of ADH secretion.
*ADH release by fall in blood volume may override osmotic changes tending to inhibit release.

2. Increased sensitivity to ADH, e.g. chlorpropamide, carbamazepine
3. Ectopic source of ADH, e.g. bronchogenic carcinoma.

> **Criteria for diagnosis of inappropriate ADH syndrome** ✔
> (Hypo-osmotic overhydration; p. 197). Water retention occurs with an expansion of the ECF volume.
> Oedema does not occur because aldosterone secretion is suppressed, which in turn causes increased urinary sodium excretion.
> 1. Hyponatraemia and low plasma osmolality: <270 mosmol/l.
> 2. Urine sodium output inappropriately high at 50 mmol/day.
> 3. Urine osmolality inappropriately high relative to serum osmolality: 350–400 mosmol/l.
> 4. No evidence of hypovolaemia.
> 5. Increasing plasma osmolality in response to a restricted intake of water.

Causes of ADH deficiency

1. Cranial diabetes insipidus: inherited (autosomal dominant or recessive) and acquired (hypothalamic disorders). Distinguished from nephrogenic diabetes insipidus by injecting exogenous vasopression which fails to improve urinary concentration in the nephrogenic type.
   Treatment: nasal lysine vasopressin, oral hypoglycaemic agents, thiazide diuretics, carbamazepine and clofibrate
2. Nephrogenic diabetes insipidus
   Inherited (sex-linked recessive) and acquired, e.g. chronic renal disease, metabolic disorders (hypercalcaemia, hypokalaemia), drugs (lithium, demeclocycline) and osmotic diuresis (diabetes mellitus, mannitol)
   Treatment: thiazide diuretics
3. Primary polydipsia associated with psychiatric disorders.

RESPIRATORY PHYSIOLOGY

LUNG VOLUMES AND CAPACITIES (Fig. 5.8)

The resting expiratory level is the most constant reference point on the spirometer trace.

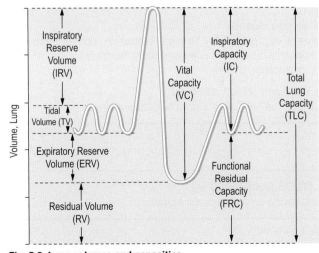

Fig. 5.8 Lung volumes and capacities.

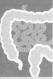

VOLUMES

Tidal volume (TV): 500 ml in males; 340 ml in females
Volume inspired or expired with each breath at rest.

Inspiratory reserve volume (IRV): 3000 ml
Maximum volume of air that can be inspired at the end of a normal tidal inspiration.

Expiratory reserve volume (ERV): 1000 ml
The maximum volume of air that can be forcibly expired after a normal tidal expiration.

Residual volume (RV): 1500 ml
Volume of air remaining after maximal voluntary expiration. Cannot be measured by spirometry. 25% of total lung capacity and increases with age.

RV = FRC (see below) **– ERV**

CAPACITIES

Inspiratory capacity (IC): 3500 ml
Maximum volume of air that can be inspired at the end of a normal tidal expiration.

IC = TV + IRV

Vital capacity (VC): 4500 ml in males, 3500 ml in females
Maximum volume of air that can be expired after a maximal inspiration. Values increase with size and decrease with age. Approx. 80% of total lung capacity.

VC = IC + ERV

Causes of decreased VC
1. Severe obstructive airways disease
2. Decreased lung volume, e.g. pulmonary fibrosis, infiltration, oedema and effusions, skeletal abnormalities and weak respiratory muscles (Guillain–Barré and myasthenia gravis).

Functional residual capacity (FRC): 2500 ml
Volume of gas remaining in the lung after a normal tidal expiration.

FRC = ERV + RV

Total lung capacity (TLC): 5500–6000 ml
Total volume of the lung following a maximal inspiration.

TLC = IRV + TV + ERV + RV = VC + RV

Causes of decreased TLC and RV
1. 'Stiff lungs': i.e. reduced lung compliance, e.g. pulmonary fibrosis, pneumoconiosis, pulmonary infiltration and pulmonary oedema.
2. Chest wall disease, e.g. deformity of thoracic spine, respiratory muscle weakness (myopathies, neuropathies and myasthenia gravis).

Causes of increased TLC and RV
1. Increased lung compliance, e.g. emphysema.
2. Airways obstruction and gas trapping, e.g. chronic bronchitis, emphysema and asthma ($\uparrow$ in RV > $\uparrow$ in TLC).

SPIROMETRIC MEASURES

Forced vital capacity (FVC)
The vital capacity when the expiration is performed as rapidly as possible.

Forced expiratory volume in one second (FEV_1)
Volume expired during 1st second of FVC. It is relatively independent of expiratory effort because of the dynamic collapse of the airways and the fact that expiratory flow is determined by the elastic recoil pressure of the lung and the resistance of airways proximal to the collapsing lung. Normally greater than 80% of the FVC (Fig. 5.9a).

- Patients with restrictive lung disease have a reduced VC and TLC due to decreased lung compliance. $FEV_1/FVC > 80\%$ (Fig. 5.9b).
- Patients with obstructive lung disease have a large TLC and a reduced VC, because their RV is increased. $FEV_1/FVC < 80\%$ (Fig. 5.9c).

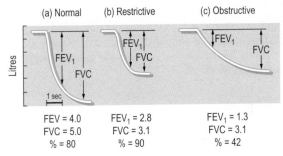

(a) Normal	(b) Restrictive	(c) Obstructive
FEV = 4.0	FEV$_1$ = 2.8	FEV$_1$ = 1.3
FVC = 5.0	FVC = 3.1	FVC = 3.1
% = 80	% = 90	% = 42

Fig. 5.9 Spirometry.

Effect of bronchodilators:
A 10% increase in either FEV_1, FVC or VC is significant, or >15–20% increase in FEV_1/FVC.

Peak flow
Maximum expiratory flow rate achieved during a forced expiration. Normal range varies with gender and height. Closely related to FEV_1.

FVC, FEV_1 and peak flow are spirometric measures. Spirometry cannot be used to calculate the RV, FRC and TLC. Helium dilution or total body plethysmography may be used.

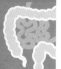

Flow volume loops (Fig. 5.10)

- Obstruction may be so severe that spirometry no longer shows the typical pattern.
- Flow volume loops measure peak flows at various lung volumes.
- Flows are most affected at low volumes in distal obstruction (e.g. asthma), and at high volumes in proximal airways or extrathoracic obstruction (e.g. trachea).

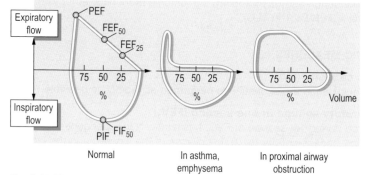

Fig. 5.10 Flow volume loops.
PEF = peak expiratory flow, PIF = peak inspiratory flow, FEF = forced expiratory flow, FIF = forced inspiratory flow.

Minute ventilation (or minute volume)

This is the volume of gas expired per minute
= Tidal volume × respirations/min = 500 × 12 = 6 l/min at rest.
May increase 20–30-fold on exercise.

Alveolar ventilation

This equals the minute ventilation minus the ventilation of the dead space, i.e. it represents the part of the minute ventilation that reaches the gas exchanging part of the airways. Approximately 5.25 l/min.

Dead space ventilation

Anatomical (150 ml)
Portion of tidal volume that remains in the non-exchanging parts of the airways, e.g. mouth, pharynx, trachea and bronchi up to terminal bronchioles.

Physiological
Identical to anatomical dead space in health. May be measured using the Bohr equation. In disease, physiological dead space may exceed anatomical dead space due to disorders of ventilation/perfusion mismatch.

PULMONARY DYNAMICS

WORK OF BREATHING

1. Elastic resistance: reciprocal of compliance. Elastic recoil of lungs and thorax due to tissue elasticity and surface tension, due to the presence of pulmonary surfactant, in the lung alveoli.
   In patients with restrictive lung disease, low compliance must overcome large elastic forces during inspiration.
2. Non-elastic resistance: airways resistance (see below) and tissue resistance of lungs and thorax.

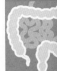

> **Pulmonary surfactant**
> A lecithin-based material which decreases the surface tension at low lung volumes, so increasing compliance. At high lung volumes it increases surface tension, decreasing compliance and facilitating expiration. Surfactant prevents alveolar collapse at end-expiratory alveolar pressures that would otherwise lead to atelectasis.

COMPLIANCE

- Change in volume produced by a unit change of pressure difference across the lungs. It is an index of lung distensibility.
- Normal value = 0.2 l/cmH$_2$O. Measured with an oesophageal catheter, which provides an estimate of the change in pleural pressure that occurs during tidal breathing.
- Static compliance reflects the elastic recoil of the lungs and expansibility of the thoracic cage.
- Dynamic compliance (i.e. compliance during respiration) is influenced by airways obstruction. Compliance is greater for expiration than inspiration due to the viscous properties of the lungs.
- Compliance is non-linear. It is greatest at mid-lung volumes and decreases at its extremes.
- *Hysteresis* is the variation of pressure depending on volume.

Causes of decreased compliance
Pulmonary oedema, interstitial fibrosis, pneumonectomy and kyphosis.

Causes of increased compliance
Emphysema and age.

AIRWAYS RESISTANCE (Raw)

- Equals the transairway pressure gradient divided by the flow rate.
- Factors which affect Raw:
  1. Flow rate and airway radius: Raw depends largely on the small peripheral airways (20%).
  2. Lung volume: increases in lung volume cause a reduction in airway resistance by dilatation of the airways.
  3. Phase of respiration: resistance greater on expiration than inspiration (hence expiratory wheeze in asthma).
  4. Autonomic effects: increased sympathetic activity results in bronchodilation; increased parasympathetic activity results in bronchoconstriction.
  5. Elastic recoil: decreased elastic recoil seen in the elderly and in patients with emphysema.
  6. Local Pco$_2$: a decrease in Pco$_2$ in expired air causes local bronchoconstriction: this mechanism is important in adjusting regional balance between ventilation and perfusion in the lungs.

Causes of increased Raw
Include chronic bronchitis, emphysema, upper airways obstruction.

INTRAPLEURAL PRESSURE
(Quiet ventilation)

- Equals the pressure in the pleural space minus the barometric pressure. Pleural pressure is less negative at the base than at the apex.
- Varies from –4 cmH$_2$O in inspiration to 1 cmH$_2$O in expiration.

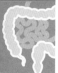

RESPIRATORY CYCLE

During inspiration, the pressure gradient from the extrathoracic to the intrathoracic veins increases and right ventricular filling and output increases. However, pulmonary venous return is decreased by the reduction in intrathoracic pressure. This produces a decrease in left ventricular stroke volume and cardiac output.

PULMONARY GAS EXCHANGE AND BLOOD GAS TRANSPORT
(see p. 273)

PARTIAL PRESSURES OF GASES IN RESPIRATION (Fig. 5.11)

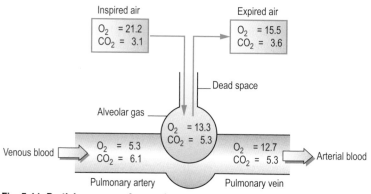

Fig. 5.11 Partial pressure of gases in respiration (kPa).

BLOOD–GAS BARRIER

Consists of:
1. Layer of pulmonary surfactant
2. Alveolar epithelium
3. Epithelium basement membrane
4. Interstitium
5. Endothelium basement membrane
6. Capillary endothelium
7. Plasma
8. Red cell membrane
9. Intracellular fluid.

DIFFUSING CAPACITY OF THE LUNG OR TRANSFER FACTOR
(T_{CO} measured in mmol/min/kPa)

- The rate at which a gas will diffuse from the alveoli into the blood.
- It is influenced by the rate of diffusion through three barriers:
  1. Alveolar–capillary wall, major determinant
  2. Plasma
  3. Cytoplasm of the erythrocyte.

- Carbon monoxide is the only gas that is used to measure the diffusing capacity, where T_{co} normally measures 25–30 ml CO/min/mmHg. The diffusing capacity for carbon dioxide is about 20-fold this value, because of greater solubility in tissue fluids.

Causes of $\downarrow T_{co}$
1. Diffuse infiltration
2. Pulmonary fibrosi
3. Pneumonia
4. Pulmonary hypertension
5. Multiple pulmonary emboli
6. Low cardiac output
7. Anaemia
8. Emphysema.

Causes of $\uparrow T_{co}$
1. Asthma/bronchitis
2. Alveolar bleeding
3. Hyperkinetic states
4. Left to right shunts
5. Polycythaemia
6. Exercise.

THE ALVEOLAR – ARTERIAL OXYGEN DIFFERENCE ($P(A - A)o_2$)

- The difference between the partial pressure of oxygen in the alveoli and the arterial partial pressure of oxygen.
- It is the best single indicator of the gas-exchange properties of the respiratory system, and is increased by any process that interferes with the diffusion of gas across the alveolar–capillary barrier, such as interstitial lung disease. It can be used to follow the progress of lung disease; an increasing gradient indicates a deterioration in lung disease.

- The mean alveolar Po_2 (PAo_2) is calculated using the alveolar gas equation.

  $$PAo_2 = Pio_2 - (Paco_2/R) + F$$ It normally varies between 0.7 and 1.0.

  where Pio_2 = the partial pressure of inspired O_2,
  $Paco_2$ = the partial pressure of arterial CO_2,
  R = the respiratory quotient (the ratio of CO_2 production and O_2 consumption),
  F = a correction factor.
  Pao_2 is obtained from arterial blood gas analysis.

- The $P(A - a)o_2$ should normally not exceed 15–20 mmHg. This difference is due to physiological shunts such as the bronchial and coronary circulations and to V–Q inequalities (see below), which exist in the lung as a function of gravity.

PULMONARY CIRCULATION

Mean pulmonary arterial pressure is 12–15 mmHg, and left atrial pressure is normally about 5 mmHg. Therefore the pressure gradient across the pulmonary circulation is 7–10 mmHg. The vascular resistance of the lung is approximately one-tenth that of the systemic circulation.

VENTILATION/PERFUSION RATIO (V/Q)

- Important in determining alveolar gas exchange.
  V   = volume of air entering alveoli = 4 l/min
  Q   = blood flow through lungs = 5 l/min
  V/Q = 0.8.
- The distribution of ventilation is determined by the pleural pressure gradient and airway closure. In erect subjects, ventilation increases *slowly* from lung apex to base (due to the diaphragm pulling the alveoli open at the bases).
- Pulmonary blood flow (perfusion) varies in different parts of the lungs because of the low pressure head, the distensibility of the vessels, and the hydrostatic effects of gravity. Perfusion increases *rapidly* from lung apex to base (mainly due to the effect of gravity).
Therefore, V/Q ratio falls from 3.3 at apex to 0.63 at base.

Causes of V/Q imbalance

- A *low* V/Q ratio indicates right to left shunting of deoxygenated blood, i.e. wasted perfusion.
- A *high* V/Q ratio indicates a large physiological dead space, i.e. wasted ventilation and is associated with CO_2 retention and a high arterial P_{CO_2}. Examples include hyaline membrane disease of the newborn, pneumothorax, bronchopneumonia and pulmonary oedema.
- Blockage of both ventilation and perfusion to one portion of a lung would maintain a constant V/Q ratio, e.g. surgical removal of a lung or a portion of a lung.

CONTROL OF BREATHING

- Coordinated activity between
  1. Central regulatory centres
  2. Central and peripheral chemoreceptors
  3. Pulmonary receptors and the respiratory muscles.
- *P_{CO_2}* is the most important variable in the regulation of ventilation, through its effect on pH. Maximal increase in CO_2 can increase alveolar ventilation 10-fold.
- *P_{O_2} and [H⁺]* play a less important role. Maximal increase in [H⁺] can increase ventilation 5-fold and maximal decrease in P_{O_2} can increase it by about one and two-thirds.
1. *Central regulatory centres* control rate and depth of respiration
   1. Medullary respiratory centre
   2. Apneustic centre (lower pons)
   3. Pneumotaxic centre (upper pons).
2. *Central chemoreceptors* respond to changes in [H⁺], i.e. an increase in [H⁺] in brain ECF stimulates ventilation.
   Peripheral chemoreceptors respond to changes in the P_{O_2}, P_{CO_2} and H⁺ concentrations of arterial blood. The carotid body chemoreceptors respond to decreases in arterial P_{O_2}, high P_{CO_2}, reduced flow and low pH. The aortic body chemoreceptors respond to increased level of P_{CO_2} and low P_{O_2}.
3. *Pulmonary receptors*
   1. Pulmonary stretch receptors are responsible for the Hering–Breuer reflex (distension of the lung results in a slowing of the respiratory rate) via the vagi. Vagotomy abolishes this reflex.
   2. Irritant receptors are stimulated by an increase in any noxious agent (e.g. histamine, bradykinin), resulting in bronchoconstriction.

3. J (juxtacapillary) receptors are stimulated by stretching of the pulmonary microvasculature.

RESPONSE TO CHRONIC HYPOXIA

For example, acclimatization to high altitude.
At high altitude (>3000 m), the partial pressure of O_2 in inspired air is reduced.
Acute and chronic adaptation to hypoxia occur.

Acute adaptation
- Increased minute ventilation (in response to hypoxia and raised CO_2 levels) by about 65%, which reduces the CO_2 level and causes an alkalosis. This is slowly corrected by renal excretion of HCO_3^-.
- Increased cardiac output and heart rate which returns to normal after two weeks at high altitude.
- Hypocapnia.
- Increased red cell 2,3,diphosphoglycerate (2,3,DPG) production stimulated by hypoxia. Causes decreased oxygen affinity for haemoglobin which facilitates O_2 release to the tissues, i.e. oxygen dissociation curve shifted to the right.

Chronic adaptation
- Further increase in ventilation by about 400%.
- Polycythaemia: erythropoietin production stimulated by hypoxia, with an increase in haemoglobin concentration and haematocrit (from 40–45% to 60–65%).
- Circulatory blood volume increases by up to 50–90%.
- Pulmonary hypertension due to pulmonary vasoconstriction caused by chronic hypoxia.

CARDIAC PHYSIOLOGY

CONDUCTING SYSTEM OF THE HEART

VENTRICULAR MUSCLE

- The resting membrane potential of cardiac cells is about –90 mV, which is maintained by movement of ions through specific ion channels in the membranes.
- A typical action potential may be divided into 5 phases (Fig. 5.12):
  Phase 0: Membrane depolarization: rapid increase in permeability to sodium.
  Phase 1: Rapid repolarization: rapid decrease in permeability to sodium, small increase in permeability to potassium.

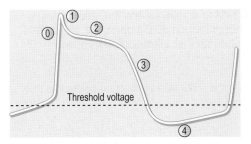
Threshold voltage

Fig. 5.12 The action potential in a Purkinje fibre.

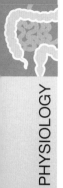

Phase 2: Slow repolarization: plateau effect due to: (i) absence of large rapid increase in permeability to K⁺; (ii) increase in Ca²⁺ permeability. Unique feature of cardiac action potential.

Phase 3: Rapid repolarization: gradual increase in potassium permeability and inactivation of slow inward Ca²⁺ channels.

Phase 4: Slow depolarization: resting potential is restored and Na⁺ and K⁺ concentrations are restored by exchange pumps.

PACEMAKER CELLS

For example, sinoatrial node.
- Slow upstroke action potential, mediated by calcium channels.
- Smaller magnitude of action potential.
- No fast sodium channels.
- Spontaneously depolarizes during diastole (phase 4 depolarization).

CARDIAC CYCLE

A cardiac cycle showing the relationship between left ventricular pressure, heart sounds, venous pulse and ECG is shown in Figure 5.13.

PHASES OF THE CARDIAC CYCLE

1. **Atrial contraction**
   The pressure in the ventricles at the end of atrial contraction is termed the ventricular end-diastolic pressure and sets the preload for the next ventricular contraction.
2. **Isovolumetric contraction**
   Pressure in the ventricular cavities rises due to the onset of ventricular contraction. This reverses the pressure gradient across the atrioventricular (AV) valves and causes closure of the AV valve. Following closure, the ventricular volume remains constant until the ventricular pressure exceeds that in the arteries, when ventricular ejection begins.
3. **Rapid ejection**
   Almost 70% of the stroke volume is ejected in the first third of systole.
4. **Reduced ejection**
   During the latter two-thirds of systole, the ejection rate declines with the ventricular and arterial pressures.
5. **Isovolumetric relaxation**
   This phase extends from the closure of the semilunar valves and ends as ventricular pressure falls below atrial pressure and the AV valves reopen.
6. **Rapid ventricular filling**
   During ventricular systole, venous filling continues and the atrial pressure reaches its peak just as the AV valves reopen. Once open, the pressure in both the atrial and ventricular cavities falls as ventricular relaxation continues.
7. **Reduced ventricular filling**
   During the later stages of diastole, the atrial and ventricular pressures rise slowly as blood returns to the heart.

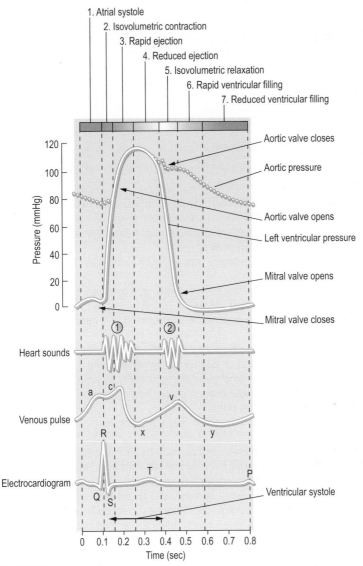

1. Atrial systole
2. Isovolumetric contraction
3. Rapid ejection
4. Reduced ejection
5. Isovolumetric relaxation
6. Rapid ventricular filling
7. Reduced ventricular filling

Aortic valve closes
Aortic pressure
Aortic valve opens
Left ventricular pressure
Mitral valve opens
Mitral valve closes

Heart sounds

Venous pulse

Electrocardiogram

Ventricular systole

Fig. 5.13 Cardiac cycle.

INTRACARDIAC PRESSURES (Table 5.4)

Table 5.4 Normal intracardiac pressures and oxygen saturation		
Chamber	Pressure (mmHg)	Oxygen saturation (%)
Right atrium	3	
Right ventricle	20/4	
Pulmonary artery	20/12	65–75
	15 (mean)	
Pulmonary capillary wedge	8 (mean)	
Left atrium	8	
Left ventricle	150/8	96–98
Aorta	130/75	
	100 (mean)	

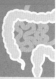

PHYSIOLOGY

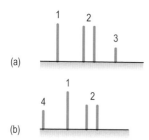

(a)

(b)

Fig. 5.14 a, Third and b, fourth heart sounds.

HEART SOUNDS (Fig. 5.14)

1. *First heart sound* is due to closure of the AV (mitral and tricuspid) valves. **Louder** sound if PR interval is abnormally long or short, as valve leaflets close from a more widely separated position, e.g. mitral stenosis, hyperdynamic circulation, tachycardia.
   Softer sound in mitral incompetence and severe heart failure. Normally split in tricuspid area on inspiration.
2. *Second heart sound* is high in frequency and is due to closure of the semilunar (aortic and pulmonary) valves.
   Physiological splitting of the second heart sound (A_2–P_2 interval; see Box below).
   Fixed splitting occurs due to pressure or volume load on the right ventricle such as in an atrioseptal defect or pulmonary hypertension.
   Paradoxical splitting occurs whenever left ventricular systole is delayed or prolonged, such as in left bundle branch block, aortic stenosis and occasionally systemic hypertension.
   Loud in systemic hypertension (in aortic area), pulmonary hypertension (pulmonary area).
   Soft in aortic stenosis (aortic area) and pulmonary stenosis (pulmonary area).
3. *Third heart sound* is due to rapid filling of the left ventricle. Best heard in children e.g. ventricular failure, constrictive pericarditis, mitral or tricuspid incompetence. Heard at apex early in diastole (Fig. 5.14a).
4. *Fourth heart sound* is due to ventricular distension caused by a forceful atrial contraction e.g. hypertension, heart block, myocardial infarction. Heard at apex early in diastole (Fig. 5.14b). Not heard in normal individuals.

Effect of respiration on murmurs
- During expiration the A_2–P_2 interval is about 0.02 seconds, and during inspiration about 0.05 seconds. This is because during inspiration the ventricular ejection period is prolonged due to increased stroke volume secondary to increased venous return.
- Respiration increases stroke volume of right ventricle and therefore increases the intensity of tricuspid stenosis, pulmonary stenosis and tricuspid incompetence.
- Respiration increases vascular volume of lungs and decreases stroke volume of left ventricle, therefore decreasing intensity of murmurs of mitral stenosis and incompetence, and aortic stenosis and incompetence.

Effect of drugs on murmurs
Vasodilators will decrease arteriolar resistance and increase systolic ejection murmurs and regurgitant murmurs at all valves. Drugs increasing arteriolar resistance will have the opposite effect.

ECG intervals (Table 5.5)

ECG intervals	Time (sec)	Event
		Table 5.5 ECG intervals (see also Fig. 5.13)
PR interval	0.12–0.2	Atrial depolarization and conduction through AV node
ORS duration	0.08–0.1	Ventricular depolarization
QT interval	0.4–0.43	Ventricular depolarization plus ventricular repolarization

VENOUS PRESSURE CHANGES (see Fig. 5.13)

- **a wave**: due to atrial systole.
  Disappears in atrial fibrillation; cannon waves are present in complete heart block. Giant 'a' waves are present in pulmonary hypertension, severe pulmonary and tricuspid stenosis.
- **c wave**: due to bulging of the AV valve during ventricular contraction. Synchronous with the pulse wave in the carotid artery.
- **v wave**: due to rise in atrial pressure before the AV valve opens during diastole.
- **x descent**: due to drawing away of the AV valve from the atrium during ventricular systole.
- **y descent**: due to fall in atrial pressure as blood rushes into ventricle when the AV valve opens. Deep 'y' descent occurs with any condition causing a high jugular venous pressure (JVP), such as constrictive pericarditis. A slow 'y' descent is seen with tricuspid stenosis.

CARDIAC PERFORMANCE

VENTRICULAR END-DIASTOLIC VOLUME (VEDV)

- The volume of blood in the ventricular cavity just prior to the first heart sound, i.e. at the end of atrial contraction. The normal LVEDV is about 120 ml.
- Influenced by the ventricular filling pressure, compliance and heart rate.
  RV filling pressure = central venous pressure (CVP).
  LV filling pressure = pulmonary wedge pressure.

CENTRAL VENOUS PRESSURE

- Normal pressure = –2 cmH$_2$O to +12 cmH$_2$O.
- Varies with cardiac cycle, respiration and position of patient.

Causes of ↓ CVP
Non-cardiogenic shock.

Causes of ↑ CVP
Heart failure
Positive end-expiratory pressure ventilation and Valsalva manoeuvre impedes venous return
Expansion of blood volume.

VENTRICULAR END-SYSTOLIC VOLUME

- The volume of blood remaining in the ventricle at the end of ejection.
- The normal left ventricular end-systolic volume is 40 ml.

STROKE VOLUME (SV)

- The volume of blood ejected with each beat.
- Equal to the difference between the ventricular end-diastolic and end-systolic volumes.
- Approximately 70–80 ml.

EJECTION FRACTION

- Ratio of stroke volume to end diastolic volume (SV/EDV)
- Normal range 50–70%
- Useful index of overall left ventricular function (measured by gated blood pool scanning and 2-D echocardiography)
- Stroke volume and ejection fraction increase with contractility.

CARDIAC OUTPUT (CO)

- Volume of blood expelled from one side of the heart per minute.
- Determined by the heart rate (HR) and stroke volume (SV).

$$CO = HR \times SV$$
$$= \frac{72 \times 70 \text{ ml}}{1000}$$
$$= 5 \text{ l/min in average resting man; 20\% less in women.}$$

- May increase 4–5 times on strenuous exertion. Varies with body surface area.
- The cardiac index is the cardiac output per square metre of body surface and averages about 3.2 l.

Measurement of cardiac output

Techniques used:

1. *Fick method*
   Principle:
   Amount of oxygen delivered to the tissues must equal the oxygen uptake by the lungs, plus the oxygen delivered to the lungs in the pulmonary artery.

$$CO = \frac{\text{oxygen consumption rate by the body (ml/min)}}{\text{arterial oxygen content} - \text{venous oxygen content}}$$
$$= \frac{250 \text{ ml } O_2/\text{min}}{190 \text{ ml } O_2/\text{l blood} - 140 \text{ ml } O_2/\text{l blood}}$$
$$= 5 \text{ l/min}$$

2. *Dye dilution*
   Principle:
   If a known amount of indicator dye is mixed into an unknown volume of blood, and its concentration is measured, the volume of blood can be calculated from the factor by which the indicator has been diluted. The flow of blood can be measured if the mean concentration of the indicator is determined for the time required for that indicator to pass a given site.

3. *Thermodilution*
   Principle:
   Cold saline injected at the proximal end of a catheter in the right ventricle, mixes with blood in the right ventricle and the temperature change is measured by a distal thermistor downstream in the pulmonary artery.

Factors modifying cardiac output

- Heart rate
  1. Intrinsic rhythmicity
  2. Extrinsic factors: e.g. autonomic nervous system.
- Stroke volume
  1. Contractility
  2. Preload (venous pressure)
  3. Afterload (arterial blood pressure).

1. Contractility

The force which the heart muscle generates as it contracts. Influenced by inotropic factors.

Causes of an **increase** *in contractility*, i.e. positive inotropic factors:
1. Sympathetic nerve stimulation and catecholamines
2. Increase in extracellular $[Ca^+]$
3. Decrease in extracellular $[Na^+]$
4. Drugs, e.g. digoxin, glucagon, L-thyroxine.

Causes of a **decrease** *in contractility*, i.e. negative inotropic factors:
1. Drugs, e.g. β-blockers, anaesthetic agents, antiarrhythmic drugs
2. Heart failure
3. Hypoxia, hypercapnia and acidosis.

2. Preload (central venous pressure)

- The ventricular end diastolic volume (LVEDV) or pressure.
- Determined by
  (i)   Blood volume
  (ii) Venous tone
  (iii) Gravity
  (iv) Respiratory and muscle pumps.

Frank–Starling law (Fig. 5.15)   ✓
- The relationship between the preload (left ventricular end-diastolic volume) and stroke volume is described by the *Frank–Starling law*, which states that the force developed in a muscle fibre depends on the degree to which the fibre is stretched.
- Applied to cardiac dynamics, the initial fibre length is equivalent to the left ventricular end-diastolic volume (LVEDV).

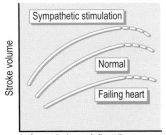

Fig. 5.15 **Frank–Starling law.**

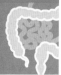

– In congestive heart failure, the set point for cardiac output is reduced and stroke volume cardiac output falls. Positive inotropic agents increase cardiac output.
– The LVEDV increases with venous return. Exercise, overtransfusion and sympathetic venoconstriction increase venous return, while haemorrhage, diuretics and venodilatation decrease venous return.
– The LVEDV fails to increase normally with decreasing contractility.

3. Afterload (arterial blood pressure)
- Determined by cardiac output and total peripheral resistance.
- Tension or force in the ventricular wall during ventricular ejection.
- Total peripheral resistance determined by:
  1. Aortic pressure
  2. Aortic valve resistance
  3. Ventricular cavity size.
- At constant preload and contractility, the stroke volume is inversely related to the afterload, i.e. decreasing the peripheral resistance with a vasodilator increases the stroke volume.

BLOOD PRESSURE

- BP = cardiac output × peripheral resistance
- Pulse pressure = systolic pressure – diastolic pressure
- Mean arterial pressure = diastolic pressure + 1/3rd of the pulse pressure.

Control
1. Autonomic nervous system via baroreceptors in aortic arch via vagus and carotid sinus and medullary and hypothalamic cardiorespiratory centres.
2. Renin–angiotensin system.

Main determinants of blood pressure
1. *Heart rate:* increase in heart rate increases arterial pressure by reducing time for diastolic run-off to the periphery. This increases the mean arterial volume and so the diastolic blood pressure.
2. *Peripheral resistance:* an increase in peripheral resistance raises the diastolic arterial volume by reducing peripheral run-off.
3. *Stroke volume:* an increase in stroke volume at a constant heart rate increases mean arterial volume and pressure and pulse pressure.
4. *Aortic elasticity:* an increase produces a greater pulse pressure ($\uparrow$ in systolic and $\downarrow$ in diastolic pressures).

PERIPHERAL RESISTANCE (PR)

- Resistance to flow of blood through arterioles.

$$PR = \frac{\text{mean arterial pressure}}{\text{cardiac output}}$$
$$= \frac{100}{5 \text{ l/min}}$$
$$= 20 \text{ mmHg/l/min}$$

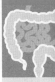

- *Control* of peripheral resistance is exerted by controlling vessel calibre. Arteriolar vasoconstriction causes an increase in peripheral resistance. Venous vasoconstriction causes an increase in stroke volume and cardiac output.
- Regulation of vascular tone involves both perivascular nerves at adventitial-medial border and endothelium. New chemical messengers identified include nitric oxide, monoamines and polypeptides.

Factors affecting the calibre of the arterioles and vascular tone ✓

Constriction
1. Increased sympathetic activity
2. Circulating catecholamines
3. Circulating angiotensin II
4. Locally released serotonin
5. Decreased local temperature
6. Endothelium-dependent vasoconstriction (in response to mechanical and chemical stress, e.g. hypoxia, stretch, extracellular K^+). Calcium channels open raising intracellular Ca^{2+}, leading to release of vasocontrictors such as endothelin-1

Dilatation
1. Decreased sympathetic activity
2. Increased Pco_2, decreased pH and Po_2 Lactic acid, histamine and prostaglandins
3. Increased local temperature
4. Endothelium-dependent vasodilatation (in response to ACh, ATP, ADP, substance P, 5-HT)
5. Endothelium-derived relaxing factors (found in nerve fibres around cerebral, mesenteric and skin vessels). Can produce endothelium dependent and independent vasodilatation

---

THE CIRCULATION

Table 5.6 Distribution of blood volume

Vessel	Function	% distribution of total blood volume
Artery	} Damping/resistance	12
Arteriole		
Capillary	} Exchange	7
Venule		
Vein	} Capacitance	64
Venous sinuses		
Pulmonary circulation		9

CIRCULATION THROUGH SPECIAL AREAS

Cerebral circulation
- Cerebral blood flow = 0.75 l/min.

- Depends on:
    1. Perfusion pressure (i.e. the arterial–venous pressure difference at the brain level)
    2. Cerebral vascular resistance, which is a function of intracranial pressure, the calibre of cerebral arterioles and blood viscosity. The vascular diameter is regulated by local factors, e.g. a local increase in Pco_2 or a local decrease in Po_2 or pH causes vasodilatation.

- Considerable degree of autoregulation to maintain an overall constant cerebral blood flow. Cerebral blood flow is not reduced until BP falls to <60 mmHg or exceeds 150 mmHg.

The *Cushing reflex* is a systemic vasoconstriction in response to an increase in the systemic blood pressure and CSF pressure, in order to maintain blood flow to the brain.

Coronary circulation

• Coronary blood flow = 200 ml/min at rest.

• Depends on:
  1. Pressure in the aorta
  2. Length of diastole.

• In the left ventricle, ventricular pressure is slightly greater than aortic pressure during systole, but much less than the aortic pressure during diastole. Therefore coronary flow to the left ventricle only occurs during diastole.
• In the right ventricle and atria, aortic pressure is greater than right ventricular and atrial pressure during systole and diastole, therefore coronary flow to these parts continues throughout the cardiac cycle.
• Oxygen consumption = 7.9 ml/min/100 g.

CIRCULATORY ADAPTATIONS

1. **Postural changes from supine to upright position:**
   • ↓ venous return and ↓ CVP → ↓ stroke volume → ↓ cardiac output → ↓ BP.
   • Compensatory ↑ heart rate and ↑ peripheral resistance. (Heart rate decreases on reversal of movement.)
2. **Severe haemorrhage:**
   • ↓ BP → vasoconstriction → ↓ in renal blood flow.
   • ↑ heart rate (4-fold) → ↑ stroke volume (1.5-fold) and ↑ cardiac output.
3. **Exercise**
   • ↑ heart rate (4-fold) and stroke volume (2-fold).
   • ↑ cardiac output (up to 30 l/min) which is redistributed to working muscles.
   • ↑ O_2 consumption (up to 20-fold) in blood to skeletal muscles and coronary circulation.
   • Peripheral vasoconstriction → ↑ systemic arterial pressure.
   • Pulmonary vessel dilatation → ↓ pulmonary vascular resistance.
4. **Altitude** (see p. 209).
5. **Valsalva manoeuvre** (or positive end-expiratory pressure):
   • Increase in intrapulmonary and intrathoracic pressures, so that venous return impeded (Fig. 5.16).
   • ↓ heart rate, stroke volume and BP.
   • On release – ↑ in peripheral volume → overshoot of BP and ↓ HR.

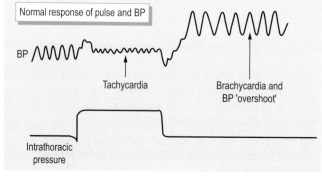

Normal response of pulse and BP

BP

Tachycardia

Brachycardia and BP 'overshoot'

Intrathoracic pressure

Fig. 5.16 Valsalva manoeuvre.

GASTROINTESTINAL POLYPEPTIDE HORMONES (Table 5.7)

Table 5.7 Principal gastrointestinal polypeptide hormones

Hormone and location	Stimulus for release	Actions
Gastrin G cells in gastric antrum	1. Amino acids in antrum 2. Distension of antrum by food 3. Vagal action Inhibited by pH <1.5	1. Stimulates gastric acid, pepsin and intrinsic factor secretion 2. Stimulates gastric emptying 3. Stimulates pancreatic bicarbonate secretion and secretin
Secretin Duodenum and jejunum	1. Intraluminal acid (vagus has no direct action on secretin secretion)	1. Stimulates pancreatic bicarbonate secretion 2. Inhibits gastric acid and pepsin secretion 3. Delays gastric emptying
Cholecystokinin-pancreozymin (CCK-PZ) Duodenum and jejunum	1. Intraluminal fat, amino acids, peptides and certain cations, e.g. Ca^{2+} and Mg^{2+}	1. Stimulates pancreatic enzyme and bicarbonate secretion 2. Stimulates gall bladder contraction (and relaxation of the sphincter of Oddi) 3. Inhibition of gastric emptying and motility of the small intestine
Gastric inhibitory peptide (GIP) Duodenum and jejunum		1. Inhibits gastric acid secretion and motility 2. Stimulates postprandial insulin secretion
Motilin Duodenum and jejunum		1. Stimulates gastric and intestinal motility
Pancreatic polypeptide (PP)* Pancreas		1. Inhibits pancreatic enzyme secretion 2. Relaxes gall bladder
Vasoactive intestinal peptide (VIP)* Small intestine		1. Inhibits gastric acid and pepsin secretion 2. Stimulates pancreatic and intestinal secretion

* Neurocrine system: VIP, substance P and endorphins.

STOMACH

GASTRIC SECRETION

- Approximately 3 l/day
  1. Parietal (oxyntic) cells produce hydrochloric acid, Na^+, Ca^{2+}, Mg^{2+} and intrinsic factor
  2. Surface mucosal cells produce mucus and bicarbonate
  3. Chief (peptic) cells secrete pepsinogen, the inactive precursor of pepsin.

Control of gastric secretion

Stimulation of gastric acid secretion
1. Neural: vagal stimulation increases both pepsin and acid output directly, as well as indirectly by causing secretion of gastrin. Vagotomy reduces basal acid secretion, and secretion in response to histamine or pentagastrin.
2. Hormonal: gastrin.

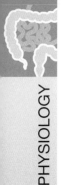

3. Histamine: via interaction with H_2 receptors on oxyntic cells. Blockage of histamine H_2 receptors by drugs such as cimetidine inhibits both the gastrin-induced and vagally mediated acid secretion.

All of these mechanisms act ultimately via the 'proton pump'.

Inhibition of gastric acid secretion
1. Higher centres, e.g. nausea, and fear through activation of the sympathetic nervous system.
2. Low gastric juice pH.
3. Small intestinal peptides, e.g. cholecystokinin-pancreozymin (CCK-PZ), secretin, and gastric inhibitory peptide (GIP).
4. Drugs blocking acetylcholine receptors, histamine H_2 receptors and the proton pump.

Gastric emptying (Table 5.8)

Table 5.8 Factors affecting gastric emptying	
Increased	*Reduced*
Distension of stomach and antrum	Fatty acids
Gastrin	Hyperosmolar solution (e.g. amino acids and polypeptides)
Cold	Acid in duodenum
Emotion	Secretin, CCK-PZ
	Heat and emotion

PANCREAS

PANCREATIC SECRETION

- Alkaline fluid (pH 8.0) containing electrolytes and digestive enzymes in the form of their proenzymes.
- 1200–1500 ml/day.
- Neutralizes gastric juice together with bile and duodenal juice and so creates the optimal pH for intestinal enzymes.
- Acinar cells produce a secretion rich in enzymes and electrolytes for the digestion of carbohydrates, proteins, fats and nucleic acids.
- The principal enzymes are: maltase, amylase, lipases, nucleases; and the proenzymes are trypsinogen, chymotrypsinogens, proaminopeptidase and procarboxypeptidases.
- Ductule cells produce water and electrolytes.

Control of pancreatic juice secretion
1. Gastric: food in the stomach stimulates the vagus, resulting in gastrin and acid release. Gastrin stimulates enzyme secretion by the acinar cells.
2. Intestinal: peptides, amino acids, fatty acids and H^+ in the duodenum cause release of:
   (i) Secretin, which stimulates a secretion, rich in bicarbonate, by the acinar cells.
   (ii) Cholecystokinin–pancreozymin (CCK-PZ), which stimulates the acinar cells to increase enzyme secretion.

BILIARY SYSTEM

- 250–1100 ml of bile are secreted daily by the liver. Bile is stored in the gall bladder and released into the duodenum through contraction of the gall bladder stimulated by CCK.

Composition of bile

Bile acids	Bile pigments (bilirubin and biliverdin)
Phospholipids	Protein.
Cholesterol	

✓

Bile acids

- *Primary bile acids*: Cholic acid and chenodeoxycholic acid. Formed in the liver from cholesterol by the addition of hydroxyl and carboxyl groups.
- *Secondary bile acids*: Deoxycholic acid and lithocholic acids. Formed from the primary bile salts through the action of intestinal bacterial enzymes.

Functions of bile acids
1. Solubilize cholesterol by incorporation into micelles.
2. Aid emulsification of fats with phospholipids and fatty acids.
3. Aid absorption of fat-soluble vitamins.
4. Stimulate pancreatic secretion by releasing CCK-PZ.

HAEM AND BILIRUBIN CATABOLISM

- Worn out red blood cells are phagocytosed by reticuloendothelial cells in the spleen. The free haemoglobin released is bound to haptoglobin. This complex is transported in the bloodstream to the liver where hepatic reticuloendothelial cells split off the haemoglobin portion, converting it to its haem and globin moeties.
- The globin is hydrolysed into its component amino acids, which are added to the hepatic pool for reuse.
- Bilirubin is formed from the catabolism of the haem moeity and is transported to the liver bound to albumin. The iron released from haem in this process is stored in the liver for reuse.
- Bilirubin is conjugated with glucuronic acid catalysed by glucuronyl transferase to form water-soluble bilirubin diglucuronide which is excreted in bile. Bacterial metabolism of bilirubin in the bowel leads to the formation of urobilinogen, some of which undergoes an enterohepatic circulation and may be found in the urine.

Enterohepatic circulation (EHC)

In the intestine, both primary and secondary bile acids are deconjugated, reabsorbed in the terminal ileum and returned to the liver by the portal vein bound to serum albumin, where they are excreted. Recirculation occurs about six times a day. EHC may be interrupted by:
1. Drugs: chelating agents, e.g. cholestyramine
2. Ileal disease causing impaired reabsorption
3. Bacterial overgrowth causing increased deconjugation.

Control of biliary secretion

1. Neural: parasympathetic stimulation increases bile secretion; sympathetic stimulation decreases bile secretion.
2. Hormonal: gastrin and secretin increase the volume and bicarbonate concentration of bile. CCK increases bile output.

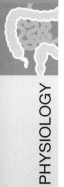

Bile pigment changes with disease (Table 5.9)

Table 5.9 Summary of urinary and faecal bile pigment changes			
	Obstructive	Hepatocellular failure with no obstruction	Haemolytic
Urinary bilirubin	↑	Normal or ↑	None
Urinary urobilinogen	↓	Normal or ↑	↑
Faecal stercobilinogen	↓	Normal	↑

SMALL INTESTINE

Digestive enzymes (Table 5.10)

Table 5.10 Digestive enzymes and products		
Digestive enzymes	Substrate	Products
Several peptidases	Polypeptides	Peptides
Amylase	Starch	Glucose, maltose and maltotriose
Lactase	Lactose	Glucose and galactose
Sucrase	Sucrose	Glucose and fructose
Maltase	Maltose	Glucose
Isomaltose	Isomaltose	Maltose and glucose
Lipases	Fats	Free fatty acids and monoglycerides
Enterokinase	Trypsinogen	Trypsin

INTESTINAL SECRETION

Approximately 2 l/day
1. Brünner's glands produce an alkaline secretion (with mucus).
2. Paneth cells at the base of the crypts of Lieberkühn produce a watery secretion.
3. Villus enterocytes (columnar cells) secrete digestive enzymes, and this is the principal site of absorption.

Control of secretion

Stimulation of secretion
1. Vagal stimulation
2. Intestinal hormones, especially CCK-PZ and secretin
3. Brünner's glands are inhibited by sympathetic stimulation.

Disorders of secretion

Causes of increased gastrin levels
1. Gastrinoma, antral G-cell hyperplasia
2. Retained and isolated antrum
3. Zollinger–Ellison syndrome with intractable peptic ulcers and high gastric acid
4. Vagotomy
5. Achlorhydria, e.g. pernicious anaemia and gastric ulcer
6. Short bowel syndrome
7. Renal failure
8. H_2 blockers and omeprazole.

Causes of decreased gastrin levels
1. Fasting states
2. Diseases causing hyperacidity, e.g. duodenal ulcer.

Causes of high VIP levels
VIPoma, resulting in the Werner–Morrison syndrome or WDHA syndrome (**W**atery **D**iarrhoea, **H**ypokalaemia and **A**chlorhydria).

Causes of high glucagon level
Glucagonoma (tumour of A cells in pancreatic islets) resulting in a necrolytic migratory erythema, diabetes, weight loss, anaemia and stomatitis.

Causes of a high somatostatin level
Somatostatinoma (flush, diabetes and hypochlorhydria).

SMALL INTESTINE MOTILITY (Table 5.11)

Table 5.11 Factors affecting small intestine motility.	
Increased	*Decreased*
Parasympathetic activity	Sympathetic activity
Cholinergic agents	Adrenergic agents
Gastrin, CCK-PZ, motilin	Secretin
Prostaglandins	
Serotonin	

DIGESTION AND ABSORPTION IN THE SMALL INTESTINE (pp. 248, 257, 267)

- Mainly occurs in the duodenum and upper jejunum, e.g. sugars, amino acids, salts, folic acid, and vitamins B and C via a passive transport system (monosaccharides and amino acids require carrier protein).
- Fatty acids, monoglycerides, cholesterol and fat-soluble vitamins A, D, E and K are released from micelles and are passively absorbed across the cell membrane.
- Little absorption takes place in the ileum except vitamin B_{12} and bile salts.
- Movement of water across the gastrointestinal mucosa is by passive diffusion and follows the transport of osmotically active solutes, e.g. Na^+, glucose, chloride and amino acids.

COLON

Functions

1. Active absorption of Na^+ and Cl^- and passive absorption following the osmotic gradient established by Na^+ and Cl^- absorption.
2. Secretion of mucus, K^+, and HCO_3^-.

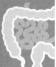

LARGE INTESTINE MOTILITY (Table 5.12)

Table 5.12 Factors affecting large intestine motility	
Increased	*Decreased*
Parasympathetic activity	Sympathetic activity
Cholinergic agents	Anticholinergic agents
Distension (gastrocolic reflex)	Inflammation
Emotion	Emotion
CCK-PZ	
Laxatives	

ENDOCRINE PHYSIOLOGY

CLASSIFICATION OF HORMONES (Table 5.13)

Table 5.13 Hormone classification		
Polypeptide	*Steroid*	*Amine*
Most hypothalamic hormones	Hormones of adrenal cortex,	Thyroid hormones
Hormones of anterior and posterior	gonads and fetoplacental unit	Catecholamines
pituitary		
Hormones of the pancreas and GI tract		
Growth factors		

MECHANISMS OF HORMONE ACTION

On cell membrane

1. Via cyclic adenosine 3′,5′-monophosphate (cAMP) as a 'second messenger', e.g. most polypeptide hormones (ACTH, ADH, TSH, LH, PTH and glucagon), many biogenic amines and some prostaglandins.
   - The first messenger is the hormone that binds to the membrane receptor and leads to the activation of the membrane-bound enzyme adenyl cyclase, which converts adenosine triphosphate to cyclic AMP (cAMP).
   - cAMP exerts biological activity via the phosphorylation of cAMP-dependent protein kinases, which can lead to the activation (e.g. via phosphorylase kinase, or phosphorylase) or the inactivation (e.g. via glycogen synthetase) of the substrate.
2. By membrane control of permeability (not via cyclic AMP). e.g. insulin-induced increased entry of glucose into cells. Other peptide hormones that may change membrane permeability include GH, ACTH, ADH and PTH.

In cytosol

Via a hormone–receptor complex, e.g. mainly steroid hormones, T3, T4 and somatomedin.

- Binding of free hormone to specific cytosol receptor proteins in target cells. The hormone–receptor complex then migrates to the nucleus, where the usual effect is to increase mRNA synthesis.

HYPOTHALAMIC REGULATORY HORMONES (Table 5.14)

- Neurons from the supraoptic and paraventricular nuclei of the hypothalamus send axons to the posterior pituitary (neurohypophysis) (Fig. 5.17).
- The portal hypophyseal vessels form a vascular connection between the median eminence of the ventral hypothalamus and the anterior pituitary.

Table 5.14 Hypothalamic regulatory hormones

Hypothalamic hormone	Pituitary hormone released
Releasing hormones	
Thyrotrophin-releasing hormone (TRH)	Thyroid-stimulating hormone (TSH) and prolactin Follicle-stimulating hormone (FSH) in men
Growth hormone-releasing hormone (GHRH)	Growth hormone (GH) Insulin, glucagon and gastrin release
Prolactin-releasing hormone (PRH)	Prolactin
Corticotrophin-releasing hormone (CRH)	ACTH
Gonadotrophin-releasing hormone (GnRH)	Luteinizing and follicle-stimulating hormone (LH and FSH)
Inhibiting hormones	*Suppresses release of*:
Prolactin-inhibiting factor or dopamine (PIF)	Prolactin, luteotrophin
Growth hormone-inhibiting hormone or somatostatin	GH, TSH, FSH

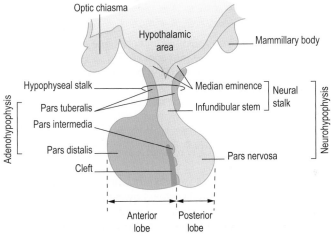

Fig. 5.17 Hypothalamo-pituitary anatomy.

ANTERIOR PITUITARY HORMONES

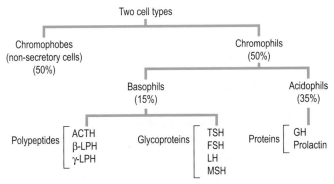

Fig. 5.18 Cells and hormones of the anterior pituitary.

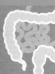

ADRENOCORTICOTROPHIC HORMONE (ACTH)

Structure (Fig. 5.19)

- Single-chain polypeptide (39 amino acids: first 24 essential for biological activity). ACTH, β-lipotrophin (β-LPH) and pro-γ-melanocyte-stimulating hormone (pro-γ-MSH) originate from a common precursor molecule, pro-opiocortin, which is synthesized in the hypothalamus and broken down in the anterior pituitary.

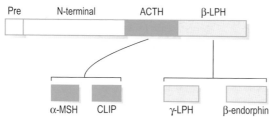

Fig. 5.19 ACTH and related peptides.

ACTH-related peptides

- These include β-LPH, γ-LPH, corticotrophin-like intermediate peptide (CLIP), endorphins (α β γ), met-enkephalin and leuenkephalin (Fig. 5.19).
- Endogenous opiates: endorphins and enkephalins bind to morphine (opiate) receptors. They have an analgesic action and possibly function in certain areas as synaptic transmitters. Their action can be blocked by morphine antagonists (e.g. naloxone).

Secretion

- Secretion controlled by hypothalamic CRH release, which is subject to negative feedback control from cortisol.
- Striking circadian rhythm in ACTH output by pituitary which in turn causes a diurnal secretion of cortisol by the adrenal cortex. Lowest levels occur at midnight and maximum levels at 8.00 a.m. Loss of rhythm occurs in Cushing's syndrome, depression, heart failure and stress.

Stimuli for release
Stress, e.g. hypoglycaemia, surgery, exercise, fever.

Actions

Acts via cAMP.
1. ↑ Secretion of cortisol by the adrenal cortex
2. ↑ Adrenal blood flow
3. ↑ Cholesterol concentration → cortisol
4. ↑ Protein synthesis in the adrenal cortex.

THYROID-STIMULATING HORMONE (TSH)

Structure

- Glycoprotein 209 amino acids and two subunits: α and β.
- α-Subunit common to LH, FSH and human chorionic gonadotrophin (HCG); β-subunit confers biological specificity and immunological properties.

Secretion

- Secreted in response to hypothalamic TRH, and subject to negative feedback that depends on plasma thyroid hormones (free T4 and T3) acting at hypothalamic and pituitary levels.
- Circadian rhythm.

Actions

1. Stimulates growth of the thyroid gland and increased iodine uptake.
2. Synthesis and release of T3 and T4 hormones.

LUTEINIZING HORMONE (LH) AND FOLLICLE-STIMULATING HORMONE (FSH)

Structure

- Glycoproteins and each consists of two subunits: α subunit is common to FSH, LH and TSH and β-subunit is hormone-specific.

Secretion (Fig. 5.20)

- Secreted in response to gonadotrophin-releasing hormone (GnRH), and subject to feedback control from both oestrogen and androgen effects.
- **FSH** is elevated in early proliferative (follicular) phase. A fall occurs preceding ovulation; with a further brief rise at ovulation. Levels fall again in secretory (luteal) phase.
- **LH**: pattern of secretion similar to FSH.
- **Both** peak at mid-ovulatory cycle. LH peak higher than FSH. Triggered by rise in plasma oestradiol.

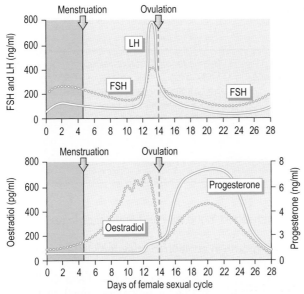

Fig. 5.20 Oestradiol, FSH and LH secretion.

High levels of FSH and LH in:	Low levels in:	
Postmenopausal women	Hypopituitarism.	
Primary gonadal failure		
Kleinfelter syndrome.		

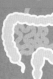

Actions

- **FSH** via FSH receptor on Sertoli cells
    1. Females: controls the development and maturation of the Graffian follicle.
    2. Males: influences growth of seminiferous tubules and spermatogenesis. Induces responsiveness to LH.
- **LH** via LH receptor on Leydig cells
    1. Females: controls development of corpus luteum and secretion of progesterone.
    2. Males: increases production of testosterone by the Leydig cells.

MELANOCYTE-STIMULATING HORMONE (γ-MSH)

Structure

- Pro-opiocortin contains three components with MSH activity, α-MSH (in ACTH component); β-MSH (in LPH component); α-MSH.
- Formed by enzyme degradation of pro-opiocortin and its ACTH and LPH components. Function unclear.

GROWTH HORMONE (GH, SOMATOTROPIN)

Structure

- Most abundant hormone in the pituitary.
- Structurally similar to prolactin and placental lactogen.

Secretion

- Under hypothalamic control through GHRF and GHRIF (somatostatin).
- Somatomedins exhibit negative feedback control of GH secretion.
- Basal secretion low during the day with increased secretion during the first few hours of sleep.

Stimuli for release	Stimuli for inhibition of release	
Stress (emotion, fever and surgery)	Fatty acids	
Vigorous exercise	Somatostatin	
Insulin-induced hypoglycaemia	Hyperglycaemia	
↑ Circulating amino acids,	↑ Cortisol.	
e.g. protein meal, arginine infusion		
Sleep		
Glucagon		
Bromocriptine.		

Somatomedins

- Family of small peptides synthesized in the liver and other sites in response to growth hormone.
- Responsible for overall body growth in addition to other growth factors which affect individual tissues or organs.
- Primary somatomedins include insulin-like polypeptides (IGF-I and IGF-II). Other growth factors include nerve growth factor, epidermal growth factor, ovarian growth factor, fibroblast growth factor and thymosin. They also have insulin-like actions on carbohydrate and fat metabolism.

Actions

Mostly mediated by the somatomedins.
1. Raises blood sugar.
2. Stimulates lipolysis.

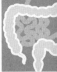

3. Stimulates protein synthesis and cell proliferation: promotes positive nitrogen balance.
4. Stimulates growth of bone, cartilage and connective tissue.

PROLACTIN (PRL; LUTEOTROPIC HORMONE, LTH)

Structure
Single-chain polypeptide of 198 amino acids. Similar in structure to GH.

Secretion
- Under inhibitory control of PIF synthesized in the hypothalamus.
- Dopamine is physiologically the most important prolactin inhibiting factor (PIF).
- Secreted intermittently in pulses lasting about 90 min. Secretion highest at night and falls during the morning.

Stimuli for release
PRH, TRH
Exercise
Sleep (circadian rhythm)
Stress, e.g. surgery, myocardial infarction
Pregnancy/oestrogens
Suckling/lactation
Puberty in girls.

Pathological causes
Hypothalamic/pituitary diseases
Hypothyroidism
Renal failure
Drugs, e.g. L-dopa and dopamine agonists (bromocriptine).

Causes of decreased secretion
Reversal of above factors
PIF, i.e. dopamine
Drugs, e.g. L-dopa and dopamine agonists (bromocriptine).

Actions
1. Milk synthesis: induces and maintains lactation postpartum.
2. Responsible for inhibitory effect on ovaries and normal breast development.

POSTERIOR PITUITARY HORMONES

Produces two important hormones.
1. **Vasopressin (antidiuretic hormone, ADH)**
2. **Oxytocin**
Both synthesized in paraventricular and supraoptic nuclei, and transported via the hypothalamoneurohypophyseal tracts to the posterior pituitary. Secretion is through stimulation of cholinergic nerve fibres.

ANTIDIURETIC HORMONE (ADH)

See pages 199–201.

OXYTOCIN

Structure
Nonapeptide.

Secretion

Stimuli for release
1. Milk-ejection reflex
2. Coital reflex
3. Labour (2nd stage).

Actions
1. Uterine contraction
2. Milk ejection due to contraction of myoepithelial cells.

ADRENAL CORTEX

Structure of steroid hormones
- Basic structure for all steroid hormones is the cyclopentanoperhydrophenanthrene nucleus (Fig. 5.21).

Oestrogens: C_{18} steroids
Androgens: C_{19} steroids
Glucocorticoids
Mineralocorticoids $\Big\}$ C_{21} steroids
Progestogens

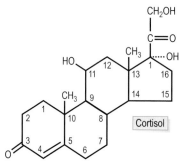

Fig. 5.21 Structure of cortisol.

Biosynthesis of adrenal steroids

Table 5.15 Secretion of steroid hormones	
Site of production	*Hormone*
Zona glomerulosa	Mineralocorticoids – aldosterone – deoxycorticosterone – corticosterone (also a glucocorticoid)
Zone fasciculata	Glucocorticolds (cortisol) Androgens (dehydroepiandrosterone, androstenedione, testosterone)
Zona reticularis	Oestrogens (oestradiol) Progestogens

- Occurs in adrenal cortex, testis and ovary (Table 5.15).
- The rate-limiting step in the biosynthesis of adrenal steroids is the mitochondrial conversion of cholesterol to pregnenolone (Fig. 5.22).
- About 75% of plasma cortisol is bound to cortisol-binding globulin; 15% is bound to plasma albumin and 10% is unbound, which represents the physiologically active steroid.

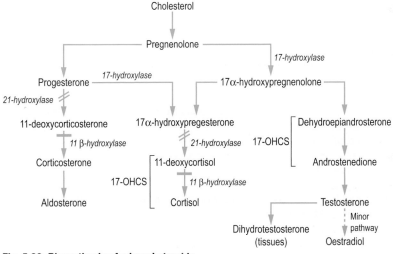

Fig. 5.22 Biosynthesis of adrenal steroids.
17-OHCS = 17-hydroxycorticosteroids, 17-OS = oxysteroids.

Urinary metabolites
1. Urinary free cortisol.
2. Urinary 17-hydroxycorticosteroids (17-OHCS). Increased levels with Cushing's disease and pregnancy.
3. Urinary 17-oxysteroids (17-OS)/17-ketosteroids (17-KS). Group of metabolites formed mainly from androgens, (adrenal, testicular or ovarian in origin). Increased levels with Cushing's syndrome, congenital adrenal hyperplasia, polycystic ovaries and some testicular tumours.

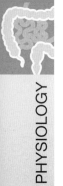

Disorders of secretion: Congenital adrenal hyperplasia

(i) *11β-hydroxylase defect: autosomal recessive*
- Principal steroids excreted are androgens and 11-deoxycortisol metabolites.
- Clinical features include hypertension with virilization.

(ii) *21-hydroxylase defect: autosomal recessive*
- Increased excretion of androgens: 17-ketosteroid and 21-deoxysteroids in the blood and urine.
- Two types:
  1. Severe, with salt-losing syndrome in infancy.
  2. Mild, with virilism in female and pseudoprecocious puberty in male.

GLUCOCORTICOIDS

- Cortisol and corticosterone (secreted at 1/10th amount of cortisol).
- Bound to corticosteroid-binding globulin (CBG) or transcortin; 10% free in plasma, which is the biologically active fraction.

Secretion
- Circadian rhythm: negative feedback control on ACTH, but can be overridden by stress, e.g. severe trauma, acute anxiety, infections and surgery.
- Highest in the morning (around 8.00 a.m.) and lowest around midnight.

Actions

Anti-insulin actions
1. Glycogenolysis (liver)
2. Gluconeogenesis from protein (liver)
3. Increased protein catabolism
4. Lipolysis, increased free fatty acid mobilization, oxidation and increased ketone production
5. Increased plasma glucose
6. Anti-inflammatory and antiallergic properties
7. Increased resistance to stress
8. Some mineralocorticoid action
9. Decreased lymphocytes and eosinophils; increased neutrophils, platelets and red blood cells
10. Decreased protein matrix in bone; increased urinary calcium
11. Increased secretion of hydrochloric acid and pepsin.

MINERALOCORTICOIDS

Aldosterone
See pages 193–194.

SEX HORMONES

Androgens: testosterone, androstenedione and dehydroepiandosterone
Oestrogens: oestradiol
Progesterone.

ADRENAL MEDULLA

- Consists of chromaffin cells which are derived from the primitive neuroectoderm, and have a common origin with ganglion cells of sympathetic nervous system.

CATECHOLAMINES

- Adrenal cells contain two catecholamines: noradrenaline (20%) and adrenaline (80%).
- Bound to ATP and protein and stored as membrane-bound granules, called chromaffin granules.

Synthesis and metabolism of catecholamines (Fig. 5.23)

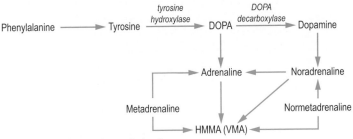

Fig. 5.23 Synthesis of catecholamines.
DOPA = dihydroxyphenylalanine, HMMA = hydroxymethoxymandelic acid.

- The plasma half-life of the catecholamines is 1–3 minutes.
- Sympathetic nerve endings take up the catecholamines from the circulation, which leads to non-enzymatic inactivation by intraneuronal storage and to enzymatic inactivation in the synaptic cleft.
- These transmitters are destroyed by the enzymes, monoamine oxidase (MAO) and catechol-o-methyltransferase (COMT).

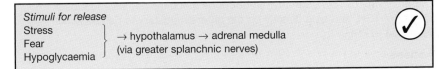

Stimuli for release
Stress
Fear   → hypothalamus → adrenal medulla
Hypoglycaemia (via greater splanchnic nerves)

Actions (see p. 278)
Mediated principally by adrenaline.
1. Increased glycogenolysis (liver, muscle)
2. Increased gluconeogenesis
3. Increased lipolysis (fat cells).

THYROID

- Consists of colloid-filled follicles containing the thyroid hormones stored as thyroglobulin, surrounded by a layer of cubical epithelial cells.
- Parafollicular (C) cells are also found between the acini. Secrete calcitonin, which prevents calcium mobilization from bone and so lowers the calcium level in the blood.

THYROID HORMONE

Structure

Thyroid hormone secreted in two forms:

1. *Thyroxine* (T_4): 90% of active thyroid hormone. Mainly protein bound: 75% to thyroxine-binding globulin (TBG), 15% to thyroxine-binding prealbumin (TBPA) and 10% to albumin. 0.05% exists as the free hormone which is the physiologically active form.
2. *Tri-iodothyronine* (T_3): 0.5% exists as the free hormone. Five times as potent as T_4, with a shorter half-life and less strongly bound. T_3 is active hormone at tissue level. Approximately 1/3rd of T_4 is converted to T_3 in tissues.

Thyroid hormone biosynthesis (Fig. 5.24)

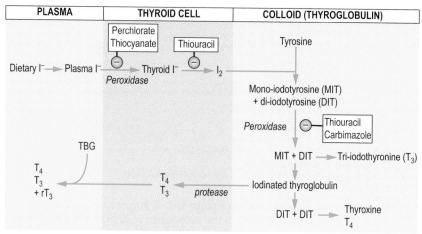

Fig. 5.24 Synthesis of thyroid hormones.
rT_3 = reverse T_3.

Secretion

Under control of TSH. Free thyroid hormone mediates negative feedback control of TSH, and acts directly on the anterior pituitary to decrease cell response to TRH.

Actions

1. Increases metabolic rate: increases O_2 consumption and metabolic rate of almost all metabolically active tissues.
2. Essential for skeletal growth and sexual maturation.
3. Essential for brain development and function.
4. Stimulates glucose absorption from the intestinal tract.
5. Lowers blood glucose.
6. Converts carotene to vitamin A.
7. Lowers circulating cholesterol level.
8. Potentiates the action of catecholamines on the heart (due to upregulation of β-receptors).

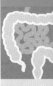

PANCREAS

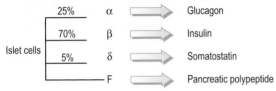

Fig. 5.25 Pancreatic islet cells.

INSULIN

Structure
Soluble protein (51 amino acids) with two chains (α chain and β chain) linked by disulphide bridges.

Synthesis
Folded proinsulin (Fig. 5.26)
- Synthesized in ribosomes of endoplasmic reticulum of β-cells of pancreatic islets as proinsulin (81 amino acids).
- The C-peptide (30 amino acids) is removed by enzyme hydrolysis and secreted in equimolar amounts with insulin.

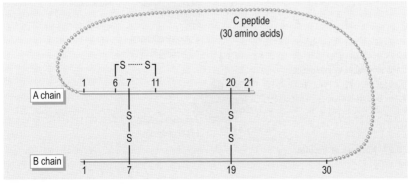

Fig. 5.26 Synthesis of insulin.

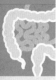

- Stored in granules prior to secretion which is initiated by Ca^{2+} influx into cells.
- Glucose stimulates entry of Ca^{2+} into β cells, synthesis of proinsulin and secretion of insulin, C-peptide and small amounts of proinsulin.
- 80% of insulin is degraded in the liver and kidneys.

Secretion

Stimuli for release
Glucose
Fatty acids and ketone bodies
Vagal nerve stimulation
Amino acids, especially leucine and arginine
Gut hormones: gastrin, CCK-PZ, secretin, glucagon and GIP
Drugs, e.g. sulphonylureas, β-adrenergic agents
Prostaglandins.

Stimuli for inhibition of release
Sympathetic nerve stimulation
α-Adrenergic agents, e.g. adrenaline (epinephrine)
β-Blockers
Dopamine
Serotonin
Somatostatin.

Insulin antagonists: include cortisol, adrenaline, glucagon, growth hormone, oestrogens and T_4.

Actions (see Fig. 5.27 and p. 278)

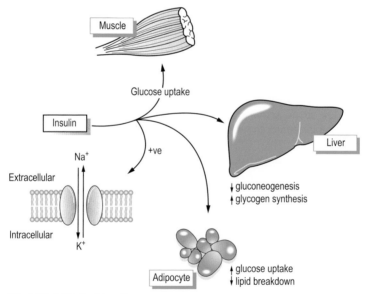

Fig. 5.27 Actions of insulin.

> *Adipose tissue*
> 1. ↑ Glucose entry
> 2. ↑ Fatty acid synthesis and lipid storage
> 3. Inhibition of lipolysis
> 4. Activation of lipoprotein lipase and hormone-sensitive lipase.
>
> | *Muscle* | *Liver* |
> |---|---|
> | 1. ↑ Glucose uptake | 1. ↑ Glucose uptake |
> | 2. ↑ Glycogen synthesis | 2. ↑ Glycogen synthesis |
> | 3. ↑ Amino acid uptake | 3. Inhibition of gluconeogenesis |
> | 4. ↑ Protein synthesis | 4. ↑ Lipogenesis |
> | 5. ↓ Protein catabolism. | 5. Inhibition of ketogenesis. |

Effect of insulin on glucose transport
- Glucose influx increased by 15–20-fold by insulin.
- Transport is by means of facilitated diffusion carrier mechanism down a concentration gradient (*not* active transport), since intracellular glucose concentration is lower than extracellular.
- Insulin has no effect on glucose transport in brain, renal tubules, intestinal mucosa and red blood cells.

Insulin resistance

Causes of insulin resistance
1. Obesity, pregnancy, polycystic ovary syndrome
2. Renal failure
3. Acromegaly
4. Drugs, e.g. isoniazid, rifampicin
5. Asian origin
6. Cystic fibrosis
7. Werner's syndrome
8. Syndrome X (association of peripheral insulin resistance with hyperinsulinaemia (fasting insulin >89.4 pmol/l), central obesity, hypertriglyceridaemia and increased risk of Alzheimer's disease).

Mechanisms
1. Obesity causes resistance by increased release of non-esterified fatty acids causing post-receptor defects in insulin's action.
2. Mutation of gene encoding insulin receptor.
3. Circulating autosomal bodies to extracellular domain of insulin receptor.

GLUCAGON
Structure
- Polypeptide (29 amino acids). Secreted by α cells of the pancreatic islets.
- Glucagon, secretin, VIP and GIP have some homologous amino acid sequences.
- Rapidly degraded in the tissues (especially in the liver and kidney) and by kallikrein in plasma.

Secretion

> | *Stimuli for release* | *Stimuli for inhibition of release* |
> |---|---|
> | Amino acids | Glucose |
> | β-Adrenergic stimulation | Somatostatin |
> | Fasting, hypoglycaemia | Free fatty acids |
> | Exercise | Ketones |
> | Gastrin, CCK and cortisol. | Insulin. |

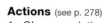

Actions (see p. 278)
1. Glycogenolytic, gluconeogenic, lipolytic, ketogenic.
2. Stimulates secretion of GH, insulin and somatostatin.
3. Reduces intestinal motility and gastric acid secretion.

SOMATOSTATIN

- Synthesized as a large precursor molecule, and then cleaved to produce a prohormone, which undergoes further modification to produce the biologically active products, somatostatin 14 and 28.
- Somatostatin inhibits the release of thyrotropin from the pituitary gland and growth hormone release.
- It also acts as a neurotransmitter in other areas of brain, and has a wide range of inhibiting effects on the gastrointestinal tract.
- Octreotide is a structural analogue of somatostatin and has been used in treatment of acromegaly, thyrotropin-secreting adenomas and non-secreting pituitary adenomas.

PHYSIOLOGICAL RESPONSE OF MOTHER TO PREGNANCY

1. Cardiovascular changes
- ↑ CO, HR and SV
- ↑ Blood flow to many tissues and organs
- Compression of vena cava in supine position → ↓ VR, CO and BP (supine hypotensive syndrome).

2. Respiratory changes
- ↑ Minute volume by 30–50%
- ↑ Oxygen consumption by 20–30%
- ↑ Basal metabolic rate
- ↑ Lung volumes (cf: for restrictive lung disease).

3. Renal
- ↑ Renal blood flow by 25%
- ↑ GFR by 50%
- ↑ Clearance of urea, uric acid and creatinine (glucose and amino acids may be lost in urine).

4. Blood
- ↑ Red cell mass and plasma volume
- ↓ Plasma [Hb], [iron]: ↑ plasma [transferrin] and total iron-binding capacity
- ↓ [Plasma protein]
- ↑ β-Globulin and fibrinogen.

5. Endocrine
- ↑ Placental hormone production
- ↑ Plasma throxine and TBG.

6. Nutrition
- ↑ 15% calorie requirement
- ↑ 50% protein requirement
- ↑ Requirement for folate, calcium, phosphorus, Mg^{2+}, iron, vitamins A and C, zinc and iodine.

6

BIOCHEMISTRY, CELL BIOLOGY AND CLINICAL CHEMISTRY

BIOCHEMISTRY AND CELL BIOLOGY 240

MAJOR METABOLIC PATHWAYS AND CYCLES 240
Interrelationship of carbohydrate, fat and protein metabolism 240
Tricarboxylic–citric acid cycle 240
Electron transport and oxidative phosphorylation 242

CELL BIOLOGY 242
Cell cycle 242
Cell signalling 244
Cellular interaction and adhesion molecules 244
Signal transduction 244
Second messenger systems 246

CARBOHYDRATES AND METABOLISM 247
Types of carbohydrate 247
Digestion of three main carbohydrates 248
Carbohydrate metabolism 248
Glycolytic pathway 248
Gluconeogenesis 249
Lactate production 250
Pentose phosphate pathway 250
Glycogen and glycogen metabolism 251
Glycogenesis 251
Glycogenolysis 252
Abnormal states of carbohydrate metabolism 252
Inborn errors of carbohydrate metabolism 252

Starvation and ketogenesis 252
Diabetic ketoacidosis 255
Spontaneous hypoglycaemia 255

LIPIDS AND METABOLISM 256
Main classes of lipids 256
Fatty acids 256
Triglycerides 256
Phospholipids 256
Cholesterol 257
Others 257
Digestion of fats 257
Lipid transport: lipoproteins 258
Lipid metabolism 260
Lipolysis 260
Lipogenesis 260
Cholesterol metabolism 260
Prostanoid (eicosanoid) metabolism 261
Pathways of synthesis and metabolism 261
Pharmacological and physiological effects 262
Disorders of lipoprotein metabolism 263
Hyperlipidaemias 263
Hypolipoproteinaemias 264
Sphingolipidoses and mucopolysaccharidoses 264

PROTEINS AND METABOLISM 266
Amino acids 266
Proteins 266
Digestion of proteins 267
Protein metabolism 267
Disorders of amino acid metabolish 268

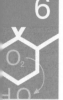

Inborn errors of amino acid metabolism 268
Amino acid transport defects   270

SPECIALIZED PROTEINS   271
Haemoglobin   271
Porphyrin and haem synthesis   271
Oxygen dissociation curve   272
Disorders of haem synthesis   273
Abnormal derivatives of haemoglobin 275
Disorders of globin synthesis   275
Collagen   276
Disorders of metabolism of collagen   276
Purines and pyrimidines   276
Metabolism   276
Disorders of purine and pyrimidine metabolism   277

HORMONAL CONTROL OF METABOLISM   278

CLINICAL CHEMISTRY   278
Vitamins   278

MINERALS   284
Sodium   284
Potassium   284
Iron   285
Calcium   286

Phosphate   288
Chloride   289
Magnesium   289
Trace elements   289

NUTRITIONAL DEFICIENCIES IN SPECIFIC DISEASES/STATES   291
Daily dietary requirements   291

PLASMA PROTEINS   291
Constituents and functions   291
Use in diagnosis   293
Changes in plasma protein concentrations   293

PLASMA ENZYMES   295

TUMOUR PRODUCTS   297

BIOCHEMISTRY OF COAGULATION/ FIBRINOLYSIS   298
Coagulation cascade and fibrinolytic pathway   298
Abnormalities of coagulation   299

INTERPRETATION OF LABORATORY FINDINGS   300
Blood   300
Cerebrospinal fluid   301
Urine biochemistry   302
Synovial fluid   304

BIOCHEMISTRY AND CELL BIOLOGY

MAJOR METABOLIC PATHWAYS AND CYCLES (Summarized in Fig. 6.1)

Cell compartments and organelles

Nucleus:	gene expression
Cytoplasm:	metabolism and protein synthesis
Mitochondrion:	energy production. Has its own genome.
Golgi apparatus:	protein processing
Endoplasmic reticulum:	protein modification
Lysosome:	protein degradation
Peroxisome:	oxidation reactions.

INTERRELATIONSHIP OF CARBOHYDRATE, FAT AND PROTEIN METABOLISM (Fig. 6.1)

Amino acids and lipids feed into the pathways of carbohydrate metabolism and the citric acid cycle, where they are degraded to hydrogen and carbon dioxide. The hydrogen ions are then oxidized to water by enzymes of the electron transport chain, and adenosine triphosphate (ATP) is generated.

TRICARBOXYLIC ACID (TCA) – CITRIC ACID CYCLE (Fig. 6.1)

- Final common pathway for the oxidation of carbohydrate, fat and some amino acids to CO_2 and H_2O.

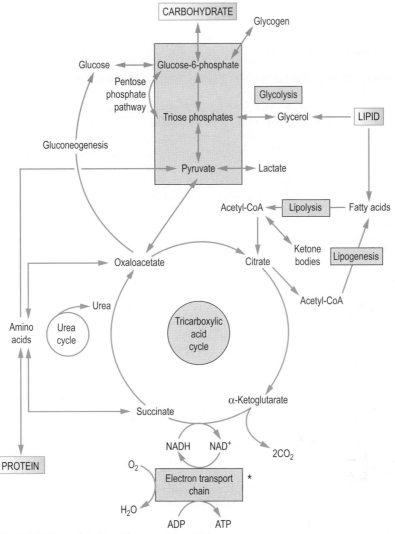

Fig. 6.1 Major metabolic pathways and cycles.
ATP = adenosine triphosphate, ADP = adenosine diphosphate, * = present in mitochondria.

- Takes place in the mitochondria.
- Oxaloacetate and acetyl-CoA condense to form citrate, which is then converted to oxaloacetate by a series of nine reactions. The net result is the conversion of the acetyl residues to two molecules of CO_2 and eight hydrogen atoms per turn of cycle, which enter the electron transport chain with the generation of two ATP molecules and oxaloacetate.
- Regulated by the availability of acetyl-CoA, oxaloacetate, NADH and FAD^+. The control enzymes are pyruvate dehydrogenase, citrate synthase, isocitrate dehydrogenase and α-ketoglutarate dehydrogenase.
- It is an amphibolic pathway, i.e. it is involved in both anabolic and catabolic processes. Some of the cycle components serve as entry or exit points for other pathways, e.g. gluconeogenesis, transamination, deamination and lipogenesis.

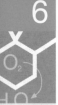
BIOCHEMISTRY, CELL BIOLOGY AND CLINICAL CHEMISTRY

- Occurs in any type of cell, except the mature erythrocyte. Only active under aerobic conditions.

ELECTRON TRANSPORT AND OXIDATIVE PHOSPHORYLATION

- The final stage in the oxidation of glucose, fatty acids and amino acids.
- Takes place in the mitochondria.
- Formation of adenosine triphosphate (ATP) from adenosine diphosphate (ADP) and inorganic phosphate (Pi) while electrons (hydrogen ions) are transferred through a series of sequential oxidation-reduction reactions by enzymes of the electron transport chain (NAD-linked dehydrogenases, flavoproteins and cytochromes) in the mitochondria. These two processes of electron transport and phosphorylation are said to be *coupled*. When electron transport proceeds without concomitant ATP production, the reactions are said to be *uncoupled*; 2,4-dinitrophenol (DNP) is an uncoupling agent.
- The net result is the transfer of electrons from NADH and $FADH_2$ to oxygen, forming water.
- Cytoplasmic reducing equivalents, NADH and NAD^+ are transported into the mitochondria by the glycerol-phosphate and the malate-aspartate shuttle.
- Main function is to regulate the ratio of $NADH/NAD^+$ and ATP/ADP for the activation or inhibition of the pathways of the cell according to functional requirements.

Energy yield

- The complete oxidation of one molecule of *glucose* to CO_2 and H_2O produces 38 ATP. (Two during glycolysis, two in the TCA cycle and 34 by oxidative phosphorylation.)
- The complete oxidation of *palmitic acid* produces 129 ATP molecules.

High-energy phosphate compounds

- Compounds which on hydrolysis result in the transfer of a large quantity of energy.
- Most important is adenosine triphosphate (ATP). On hydrolysis to adenosine diphosphate (ADP) it liberates energy directly to processes such as muscle contraction, active transport and the synthesis of many chemical compounds.
- Other high-energy phosphate compounds include creatine phosphate, guanosine triphosphate (GTP), uridine triphosphate (UTP) and cytidine triphosphate (CTP).

CELL BIOLOGY

CELL CYCLE

The sequence of events leading to cell reproduction (Fig. 6.2). Divided into two phases.

1. Mitosis (or cell division) which results in the production of two daughter cells.
2. Interphase (prophase, prometaphase, metaphase, anaphase, telophase) is the interval between divisions during which the cell undergoes its functions and prepares for mitosis.
   Divided into G1, S and G2 phase (Fig. 6.2).
   Non-dividing cells, e.g. neurons, do not go through this cycle and remain in a resting G0 state.

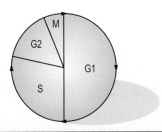

- G1 (6–12 hours): RNA and protein is synthesized; there is no DNA replication
- S (6–8 hours): period of DNA replication
- G2 (3–4): during this period the cell has two complete diploid sets of chromosomes
- M (1 hour): mitosis, the period of actual cell division

Fig. 6.2 The cell cycle.

Regulation of the cell cycle

Three points of control in the cell cycle:
1. At end of G1 when cell becomes committed to completing a cycle of division. Requires adequate nutrients and growth factors.
2. Beginning of mitosis M phase. Will not progress if there is DNA damage.
3. End of mitosis.

Cyclins are proteins that govern the transition from one stage to another by regulating cyclin-dependent kinases (CDKs). These become active when they bind and form a complex with cyclin proteins, e.g. maturation-promoting factors (MPF).

Human cyclins are designated A, B, D and E and each one accumulates at a different time in the cell cycle. Cell cycle also influenced by growth factors, hormones and cell–cell interactions.

Cell cycle and cancer

Malignancy occurs as a result of DNA mutations that cause increased or decreased expression of genes associated with cell cycle control.

Causes of altered gene expression:
1. Chemical damage, e.g. nitrosamines
2. Radiation, e.g. UV light
3. Integration of new DNA into host genome
4. Inherited defects.

DNA mutations associated with cancer
1. Oncogenes (e.g. *ras*, *fos*, *myc*): mutated or upregulated versions of normal cellular genes (proto-oncogenes) that induce uncontrolled growth (see also p. 33).
2. Tumour suppressor genes (e.g. *p53*, *Rb*, *GAB*): genes expressed in normal cells. Loss of their activity results in uninhibited growth (see also p. 34).

---

p53 (see also p. 34)
1. Main function is to restrict the entry of cells with damaged DNA into S phase. Cells with mutant *p53* are not arrested at this point and progress through the cell cycle with damaged DNA.
2. *p53* gene lies on chromosome 17.
3. Main roles of *p53* include as a transcription activator (i.e. regulating certain genes involved in cell division); as an inhibitor of cell division if there has been excess DNA damage; and participation in the initiation of apoptosis.

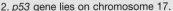

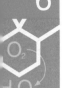

BIOCHEMISTRY, CELL BIOLOGY AND CLINICAL CHEMISTRY

CELL SIGNALLING

> **Summary of mechanisms for cell-to-cell signalling**
> 1. *Direct signalling*
>   - Gap junctions
>   - Cell adhesion via adhesion molecules.
>
> 2. *Indirect signalling*
>   - Chemical messengers that utilize a specific receptor.

CELLULAR INTERACTION AND ADHESION MOLECULES

- Interactions between cells and with extracellular matrix (ECM) facilitate cell–cell communication in several biological processes, e.g. migration, growth, immunological functioning, permeability, cell recognition, tissue repair, differentiation and embryogenesis.
- These physical interactions are mediated by several families of membrane-spanning proteins, called adhesion molecules.
- There are 4 major cell adhesion molecule families (Table 6.1).

Table 6.1 Adhesion molecule families

Families	Members	Function
Cadherins	E-CAD, N-CAD	Mediate communication and adhesion
Immunoglobulin (Ig) superfamily	ICAM-1, ICAM-2 (intracellular) VCAM-1 (vascular) NCAM (neural)	Involved in adhesion, signalling, axonal growth and fasciculation
Selectins (blood and endothelial cells only)	P-selectin E-selectin	Expressed during inflammatory responses, and expression activated by local chemical mediation, e.g. F-selectin activated by TNF, IL-1 and endotoxin
Integrins*	LF-1, MAC-1	Binding to ECM and cell–cell interactions

* The *integrin* gpIIa/IIIb, which is expressed on the surface of platelets, acts as a receptor for fibrinogen and von Willebrand factor, and mediates platelet aggregation. An anti-gpIIb/IIIa antibody is a powerful antithrombotic and is used in the prevention of ischaemic complications following coronary angioplasty.
Dystrophin: In skeletal muscle, the major link between the actin cytoskeleton and the ECM involves dystroglycan, a glycoprotein – an adhesion receptor for laminin. Dystroglycan forms part of a membrane complex of proteins that are connected to actin by a cytoplasmic plaque protein, dystrophin. Duchenne muscular dystrophy results from mutations that affect the stability of dystrophin.

SIGNAL TRANSDUCTION

Universal pathway by which cells are directed to divide, differentiate, migrate and degranulate. Most molecules transmit their signal by binding cell surface receptors, which then convert this binding into intracellular signals that alter the cell's behaviour.

- A ligand is a molecule, e.g. hormone, that binds the receptors, and is termed the *first messenger*.
- The *second messenger* system is a set of intracellular molecules that are activated by cell surface receptors and produce a physiological response, e.g. AMP, GMP, DAG. These systems produce a signal cascade that amplifies the initial system and facilitates a variety of cellular responses.

Mechanisms

- Some hydrophobic molecules, e.g. steroid and thyroid hormones, are able to cross the plasma membrane and interact with intracellular receptors and produce an effect.
- Most other signalling molecules are hydrophilic and must interact with specific receptors at the cell surface to transduce an extracellular signal into an intracellular event.

1. Membrane-bound receptors with integral ion channels

Drugs, hormones, growth factors, metabolites and physical stimuli such as photons of light interact with cell receptors to stimulate second messenger systems to produce changes in the state of cells.

Voltage-gated ion channels, e.g. skeletal muscle sodium channel responds to changes in local membrane potentials.

Ligand-gated ion channels, e.g. nicotinic acetylcholine (ACh) receptor. Binding of ACh results in a conformational change in the receptor and the rapid influx of sodium ions and depolarization of the cell membrane.

Ion channel associated diseases ✓

Voltage-gated channels
- Long QT syndrome: mutation in potassium channel genes
- Myotonia congenita: skeletal muscle chloride channel
- Hyperkalaemic periodic paralysis: skeletal muscle sodium channel
- Hypokalaemic periodic paralysis: skeletal muscle calcium channel.

Ligand-gated channels
- Cystic fibrosis: ATP-gated chloride channel
- Nocturnal frontal lobe epilepsy: neuronal nicotinic acetylcholine receptor
- Startle disease: glycine receptor.

---

2. Membrane-bound receptors with integral enzyme activity

Tyrosine kinase (TK) receptors

Catalytic receptors that signal directly to the cell, and phosphorylate target proteins. Binding of ligand induces dimerization and autophosphorylation at a tyrosine residue. The tyrosine kinase activity intrinsic to the receptor is then activated and the result is the phosphorylation of cytoplasmic proteins and initiation of an intracellular cascade of second messengers.

Examples
- Epidermal growth factor (ECF) receptor. In inflammatory disease such as pancreatitis, there may be upregulation of receptors leading to abnormal growth and possibly carcinoma.
- Insulin growth factor (IGF) receptor, fibroblast growth factor (FGF) receptors. Important in angiogenesis and abnormalities of this receptor are seen in some carcinomas.

3. Membrane-bound receptors that use transducing molecules (G-proteins) or guanine nucleotide-binding proteins

Heterotrimeric G-proteins are associated with seven-helical membrane receptors. On ligand binding the conformational change in the receptor leads to the activation of the G-protein which swaps GDP for GTP. Second messenger systems such as adenylate cyclase are then activated. G-proteins can be inhibitory or facilitatory.

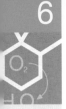

Clinical examples
- In *V. cholera* infection, G-protein activity is increased. The resulting increase in cAMP levels causes secretory diarrhoea.
- In Albright's hereditary osteodystrophy. 50% reduction in activity of one of the G-proteins results in a generalized resistance to action of several hormones and dysmorphic characteristics.

4. Intracellular receptors

Nuclear hormone superfamily: corticosteroids, vitamin D, retinoic acid, sex steroids. The lipophilic hormone crosses the plasma membrane and binds to intracellular receptors. The complex then travels to the nucleus where the receptor acts as a transcription factor by binding to recognition elements in the 5′ end of genes.

Three mechanisms of cell signalling to surface receptors

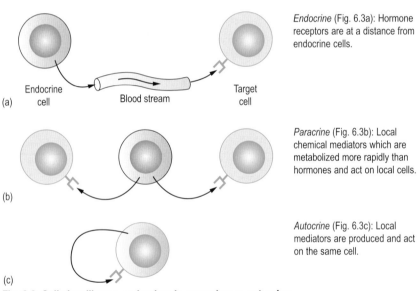

Endocrine (Fig. 6.3a): Hormone receptors are at a distance from endocrine cells.

Paracrine (Fig. 6.3b): Local chemical mediators which are metabolized more rapidly than hormones and act on local cells.

Autocrine (Fig. 6.3c): Local mediators are produced and act on the same cell.

Fig. 6.3 Cell signalling: a, endocrine; b, paracrine; c, autocrine.

SECOND MESSENGER SYSTEMS

1. Cyclic AMP activation or inhibition of adenylate cyclase (Fig. 6.4)

Hormones that affect cAMP levels in appropriate target cells by altering adenyl cyclase activity include:

Stimulatory: ACTH, FSH, glucagons, LH, PTH, TSH, ADH
Inhibitory: Angiotensin II, somatostatin.

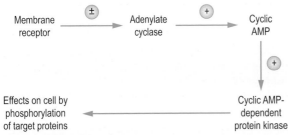

Fig. 6.4 Cyclic AMP activation.

2. Cyclic GMP

Components similar to those of cyclic AMP and include cyclic GMP-dependent protein kinase (protein kinase G) and phosphoprotein phosphatases.

3. Calcium

Several hormones exert their action in part by affecting intracellular calcium levels, e.g. ACTH, angiotensin II, gastrin, histamine (H_1), TRH, ADH.

4. Diglyceride system (Fig. 6.5)

Both protein kinase C and inositol triphosphate act as second messengers in important cellular pathways.

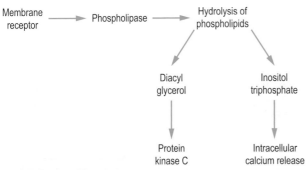

Fig. 6.5 Diglyceride system.

TYPES OF CARBOHYDRATE

Dietary carbohydrate consists mainly of starch, amylose, and amylopectin (polysaccharides), cellulose, sucrose, lactose and maltose (disaccharides), with small amounts of free glucose and fructose (monosaccharides). Most of the monosaccharides occurring in the body are D-isomers.

Complex carbohydrates include:

1. Glycoproteins: proteins which have oligosaccharides covalently attached to the protein chain, e.g. most membrane and plasma proteins. Sugars found in glycoproteins include glucose, galactose, mannose, galactosamine, arabinose, *N*-acetyl neuraminic acid or sialic acid.
2. Glycolipids: lipids containing a covalently attached oligosaccharide, e.g. many cell surface antigens.

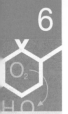
3. Proteoglycans: complex molecules composed of a core protein with covalently attached glycosaminoglycans, e.g. chondroitin sulphate, hyaluronate and dermatan sulphate.
4. Glycosaminoglycans (GAGs): linear polysaccharides generally composed of alternating hexosamine and either uronic acid and/or galactose. Usually found as constituents of proteoglycans. The sugars found include N-acetylglucosamine, galactosamine, glucuronic acid and iduronic acids.

DIGESTION OF THREE MAIN CARBOHYDRATES

1. Carbohydrates are partially hydrolysed by salivary and pancreatic α-amylase to limit dextrans and oligosaccharides, maltose and maltotriose.
2. These are then hydrolysed by disaccharidases on the intestinal mucosal membrane to monosaccharides (glucose, fructose and galactose) (Fig. 6.6).
3. In the small intestine, the monosaccharides are absorbed either by an active cellular process, coupled to Na^+ transport using a common carrier protein (specific for glucose and galactose) or via Na^+ independent, facilitated diffusion (specific for fructose) and transported to the liver.
4. They are removed from the circulation by the hepatic cells and immediately phosphorylated.
5. Their ultimate fate depends totally on the body's needs.

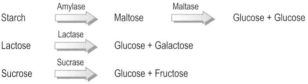

Fig. 6.6 Hydrolysis of carbohydrates.

CARBOHYDRATE METABOLISM

Fate of glucose

Glucose may be:
- Oxidized to give energy, or
- Stored as glycogen (muscle), or
- Converted to triglycerides, amino acids and proteins.

GLYCOLYTIC PATHWAY (EMBDEN–MEYERHOF) (Fig. 6.7)

- The oxidation of glucose to pyruvate with generation of ATP in muscle, fat and non-gluconeogenic tissue. The pathway also metabolizes glucose derived from glycogen, galactose and fructose.
- May also occur in the absence of oxygen (i.e. anaerobic), when pyruvate is converted to lactate.
- Takes place in the cytoplasm.
- The net yield is two moles of ATP and NADH per glucose molecule.

Control of glycolysis
Control of glycolysis is through three regulatory enzymes:
1. Hexokinase (glucokinase in the liver)
2. Phosphofructokinase
3. Pyruvate kinase.

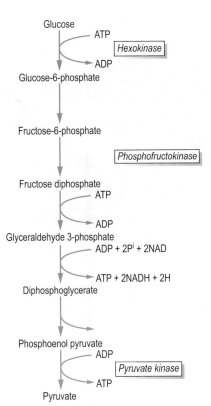

Fig. 6.7 Glycolytic pathway.

Pyruvate kinase deficiency
Inadequate production of ATP reduces the activity of the Na^+/K^+-stimulated ATPase pump in the red blood cell. The cells swell and lyse resulting in a haemolytic anaemia.

Pyruvate is an intermediary product of glucose metabolism in the cytoplasm, that links together glycolysis, the TCA cycle, amino acid metabolism and fatty acid oxidation. It crosses the mitochondrial membrane and may:
1. React with coenzyme A to produce acetyl-CoA and NADH (*pyruvate dehydrogenase*), which can then enter the TCA cycle or lipid metabolism.
2. Condense with CO_2 to form oxaloacetate (*pyruvate carboxylase*).
3. Form alanine (*transamination*).
4. Be reconverted to glucose (*gluconeogenesis*).
5. Be reduced to lactate in the absence of oxygen (*lactate dehydrogenase*), with net synthesis of two molecules of ATP per molecule of glucose.

GLUCONEOGENESIS

- Synthesis of glucose from non-glucose precursors, especially amino acids (except leucine and lysine) and glycerol in the liver, kidney or intestinal epithelium, but also from any of the intermediates of glycolysis or the TCA cycle e.g. pyruvate, oxaloacetate, lactate (Cori cycle, see Note) and fructose.
- Takes place in the cytoplasm.
- Generally the enzymatic reactions of glycolysis are reversible, but in addition there are four unique enzymic steps (Fig. 6.8).

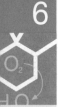

BIOCHEMISTRY, CELL BIOLOGY AND CLINICAL CHEMISTRY

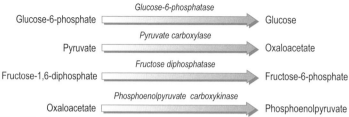

Fig. 6.8 Glycolytic enzymes.

- The net result of the conversion of pyruvate to glucose is the consumption of six moles of ATP and two moles of NADH.

Note: Cori cycle. Lactate is released into the blood and travels to the liver, where it is converted to pyruvate, and finally to glucose, by the gluconeogenic pathway. The glucose is released into the circulation where it is taken up by muscle. Therefore, lactic acid production occurs temporarily in contracting muscles.

Functions
1. Important during starvation and interdigestive periods (especially at night) to maintain a steady blood glucose for brain cell metabolism. During fasting, protein is the most important glucose source.
2. During severe exercise, gluconeogenesis allows the use of lactate from anaerobic glycolysis and of glycerol from fat breakdown.
3. Allows the use of dietary protein in carbohydrate pathways after disposing of the amino acid nitrogen as urea.

LACTATE PRODUCTION

During strenuous muscular activity, glycogenolysis is stimulated and the resulting glucose-6-phosphate (G-6-P) is further metabolized by the glycolytic pathway and then by oxidation within the TCA cycle to supply the necessary energy. When the rate of glycolysis exceeds the availability of oxygen, glucose is converted to lactate by the muscle *anaerobic* glycolytic pathway.

$$\text{Glucose} \rightarrow 2\text{Lactate} + 2\text{H}^+$$

Pathological lactic acidosis
High blood lactate levels (>5 mmol) can be due to increased production (i.e. increased rate of anaerobic glycolysis, e.g. in severe illnesses) or decreased utilization (i.e. impairment of the TCA cycle or gluconeogenesis, e.g. phenformin) or both, as in tissue hypoxia.

Causes
See pages 189–190.

PENTOSE PHOSPHATE PATHWAY OR HEXOSE MONOPHOSPHATE SHUNT
(Fig. 6.9)

- Takes place in the cytoplasm. Occurs in muscle, liver, fat cells, thyroid, lactating mammary gland and erythrocytes.
- Consist of two branches, an oxidative and non-oxidative branch.
- The net result is the production of 12 NADPH, 6 CO_2 and one glyceraldehyde-3-phosphate molecule for each glucose-6-phosphate molecule passing through the pathway.

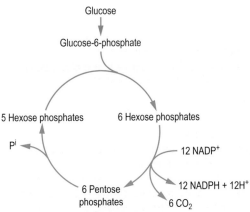

Fig. 6.9 Pentose phosphate pathway.

Main functions

1. Provides reducing equivalents, e.g. reduced nicotinamide adenine dinucleotide phosphate (NADPH) for the reductive synthesis of fatty acids, cholesterol and other steroids, and for maintenance of glutathione in a reduced form inside erythrocytes. Two dehydrogenases are involved: *glucose-6-phosphate-dehydrogenase* (*G6PDH*) and *6-phosphogluconate dehydrogenase* (Fig. 6.10).
2. Source of pentoses, e.g. ribose for nucleotide and nucleic acid synthesis.
3. Oxidizes glucose to CO_2.
4. Maintenance of integrity of red cell membrane as follows:
   (i) Production of NADPH which maintains glutathione in reduced state. The most important disease of the pathway is G6PDH deficiency.
   (ii) Glycolysis to produce 2 ATP which maintains Na^+ and K^+ distribution across the cell membrane.

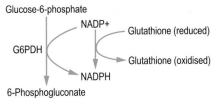

Fig. 6.10 Reduction of NADPH.

GLYCOGEN AND GLYCOGEN METABOLISM

Glycogen is an α-1,4 glucose polymer with α-1,6 branches. It is the storage form of glucose, and is found in abundance in the liver, kidney and muscle. Liver glycogen can be mobilized for the release of glucose to the rest of the body, but muscle glycogen can only be used to support muscle glycolysis.

GLYCOGENESIS

- The conversion of excess glucose to glycogen for storage.
- The synthesis of glycogen begins with the phosphorylation of glucose to glucose-6-phosphate, which is then isomerized to glucose-1-phosphate and

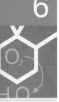

added to a glycogen primer, uridine diphosphoglucose (UDPG). Catalysed by *glycogen synthetase*, which exists in two forms:

1. An active (D or dependent) form, since the enzyme is active in the absence of glucose-6-phosphate
2. An inactive (L or independent) form, which is inactive in the absence of glucose-6-phosphate.

GLYCOGENOLYSIS

- Glycogen is degraded in two distinct steps:
  1. *Phosphorylase* splits the α-1,4 linkage, releasing glucose-1-phosphate.
  2. A debranching enzyme then splits the α-1,6 bond producing free glucose.
- The glucose-1-phosphate can then be isomerized to glucose-6-phosphate and either enter glycolysis or be hydrolysed to free glucose.
- Phosphorylase b is the inactive form of the enzyme and is converted to the active form, phosphorylase a, by phosphorylation catalysed by phosphorylase b kinase.

Regulation of glycogen synthesis and degradation by cyclic AMP

- Cyclic AMP (cyclic adenosine 3′,5′-monophosphate) activates a cAMP-dependent protein kinase, which in turn activates both phosphorylase b kinase and glycogen synthetase kinase. This results in glycogen breakdown with inhibition of glycogen synthesis. The enzymes that promote glycogenolysis are active in the phospho-forms and inactive in their dephospho-form. The reverse is true for glycogen synthetase.
- *Glycogenesis* is promoted by glycogen synthetase.
- *Glycogenolysis* is promoted by phosphorylase.
- Adrenaline or glucagon activate glycogen degradation and inhibit glycogen synthesis.
- Insulin activates glycogen synthesis and inhibits glycogen degradation (see p. 278).

ABNORMAL STATES OF CARBOHYDRATE METABOLISM

INBORN ERRORS OF CARBOHYDRATE METABOLISM

See Table 6.2.

STARVATION AND KETOGENESIS

- During fasting, endogenous triglycerides in adipose tissue are reconverted to fatty acids and glycerol by lipolysis.
- Blood glucose levels are maintained initially by increased liver gluconogenesis using glycerol (which enters the pathway at the triose phosphate stage) and amino acids (mainly from muscle).
- This is supplemented by conversion of the fatty acids to acetyl-CoA, and also into ketone bodies, via β-hydroxy-3-methylglutaryl-CoA (HMG-CoA). The ketone bodies include acetone, acetoacetate and β-hydroxybutyrate, and are used as a fuel by all cells except those of the brain.
- On prolonged starvation, brain cells can also adapt to using ketone bodies as a major source of fuel. The liver is the chief ketogenic organ.
- Ketosis occurs whenever the rate of hepatic ketone body production exceeds the rate of peripheral utilization as in severe diabetes, starvation, during anaesthesia and with a high fat, low carbohydrate diet.

Table 6.2 Inborn errors of carbohydrate metabolism (Fig. 6.11)

Disease	Enzyme defect	Clinical features	Diagnosis	Treatment
1. Glycogen storage diseases Incidence 1:60 000 births				
Type I von Gierke's	Glucose-6-phosphatase (G-6-P → glucose + P$_i$)	1. Recurrent hypoglycaemia 2. Hepatomegaly 3. Muscle weakness 4. Cardiac failure	• Liver biopsy* and liver enzyme analysis	• Frequent glucose feeds and restriction of fructose and galactose intake
Type II Pompe's	Lysosomal α-glucosidase (Glycogen → glucose)	• Usually presents in infancy, with features as above (plus metabolic acidosis, hyperlipidaemia, hyperuricaemia and ketosis) • Presents at or soon after birth, with features as above and cardiorespiratory failure	• Muscle/liver biopsy* and enzyme analysis on muscle, fibroblasts or amniotic cells	• Supportive only
Type III Cori's limit dextrinosis and Type IV Andersen's	Debranching and branching enzyme (Limit dextran → glucose)	• Types III and IV have a presentation similar to Type I, but milder	• Muscle/liver biopsy* and leucocyte enzyme levels	
Type V McArdle's	Muscle phosphorylase (Glycogen → G-1-P)	• Presents in adult life with muscle cramps on exercise, myoglobinuria, muscle weakness and wasting but no hypoglycaemia	• Muscle biopsy*, histochemistry or enzyme analysis. No normal rise in blood lactate after exertion	

* Excessive glycogen deposition.

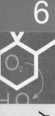
Table 6.2 (Cont'd)

Disease	Enzyme defect	Clinical features	Diagnosis	Treatment
2. Galactosaemia Incidence 1:60 000 births	Galactose-1-phosphate-uridyl transferase (Galactose → glucose)	• Presents at commencement of milk feeds with failure to thrive, vomiting, diarrhoea and jaundice. • Also hepatomegaly, ascites, cataracts and mental retardation	• Urine contains galactose (Clinitest +ve, Clinistix –ve) • Erythrocyte enzyme analysis (for prenatal and carrier state diagnosis)	• Lactose-free diet
3. Fructose intolerance Incidence 1:20 000 births	Fructose-1-phosphate-aldolase (F-1-P → DHA-P + α-glycerophosphate)	• Provoked by fructose-containing foods • Nausea, vomiting, abdominal pain, hypoglycaemia, growth retardation hepatomegaly, liver failure and aminoaciduria	• Dietary history (onset of symptoms with introduction of sucrose into the diet) • Fructosaemia and fructosuria after sucrose ingestion • Liver enzyme analysis	• Sucrose/fructose-free diet
4. Benign/essential fructosuria Incidence 1:130 000 births	Fructokinase	• Asymptomatic	• Fructosaemia and fructosuria after ingestion	

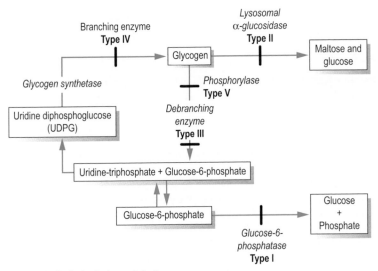

Fig. 6.11 Carbohydrate metabolism.

DIABETIC KETOACIDOSIS

The mechanism of ketosis in diabetes is the same as that in fasting, but is more severe and occurs in the presence of hyperglycaemia. In prolonged fasting the supply of glucose to the cells is insufficient for normal glycolysis or lipolysis. With insulin deficiency, there is simply an impaired uptake of glucose into the cells, resulting in an intracellular glucose deficiency. Excessive lipolysis occurs, causing ketosis and acidosis.

SPONTANEOUS HYPOGLYCAEMIA

Causes
1. Glycogen storage diseases (Types I & III)
2. Galactosaemia
3. Fructose intolerance
4. Leucine sensitivity
5. Addison's disease ⎫ due to inhibition of gluconeogenesis
6. Hypopituitarism ⎬
7. Post-gastrectomy syndrome
8. β-Cell islet tumours
9. Alcoholic cirrhosis, due to inhibition of gluconeogenesis and glycogenolysis
10. Hypothyroidism

but not in:
1. Glycogen storage diseases (Types II and V)
2. Gaucher's disease
3. Glucose-6-phosphate dehydrogenase (G6PDH) deficiency.

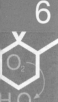

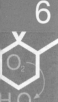

6

BIOCHEMISTRY, CELL BIOLOGY AND CLINICAL CHEMISTRY

MAIN CLASSES OF LIPIDS

FATTY ACIDS

- Long, straight chain monocarboxylic acids with an even number of carbon atoms (usually between 16 and 24). $CH_3.CH_2.CH_2.CH_2.COOH$
- Classified as:
  Saturated fatty acids (i.e. no double bonds) e.g. palmitic (C_{16}) and stearic (C_{18}) acids, or
  Unsaturated fatty acids (i.e. one or more double bonds) e.g. oleic, linoleic and arachidonic acids.
- Fatty acids may be *esterified* with glycerol to form glycerides, or they may be free fatty acids (FFA) or *non-esterified* free fatty acids (NEFA).
- *Essential fatty acids*: certain polyunsaturated fatty acids cannot be synthesized, e.g. linoleic and linolenic acids. They may function as:
  1. Precursors of prostaglandins (see Prostanoids, p. 261)
  2. Confer on membrane phospholipids many of the properties associated with membrane function.

TRIGLYCERIDES

- Major dietary lipids of nutritional value. They are degraded in the small intestine by lipases into monoglycerides, fatty acids and glycerol.
- Esters of glycerol with three fatty acids.

$CH_2.O - FA$
|
$CH_2.O - FA$
|
$CH_2.O - FA$

- Mostly resynthesized into triglycerides in mucosal cells, and transported via the lymphatic system as chylomicrons into the systemic circulation.
- Adipose tissue and liver are the major sites of endogenous triglyceride synthesis. Transported from the liver as VLDL.

PHOSPHOLIPIDS

Phosphoglycerides and sphingolipids (Fig. 6.12).
- Triglycerides with one of the fatty acid residues replaced by a nitrogenous base, e.g. choline (phosphatidylcholine or lecithin), ethanolamine (phosphatidylethanolamine), serine or inositol (phosphatidylinositol), and linked to the glycerol via a phosphate residue.

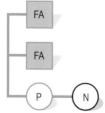

Fig. 6.12 Structure of phospholipids.

- Mainly synthesized in the mucosa of the small intestine and in the liver.
- Important constituents of biological membranes and of the plasma lipoproteins.
- Includes the sphingolipid class which are characterized by the presence of the base sphingosine and comprise the ceramides, cerebrosides, sulphatides, gangliosides and sphingomyelin; all components of white matter in the central nervous system.

CHOLESTEROL (Fig. 6.13)

- Major constituent of the plasma membrane and of plasma lipoproteins. Widely distributed in all cells, but particularly nervous tissue.
- Two sources of cholesterol: *dietary cholesterol* (mostly triglycerides) ~70 g/day, and *de novo synthesis* from acetate.

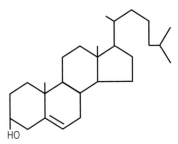

Fig. 6.13 Cholesterol.

OTHERS

Other lipids of clinical significance include carotene, vitamins A, D, E and K.

DIGESTION OF FATS: EXOGENOUS PATHWAY

- The entry of fats into the duodenum causes the release of pancreozymin-cholecystokinin, which in turn stimulates evacuation of the gall bladder.
- Hydrolysis of dietary triglycerides by pancreatic lipase takes place in the small intestine. The resulting free fatty acids, glycerol and monoglycerides are emulsified by bile salts and form micelles which are then absorbed along the brush border of mucosal cells.
- Small fatty acids enter the portal circulation bound to albumin. Larger ones are re-esterified within the mucosal cell into triglycerides which combine with lesser amounts of protein, phospholipid and cholesterol to create chylomicrons.
- Chylomicrons represent triglycerides and esters of cholesterol, with a coating of phospholipid, protein and cholesterol. These enter the lymphatic system and are transported via the thoracic duct to the bloodstream.
- The main sites for removal of chylomicrons are the muscle and liver. *Lipoprotein lipase*, an enzyme bound to the capillary endothelium of extrahepatic tissues, hydrolyses triglycerides in chylomicrons, and VLDL into free fatty acids and glycerol. After entering adipose tissue or muscle, these compounds are esterified and stored.
- The smaller remnant particles contain mainly cholesterol, and pass to the liver where they are metabolized further.

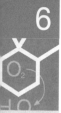
LIPID TRANSPORT: LIPOPROTEINS (Table 6.3 and Fig. 6.14): ENDOGENOUS PATHWAY

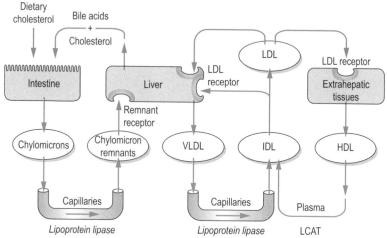

Fig. 6.14 Lipid metabolism.

- In plasma, free fatty acids (FFA) are bound to albumin. Other lipids (e.g. cholesterol, triglycerides and phospholipids) circulate with carrier apoproteins to form a series of soluble lipoprotein complexes. In general, the lipoproteins consist of a hydrophobic core of cholesterol and triglyceride esters surrounded by phospholipid and protein.

- Most endogenous cholesterol and triglycerides formed in the liver are transported from the liver as VLDL. In the peripheral tissues triglycerides are removed in the same way as chylomicrons. The smaller complex is further degraded via intermediate density lipoprotein (IDL) to form LDL, which is mainly composed of cholesterol. Most cells have surface receptors for LDL. LDL is bound and enters the cells by a process of receptor-mediated endocytosis, where the cholesterol is released and which in turn suppresses endogenous cholesterol synthesis.

- HDL carries the cholesterol formed peripherally from the peripheral tissues to the liver, to be excreted in the bile. An enzyme *lecithin-cholesterolacyl transferase (LCAT)* is associated with HDL and esterifies cholesterol. In LCAT deficiency, free unesterified cholesterol accumulates in the tissues.

Apolipoproteins

1. Apo A-I and apo A-II
   - Major components of HDL.
2. Apo B
   - Structural protein for chylomicron remnants, VLDL, LDL.
3. Apo C-I, apo C-II, and apo E-III
   - Normally stored in HDL between meals, but transfer to triglyceride-rich lipoproteins after meals.
4. Apo E-I, apo E-II, apo E-III, and apo E-IV
   - Enter plasma with nascent HDL produced in liver.
   - Transfer with cholesterol ester from HDL to triglyceride-rich lipoprotein remnants.

Table 6.3 Lipids and metabolism

	Chylomicrons (CM)	Low density or β-lipoprotein (LDL)	Very low density or pre-β-lipoprotein (VLDL)	High density α-lipoprotein (HDL)
Site of synthesis	Intestine	In blood and liver from VLDL	Liver and intestine	Liver and intestine
Function	Transport of dietary fat from the intestine to the liver and adipose tissue. The triglycerides are hydrolysed by lipoprotein lipase, and the cholesterol rich remnants are taken up by the liver	Transport of cholesterol to the tissues. LDL is removed by a receptor-mediated process	Transport of endogenous triglycerides from the liver. Degraded by lipoprotein lipase, resulting in the production of IDL*, then LDL	Transport of cholesterol from the plasma to the liver for excretion
Diameter (nm)	100–1000	25	50	10
Apoprotein[†]	A, B, C	B	B, C	A, C
% Triglyceride	85	10	50	10
% Cholesterol	4	50	20	15
% Protein	1	20	7	45

* IDL, intermediate density lipoprotein.
[†] Nine apolipoproteins: Apo A-I, A-II, A-IV, B, C-I, C-II, C-III, D and E have been isolated and characterized.

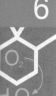

LIPID METABOLISM

LIPOLYSIS

- Adipose tissue also contains an enzyme, *hormone-sensitive lipase (HSL)*, that hydrolyses triglycerides to produce fatty acids and glycerol. HSL is activated by catecholamines, ACTH, TSH and glucagon and inhibited by insulin, which stimulates glucose uptake for lipogenesis.
- The fatty acids released from adipose tissue are either bound to plasma albumin or circulate as free fatty acids (FFA) or non-esterified fatty acids (NEFA) and are taken up by the peripheral tissues for oxidation.
- *β-Oxidation of fatty acids*: is the process of degradation of fatty acids for energy and involves the removal of two carbon units at a time. It takes place in the mitochondria of the liver and muscle and results in the formation of acetyl coA and fatty acid residue.

LIPOGENESIS

- Synthesis of triglycerides from fatty acids, glycerophosphate and non-fat materials, especially carbohydrate.
- Occurs mainly in the liver, but also in the adipose tissue within the microsomes. Takes place in the cytoplasm.
- Occurs in two stages:
  1. The transfer of acetyl CoA from the mitochondria to the cytoplasm and the formation of malonyl-CoA from acetyl-CoA, via the acetyl CoA shuttle system.
  2. The second stage involves the reaction pathway of the *fatty acid synthetase (FAS) multienzyme complex*. The control step is catalysed by acetyl-CoA carboxylase and requires NADPH. Fatty acids longer than 16 carbon atoms can be formed through the addition of two carbon units by elongation systems.

After synthesis in *adipose tissue*, they are stored as fat droplets. After synthesis in the *liver*, they are then packaged with apoprotein molecules and secreted into the blood.

CHOLESTEROL METABOLISM (Fig. 6.15)

- *Hydroxymethyl-glutaryl-CoA reductase (HMGCoA reductase)* is a key enzyme that catalyses the reduction of β-hydroxy-β-methylglutaryl-coenzyme A (HMG-CoA) to mevalonate and regulates the activity of the pathway for cholesterol synthesis from acetate.

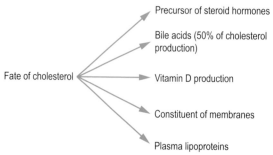

Fig. 6.15 Fate of cholesterol.

- The greater the dietary intake of cholesterol, the lower the rate of endogenous cholesterol biosynthesis in the liver and adrenal cortex. Synthesis in the peripheral tissues is regulated by the plasma LDL level. Diets high in fat or carbohydrate increase hepatic cholesterol synthesis.

PROSTANOID (EICOSANOID) METABOLISM

1. Prostaglandins (PGs) (Fig. 6.16)
   20-carbon unsaturated fatty acids containing a 5-carbon cyclopentane ring.
   Each *series* (A,B,E,F) has a different cyclopentane ring.
   Each *subset* $(_{1,2,3,4})$ denotes the degree of unsaturation of the hydrocarbon chain.

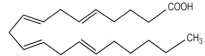

Fig. 6.16 Structure of prostaglandin.

2. Prostacyclin.
3. Thromboxanes (TX).
4. Leucotrienes (LT).

PATHWAYS OF SYNTHESIS AND METABOLISM (Fig. 6.17)

Synthesized in almost any tissue. The lung is the most important site for breakdown.

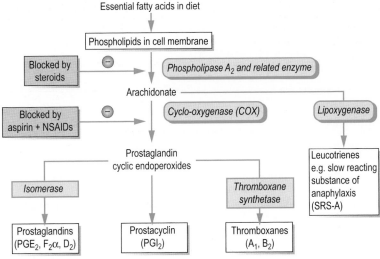

Fig. 6.17 Prostanoid metabolism.

Cyclo-oxygenase

Cyclo-oxygenase exists in two enzyme isoforms:

1. *COX-1* which is expressed in most tissues, especially platelets, gastric mucosa and renal vasculature. It is involved in physiological cell signalling. Most adverse effects of NSAIDs are caused by inhibition of COX-1.

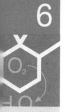
2. *COX-2*, which is induced at sites of inflammation and produces the prostanoids involved in inflammatory responses. Analgesic and anti-inflammatory effects of NSAIDs are largely a result of inhibition of COX-2. COX-2 specific inhibitors, e.g. rofecoxib and celecoxib, are now licensed for treatment of osteoarthritis and rheumatoid arthritis.

Inhibition of cyclo-oxygenase can occur by the following mechanisms:
- Irreversible inhibition, e.g. aspirin
- Competitive inhibition, e.g. ibuprofen
- Reversible, non-competitive, e.g. paracetamol.

PHARMACOLOGICAL AND PHYSIOLOGICAL EFFECTS

1. Variable effects on smooth muscle and blood vessels depending on the prostaglandin series.
2. Chemotaxis for neutrophils and eosinophils.
3. Increased vascular permeability; vasodilatation (prostacyclin).
4. Smooth muscle contraction and uterine contraction (PGE_2).
5. Stimulate or inhibit (prostacyclin) platelet aggregation.
6. Type 1 hypersensitivity reactions.

Comparison of prostacyclins and thromboxanes (Table 6.4)

Table 6.4 Prostacyclins and thromboxanes		
	Prostacyclin	*Thromboxanes*
Site of synthesis	Blood vessel wall	Platelets
Platelet aggregation	Inhibited	Stimulated
Coronary arteries	Relaxed (vasodilatation)	Constricted (vasoconstriction)
Blood pressure	Lowered	Raised
Smooth muscle	Relaxation PGE_1 and E_2 inhibits motility of non-pregnant uterus but increases contraction of pregnant uterus	Contraction

The leukotrienes

- Synthesized by leucocytes. Mediators of inflammation and allergic reactions.
- Produce arteriolar and bronchoconstriction, increase vascular permeability and attract neutrophils and eosinophils to inflammatory sites.
- Leukotriene D_4 has been identified as SRS-A which causes smooth muscle contraction.

HYPERLIPIDAEMIAS

Six inherited types identified (Table 6.5).

Table 6.5 Hyperlipidaemias (Fredrickson's classification)

Type	Lipoprotein abnormality	Biochemical feature	Causes
I	↑ Chylomicron	Marked hypertriglyceridaemia (↑ TG)	1° Usually familial (lipoprotein lipase deficiency: autosomal recessive)
IIa	↑ LDL	Hypercholesterolaemia with normal triglycerides (↑ CHOL)	1° Familial hypercholesterolaemia (absence or deficiency of normal receptor for LDL: autosomal dominant) 2° Hypothyroidism, obstructive jaundice, nephrotic syndrome, pregnancy, diabetes mellitus, obesity
IIb	↑ LDL and VLDL	Familial combined hyperlipidaemia (1° ↑ TG + CHOL)	1° Usually familial
III	Abnormal β-lipoprotein	Combined hyperlipidaemia (2° ↑ TG + CHOL)	2° Diabetes mellitus, hypothyroidism, renal disease
IV	↑ VLDL and chylomicron	Familial hypertriglyceridaemia (1° ↑ TG ± ↑ CHOL)	1° Usually familial 2° Diabetes, hypothyroidism, obesity, liver disease, alcoholism, nephrotic syndrome, pancreatitis, pregnancy, oral contraceptives, steroids, anorexia nervosa and glycogen storage diseases
V	↑ VLDL and chylomicron	Equivalent of Type I and IV	

In general:
All types except Type I have an ↑ cholesterol and all types except Type II have ↑ triglycerides.

Causes of raised HDL
1. Increasing age
2. Exercise
3. Fish diet
4. Moderate alcohol consumption.

Causes of reduced HDL
1. Smoking
2. Obesity and a high carbohydrate diet
3. Androgens and progesterone.

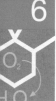
HYPOLIPOPROTEINAEMIAS

1. **Abetalipoproteinaemia**
   - Rare, autosomal recessive. LDL deficiency due to complete absence of apoprotein B. Chylomicrons, VLDL, IDL and LDL are absent from the plasma.
   - Clinical features include: steatorrhoea, failure to thrive, ataxia, nystagmus, muscle weakness, abnormal red cell morphology (acanthocytosis) and low serum lipid concentrations.
2. **Tangier disease (α-lipoprotein (HDL) deficiency)**
   - Rare; autosomal recessive.
   - Reduced HDL, LDL and very low levels of apoA due to a high rate of catabolism.

SPHINGOLIPIDOSES AND MUCOPOLYSACCHARIDOSES

Disorders of sphingolipid and mucopolysaccharide metabolism are described in Tables 6.6 and 6.7.

Table 6.6 Disorders of sphingolipid metabolism (sphingolipidoses)

Disease	Defective enzyme	Clinical features/prognosis	Laboratory features/comments
1. Tay–Sachs	Hexosaminidase A (Ganglioside $GM_1 \rightarrow GM_2$)	• Presents at 6–9 months with mental retardation, spastic motor weakness and progressive optic atrophy (cherry-red spot at the macula) • No organomegaly or bony involvement • Death aged 3–5 years	• Reduced serum hexosaminidase activity • Prenatal detection available, but 80% of cases present first appearance of disease in families • High frequency of heterozygotes in Ashkenazi Jews
2. Gaucher's	β-Glucosidase (Glucocerebroside → galactose)	• Mental retardation with spasticity, marked hepatosplenomegaly and erosion of long bones in infants • Death occurs within months in *infant* form, but almost normal lifespan in *adult* form	• Cerebroside-filled • Gaucher cells in marrow or liver biopsy • Raised serum acid phosphatase • High frequency in Ashkenazi Jews
3. Niemann–Pick	Sphingomyelinase (Sphingomyelin → ceramide + phosphorylcholine)	• Mental retardation and hepatosplenomegaly • May resemble Tay–Sachs with a cherry-red spot at the macula • Early death	• Typical foam cells in marrow and liver biopsy
4. Metachromatic leucodystrophy	Arylsulphatase-A (catabolism of sulphides)	• Mental retardation and demyelination in adults	• Reduced enzyme activity in leucocytes

Table 6.7 Disorders of mucopolysaccharide metabolism (mucopolysaccharidoses*). Accumulation of glycosaminoglycans in fibroblasts and chrondrocytes

Syndrome	Defective enzyme	Clinical features/prognosis	Laboratory features	Treatment
1. Hurler's (best recognized form) 2. Hunter's	Iduronidase and iduronate sulphatase respectively (degradation of dermatan and heparan sulphate)	• Both have similar clinical features with severe mental and growth retardation by end of first year, facial abnormalities ('gargoylism'), macroglossia, hepatosplenomegaly, heart disease, corneal opacities (Hurler's syndrome only) and conductive nerve deafness • Death occurs in childhood	• Dermatan sulphate and heparan sulphate in urine, tissues and amniotic fluid • Presence of mucopolysaccharide inclusion bodies (Alder–Reilly bodies) in white blood cells	• Plasma infusion/enzyme replacement

* Other mucopolysaccharidoses include Sanfilippo's, Morquino's and Scheie's syndromes (mental retardation absent or slight).

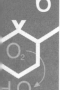

6

BIOCHEMISTRY, CELL BIOLOGY AND CLINICAL CHEMISTRY

AMINO ACIDS (Table 6.8)

- All the common amino acids (except for proline) have the same general structure: α-carbon bears a carboxy (COOH) and an amino (NH_2^-) group, but they differ with respect to their side-chain or 'R' groups.
- The 'R' groups confer their characteristic properties on each amino acid.

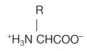

$$R$$
$$|$$
$$^+H_3N\ CHCOO^-$$

Table 6.8 The essential and non-essential amino acids

Essential (cannot be synthesized in the body, therefore must be present in the diet)	Non-essential (synthesized in the body from metabolites from other pathways)
Isoleucine — aliphatic	Alanine — aliphatic non-polar
Leucine — non-polar	Aspartic acid — acidic side chain
Valine	Hydroxyproline
Phenylalanine	Glutamic acid — acidic side chain
Tyrosine — aromatic	Glycine — aliphatic non-polar
Tryptophan	Cystine
Methionine ⎫ sulphur-containing	Proline — imino acid
Cysteine ⎭	Serine — hydroxy side chain
Arginine — basic	Tyrosine
Histidine — basic	Cysteine
Lysine — basic	Hydroxylysine
Threonine — hydroxy side chain	

Essential amino acids

Mnemonic for essential amino acids: **PVT TIM HALL**

P — phenylalanine	**T** — tryptophan	**H** — histidine
V — valine	**I** — isoleucine	**A** — arginine
T — threonine	**M** — methionine	**L** — lysine
		L — leucine

✓

PROTEINS

- Linear, unbranched polymers constructed from 20 different α-amino acids.
- The peptide bond is formed between the α-carboxyl group (C-terminal) of one amino acid and the α-amino group (N-terminal) of another.
- The *specific biological action* of the protein is determined by its primary, secondary, tertiary and quaternary structure.

  1° structure is the specific order of amino acids in the peptide chain.

  2° structure is the spatial relationships of neighbouring amino acid residues produced by twisting and turning, e.g. α-helix.

  3° structure is the spatial relationship of more distant residues produced by arrangement of the secondary structure into layers, crystals and fibres.

  4° structure is the spatial relationship between individual polypeptide chains, e.g. arrangement of subunits of haemoglobin.

Biological value

- The *biological value* of a protein is determined by its content of essential amino acids.
- A *high* biological value protein supplies all the essential amino acids in optimal proportions, e.g. most animal proteins (meat and eggs).
- A *low* biological value protein is deficient in one or more essential amino acids, e.g. rice protein is deficient in lysine and threonine.

DIGESTION OF PROTEINS

- Pepsin hydrolyses protein in the stomach (pH optimum 2.5) to produce shorter peptide chains.
- Further breakdown into free amino acids occurs through the action of the pancreatic proteolytic enzymes (endopeptidases and carboxypeptidases) and the brush border enzymes (dipeptidases and aminopeptidases).
- The gastric and pancreatic proteases are secreted into the duodenum as zymogens, or inactive precursors, e.g. pepsinogen, trypsinogen and chymotrypsinogen.
- The small intestine absorbs these free amino acids by active transport. They then enter the hepatoportal venous system and are carried to the liver.

Intestinal transport mechanisms
- Several specific intestinal transport mechanisms exist for different classes of amino acids (e.g. small neutral, large neutral, basic and acidic amino acids and proline).

The transport is tightly coupled to the entry of Na^+ into the cell, with the energy derived from the Na^+ gradient.

For defects in the transport of amino acids see page 270.

PROTEIN METABOLISM (Fig. 6.18)

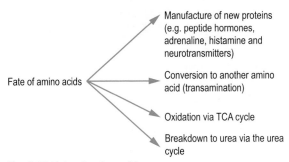

Fig. 6.18 Fate of amino acids.

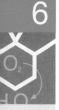

Protein catabolism

- Breakdown of protein to free amino acids. Main site of catabolism is in the liver; the kidney is a secondary site.
- The metabolic pathways of amino acid degradation include transamination, oxidative deamination, direct deamination and the urea cycle. The carbon skeletons of the amino acids can be oxidized to make glucose in the process of gluconeogenesis.

Urea cycle

- Takes place in the liver and brain and involves the condensation of ornithine with carbamyl phosphate to form citrulline which then combines with aspartic acid to form arginosuccinate. Arginosuccinate is cleaved to arginine which is then hydrolysed to urea and ornithine.
- The first two reactions are rate-controlling, catalysed by: *carbamyl phosphate synthetase* and *ornithine transcarbamylase*, both located in the mitochondria.
- The remainder of the urea cycle takes place in the cytoplasm.

Nitrogen balance

Positive nitrogen balance exists if the total daily nitrogen losses in urine, skin and faeces are less than the total daily nitrogen intake, e.g. as in healthy, growing children or convalescing adults. *Negative nitrogen balance* exists if nitrogen losses are greater than intake, e.g. in disease involving tissue wasting or in starvation.

DISORDERS OF AMINO ACID METABOLISM

INBORN ERRORS OF AMINO ACID METABOLISM (Table 6.9 and Fig. 6.19)

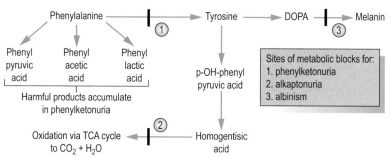

Fig. 6.19 Inborn errors of amino acid metabolism.
DOPA = dihydroxyphenylalanine.

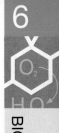

Table 6.9 Inborn errors of amino acid metabolism (see Fig. 6.19)

Disease	Site of metabolic block	Clinical features	Laboratory features	Treatment
1. Phenylketonuria (PKU) Incidence 1:12 000 births	Phenylalanine hydroxylase pathway **(1)**	• Presents in early childhood with reduced pigmentation, eczema, mental retardation (IQ usually <20) and seizures	• Raised blood phenylalanine at approx. 1 week after birth; phenylpyruvic acid in urine (phenistix +ve) • Prenatal diagnosis available	• Low phenylalanine diet • Early treatment important
2. Alkaptonuria Incidence 1:300 000 births	Homogentisic acid oxidase pathway **(2)**	• Deposition of homogentisic acid in cartilage and other tissues causing ochronosis, pigmentation of face, ears and sclera and arthritis • Urine darkens on exposure to air		
3. Albinism Three types: 1. Oculocutaneous (autosomal recessive) 2. Ocular (X-linked) 3. Cutaneous (autosomal dominant)	Tyrosinase pathway **(3)**	• White hair, photosensitive skin • Prominent red reflex from unpigmented fundus. Strabismus, nystagmus, photophobia, and loss of visual acuity		
4. Homocystinuria Incidence 1:160 000 births	Cystathione-β-synthetase (Homocysteine + serine → cystathionine)	• Mental retardation, seizures, spastic paraplegia, osteoporosis, cataractcs, and thromboembolic disease • Some features similar to Marfan's syndrome, i.e. dislocation of lens (but downwards) arachnodactyly, high arched palate, lax ligaments, kyphoscoliosis; but no dissecting aneurysm	• Elevated plasma methionine and urinary homocystine • Prenatal diagnosis and carrier detection available	• Dietary restriction of methionine with cystine supplementation
5. Maple syrup urine disease Incidence 1:175 000 births	Branched chain ketoacid decarboxylase	• Presents in 1st week of life, with mental deficiency, areflexia, dysphagia, metabolic acidosis and hypoglycaemia	• Characteristic urine smell • Leucocyte/fibroblast enzyme analysis	• Reduced intake of branched chain amino acids

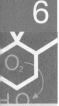

BIOCHEMISTRY, CELL BIOLOGY AND CLINICAL CHEMISTRY

AMINO ACID TRANSPORT DEFECTS

Generalized aminoaciduria

Causes
1. 'Overflow'
   Amino acid infusion, liver failure and inborn errors of metabolism, e.g. phenylketonuria, maple syrup urine, homocystinuria.
2. Renal causes
   (i) Specific transport defects, e.g. cystinuria, Hartnup's disease
   (ii) General tubular damage, e.g. Fanconi syndrome, heavy metal poisoning, drugs (neomycin), nutritional deficiencies (e.g. vitamins D and B_{12}), acute tubular necrosis, nephrotic syndrome and renal transplant rejection.

Specific transport defects

1. **Cystinuria** (not an inborn error of metabolism). Defective transport of the basic amino acids (*cystine*, *ornithine*, *arginine* and *lysine*) in the renal tubule and the gastrointestinal tract.
   Clinical features: Cystine urinary calculi and crystals in the urine. The cyanide-nitroprusside urine test is positive in cystinuria and homocystinuria.
2. **Hartnup's disease** (not an inborn error of metabolism). Defective renal and intestinal transport of neutral amino acids, especially tryptophan.
   Clinical features: Malabsorption, ataxia and pellagra rash.

General tubular damage

1. **Fanconi syndrome**
Causes:
* *Inherited*: Cystinosis, galactosaemia, hereditary fructose intolerance, glycogen storage disease Type I, and Wilson's disease.
* *Acquired*:
  – Poisoning, e.g. mercury, lead, zinc, bismuth, arsenic, Paraquat.
  – Drugs, e.g. salicylates, cisplatinum, adefovir and tenofovir.
  – Renal diseases, e.g. acute tubular necrosis, nephrotic syndrome, renal transplant rejection.
  – Nutritional deficiency, e.g. vitamins B_{12} and D, kwashiorkor.

Clinical features: Generalized aminoaciduria, glycosuria, and hyperphosphaturia, rickets or osteomalacia, *also* acidosis, hypokalaemia, polyuria and hypouricaemia.

2. **Cystinosis** (compare with cystinuria and homocystinuria (p. 269). Deposition of L-cystine crystals in the proximal renal tubule, reticuloendothelial tissue and cornea.

Clinical features: Fanconi syndrome, renal tubular acidosis, progressive renal failure and hepatosplenomegaly.

Hyperhomocysteinaemia
* *Severe*: Associated with increased risk of cerebral vascular and peripheral thromboembolism and vascular disease.
* Causes: Homozygous deficiency of cystathionine-B synthase.
* Clinical features: Mental retardation, osteoporosis, ectopic lens, skeletal abnormalities, premature vascular disease and venous thrombosis.
* *Mild/moderate*: Caused by gene defects, or acquired, e.g. nutritional deficiencies of cobalamin, folate, pyridoxine, renal insufficiency, hypothyroidism, and folate metabolism inhibitors, e.g. anticonvulsants.

SPECIALIZED PROTEINS

HAEMOGLOBIN

Structure (see also Table 6.10)

- Mol. weight = 67 000.
- Each haemoglobin molecule consists of a globin molecule and four haem groups (tetramer). Each haem group is a binding site for oxygen.
- *Haem part*: ferrous complex of protoporphyrin IX arranged in four pyrrole rings.
- *Globin part*: two pairs of polypeptide chains (α and β chains) are linked through histidine residues with one haem molecule. In both myoglobin and haemoglobin, the iron of the haem group is in the Fe^{2+} form. When in the ferric or Fe^{3+} form, the proteins are methaemoglobin and metmyoglobin.

Table 6.10 Normal human haemoglobins

Haemoglobin	% of normal adult haemoglobin	% of haemoglobin at birth	Globin structure
A	97	10–50	$\alpha_2\beta_2$
A_2	2.5	Trace	$\alpha_2\delta_2$
F (fetal)	0.5	50–90	$\alpha_2\gamma_2$

PORPHYRIN AND HAEM SYNTHESIS (Fig. 6.20)

Three main successive steps in the pathway:

1. Biosynthesis of δ-amino laevulinic acid (ALA) from the precursors, glycine and succinyl coA. The enzyme for this reaction, δ-*aminolaevulinate synthetase (ALA-S)* is the rate-controlling enzyme for porphyrin synthesis.
2. Two molecules of ALA condense to form porphobilinogen.
3. Conversion of porphobilinogen to the cyclic tetrapyrrole porphyrin ring and haem. Haem, the end-product of porphyrin synthesis inhibits ALA-synthetase.

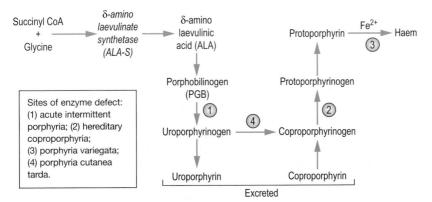

Fig. 6.20 Porphyrin and haem synthesis.

Haem pigments

Other important haem-containing compounds in the body include:
- Myoglobin: oxygen-binding pigment found in red (slow) muscle and in the respiratory enzyme cytochrome *c*
- Enzymes, e.g. catalase and peroxidase
- Cytochromes: conjugated proteins in which the prosthetic group (haem) is a porphyrin ring (see Note) containing an iron atom, e.g. cytochrome *c* and cytochrome p450 (liver microsomes).

Note: Large, flat, heterocyclic ring structures made up of four pyrrole rings linked together by $-C=$ bridges, and found in all aerobic cells.

OXYGEN DISSOCIATION CURVE OF HAEMOGLOBIN (AND MYOGLOBIN)
(Fig. 6.21)

The relationship between the percentage saturation of haemoglobin and partial pressure of oxygen in arterial blood (Pa_{O_2}).

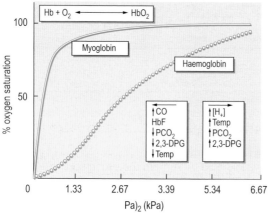

Fig. 6.21 Oxygen dissociation curve.

Haemoglobin curve
- Oxygen binds to the Fe^{2+} in haem to form oxyhaemoglobin.
- Sigmoidal-shaped curve due to positive cooperativity, i.e. the binding of one oxygen molecule facilitates the binding of the next. Similarly, the release of one oxygen molecule promotes the release of others.
- The effect of pH on the oxygen binding of haemoglobin is called the *Bohr effect*. The affinity of Hb for O_2 increases at higher pH, and decreases with a fall in pH.
- High P_{CO_2}, acidosis, raised 2,3-diphosphoglycerate (2,3-DPG) (see Note) or raised temperature are associated with a shift in the oxygen dissociation curve to the *right* (i.e. a lower O_2 saturation for a given Pa_{O_2}).
- Low Pa_{CO_2}, acute alkalosis, reduced 2,3-DPG, hypothermia, certain rare haemoglobinopathies (haemoglobins Chesapeake and Heathrow), in cells containing fetal Hb and with methaemoglobin and carboxyhaemoglobin, the oxygen dissociation curve is well to the *left* of that of normal Hb, i.e. oxygen affinity is increased, leading to tissue hypoxia.

Myoglobin curve
- One oxygen molecule bound per haem molecule, i.e. the myoglobin molecule does not alter conformation on oxygenation, and shows no Bohr effect. Follows Michaelis–Menten kinetics and produces a hyperbolic curve.

Table 6.11 Summary of binding characteristics

Myoglobin	Haemoglobin
Monomer	Tetramer, 2α and 2β chains
Binds one O_2	Binds $4O_2$
Binding kinetics hyperbolic	Binding kinetics sigmoidal

Note: *2,3-Diphosphoglycerate (2,3-DPG)* is synthesized in the red cells from metabolites of the glycolytic pathway. It binds to haemoglobin, stabilizing the deoxy form, and reduces the affinity of haemoglobin for oxygen, causing the release of oxygen. Production is stimulated by hypoxia, e.g. anaemia and altitude.

Carriage of gases

Oxygen
1. Combined with haemoglobin in the red cell: 1 g of haemoglobin carries 1.39 ml of oxygen.
2. Dissolved in plasma: at 100 mmHg, 0.3 ml oxygen is dissolved in every 100 ml of blood.

Carbon dioxide
1. In plasma, mostly as bicarbonate, but also as carbonic acid and carbamino compounds with plasma proteins.
2. In red blood cells as carbaminohaemoglobin (30%) and bicarbonate (60%).
3. Dissolved in plasma (5%).

Carbon dioxide has 20 times the rate of diffusion of oxygen. The capacity of blood and tissues for CO_2 is three times and 100 times respectively greater than for oxygen.

The CO_2 dissociation curve is relatively linear over a physiological range of oxygen tensions.

DISORDERS OF HAEM SYNTHESIS (Table 6.12)

Other causes of excessive porphyrin excretion
1. Lead poisoning: Inhibits several enzymes in haem synthesis.
   Clinical features: Intestinal colic, gingivitis, blue line on gums. Lead encephalopathy (mortality 25%), motor neuropathy. Haematological effects: anaemia (may be sideroblastic), basophilic stippling, reticulocytosis, increased serum iron. Large amounts of urinary coproporphyrin and ALA.
2. Cholestatic liver disease: Increased urinary coproporphyrin, possibly due to decreased biliary excretion.
3. Iron deficiency anaemia and sideroblastic anaemia.
4. Dubin–Johnson syndrome.
5. Gilbert's syndrome.

Precipitants of an acute porphyria attack
1. Antibiotics e.g. rifampicin, sulphonamides, chloramphenicol, tetracyclines, pyrazinamide, dapsone
2. Anticonvulsants e.g. phenytoin, phenobarbitone
3. Other drugs e.g. alcohol, oral contraceptives, methyldopa, sulphonylureas, chloroquine
4. Other causes e.g. pregnancy, stress, sepsis.

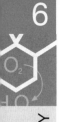

Table 6.12 Disorders of haem synthesis

	Hepatic porphyrias	**Porphyria cutanea tarda (PCT)**	**Erythropoietic porphyrias***	
	Acute intermittent porphyria (AIP) Porphyria variegata (VP) Hereditary coproporphyria (HCP)		Congenital porphyria (Gunther's disease)	Erythropoietic porphyria
Cell affected	Liver	Erythrocyte and liver	Erythrocyte	Erythrocyte
Inheritance	Autosomal recessive Increased activity of liver ALA-S	No family history Usually secondary to chronic (especially alcoholic) liver disease	Autosomal dominant Rare	Autosomal dominant
Clinical features	1. GI: abdo pain, vomiting and constipation 2. CNS: peripheral neuropathy, confusion and psychosis 3. CVS: tachycardia and hypertension 4. Fragile skin with VP 5. Acute attacks precipitated by: drugs (see p. 340), alcohol, hormonal change, diet and infection	1. Skin photosensitivity, hypertrichosis, skin pigmentation 2. Liver function test abnormal	Pink teeth, hypertrichosis and severe photosensitivity	Photosensitivity and hepatocellular damage
Accumulating materials	δ-Aminolaevulinic acid (ALA) and porphobilinogen (PBG)	Uroporphyrins	ALA and PBG excretion are normal Uroporphyrin I and coproporphyrin	ALA and PBG excretion are normal Protoporphyrin
Diagnosis	1. ↑ ALA and PBG in the urine and ↑ faecal porphyrins with VP and HCP 2. Urine turns deep red in sunlight†	Excess plasma, faecal and urinary uroporphyrins and coproporphyrins	Both compounds in erythrocytes, urine, and faeces (red urine)	↑ Erythrocyte, urine and faecal protoporphyrin

* Acute attacks do not occur.
† Porphyrinogens, ALA and PBG are colourless, but oxidize to corresponding porphyrins which are dark red and fluoresce in UV light.

ABNORMAL DERIVATIVES OF HAEMOGLOBIN

Methaemoglobin

Form of oxidized Hb (Fe^{2+} replaced by Fe^{3+}), so that ability to act as an O_2 carrier is lost.

Causes of methaemoglobinaemia
1. Haemoglobinopathies, e.g. HbM, deficiency of NADH-methaemoglobin reductase.
2. Drugs: phenacetin, primaquine, sulphonamides, nitrites, nitrates (after conversion to nitrites in the gut), and various aniline dye derivates.

Carboxyhaemoglobin (HbCO)

- Haemoglobin can combine with carbon monoxide (CO) to form carboxyhaemoglobin.
- Affinity of haemoglobin for CO is 200 times that for O_2, so CO will displace O_2 from oxyhaemoglobin.

Glycosylated haemoglobin (HbA$_{1c}$)

- Glycosylation occurs as the result of binding between adult haemoglobin A and glucose during the 120 day lifespan of the red blood cell, and is an irreversible reaction.
- Normally about 6–9% of adult HbA is glycosylated and in the diabetic about 12–21%. Useful for providing a picture of the long-term state of diabetic control (over 2–3 months). Difficult to interpret in the presence of abnormalities of red blood cells.

DISORDERS OF GLOBIN SYNTHESIS

1. Haemoglobinopathies

Abnormal polypeptide chains are produced.

Sickle cell disease
- Substitution of valine for glutamic acid at 6th position on β chain. Abnormal HbS is produced, which is less soluble in the deoxygenated state.
- Homozygotes produce HbS with HbF and HbA$_2$. Heterozygotes produce 30–40% HbS and the rest HbA.
- World distribution of HbS: Central Africa, Mediterranean and India.

2. Thalassaemias

Polypeptide chains are normal in structure but are produced in decreased amounts.

1. β-Thalassaemia
- Homozygotes (thalassaemia major) are characterized by ↓ β-chain production and ↑ HbA$_2$ and HbF production. Mild disease in heterozygotes (thalassaemia minor) with HbA$_2$ ↑.
- World distribution: Middle East.

2. α-Thalassaemia
↓ α-chain production. Severe disease in homozygotes with death in utero, e.g. Hb-Barts of HbH, but insignificant disease in heterozygotes.

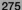

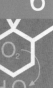

COLLAGEN

Structure and synthesis

- Collagen is formed by fibroblasts in connective tissues, osteoblasts in bone and chondroblasts in cartilage.
- Synthesized in an inactive form called procollagen which is then proteolytically processed outside the cell into tropocollagen. Three chains of tropocollagen twist around each other in a right-handed superhelix. Cleavage of the ends of tropocollagen forms collagen, which is held together by cross-links between hydroxylysine residues.
- Collagen has a unique distribution of amino acid residues with 33% glycine, 10% proline, 10% hydroxyproline and 1% hydroxylysine.
- Other examples of fibrous proteins are elastin and fibronectin.

DISORDERS OF METABOLISM OF COLLAGEN

1. Scurvy.
2. Ehlers–Danlos syndrome type VI
   - Enzyme lysyl hydroxylase is deficient and collagen with a reduced hydroxylysine content is formed.
   - Clinical features include musculoskeletal deformities, especially hypermobility of the joints and poor wound healing.
3. Homocystinuria.
4. Ehlers–Danlos syndrome type VIII
   - No proteolytic cleavage of the N-terminal peptide on procollagen.
   - Clinical features include hyperelastic skin which bruises easily and bilateral hip dislocation.

PURINES AND PYRIMIDINES

Physiologically important purines and pyrimidines
Purines: adenine, guanine, hypoxanthine and xanthine.
Pyrimidines: cytosine, uracil and thymidine.

METABOLISM

Synthesis
Most purines and pyrimidines are synthesized de novo from amino acids, especially in the liver, via complex pathways involving the incorporation of many molecules into the purine and pyrimidine structure or from the breakdown of ingested amino acids. The nucleotides of RNA and DNA are then synthesized.

Catabolism (Fig. 6.22)
- 90% of the purine and pyrimidine bases and nucleosides obtained from the breakdown of cellular polynucleotides are not catabolized, but salvaged and re-utilized. Minor amounts are excreted unchanged in the urine. The pyrimidines are catabolized to CO_2 and NH_3, and the purines are converted to uric acid.
- Two salvage pathways exist to regenerate AMP and GMP released from nucleosides:
  1. *Adenine phosphoribosyl transferase (APRT)* adds ribose phosphate from phosphoribosyl pyrophosphate (PRPP) to adenine to regenerate AMP.
  2. *Hypoxanthine guanine phosphoribosyl transferase (HGPRT)* catalyses the same reaction with guanine. In addition, adenosine may be deaminated to inosine, which then liberates its ribose forming hypoxanthine.

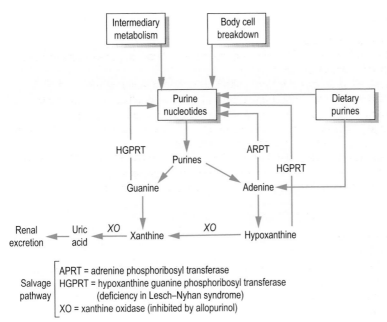

Fig. 6.22 Purine metabolism.

- Xanthine oxidase (XO) transforms hypoxanthine to xanthine and then into uric acid.

Uric acid
- Produced by breakdown of purine bases. Only 10% obtained from diet.
- Uric acid filtered at glomeruli, and 90% reabsorbed in proximal and distal convoluted tubules.
- 75% excreted via kidney.

DISORDERS OF PURINE AND PYRIMIDINE METABOLISM

Causes of hyperuricaemia
1. *Increased purine synthesis*
Primary gout (25% of cases due to increased synthesis de novo) Lesch–Nyhan syndrome (HGPRT deficiency), Type I glycogen storage disease.
2. *Increased purine turnover*
Myeloproliferative and lymphoproliferative disorders, polycythaemia, severe exfoliative psoriasis, high purine diet.
3. *Decreased excretion of uric acid*
Primary gout (75% of cases), renal failure, increased levels of organic acids, e.g. exercise, alcohol, diabetic ketoacidosis, starvation, hyperparathyroidism and lead poisoning.
4. *Drugs*
Thiazide and loop diuretics, pyrizinamide, ethambutol, salicylate in low doses, cytotoxic agents, ciclosporin and alcohol.

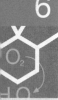

BIOCHEMISTRY, CELL BIOLOGY AND CLINICAL CHEMISTRY

HORMONAL CONTROL OF METABOLISM (Table 6.13)

Table 6.13 The principal actions of insulin, glucagon, adrenaline, cortisol and growth hormone

Action	Insulin	Glucagon	Adrenaline	Cortisol	Growth hormone
Liver					
Glycogen synthesis	↑	↓	↓	↑	↑
Glycogen breakdown	↓	↑	↑		
Gluconeogenesis	↓	↑	↑	↑	
Glucose release	↓	↑	↑	↑	↑
Ketone body production	↓	↑	↑		
Amino acid catabolism	↓	↑		↑	
Fatty acid synthesis	↑	↓	↓		
Muscle					
Fatty acid utilization			↑		↑
Glycogen breakdown	↓		↑		
Glucose uptake	↑		↓	↓	↓
Protein synthesis	↑			↓	↑
Adipose tissue					
Glucose uptake	↑	↑			
Fatty acid release	↓		↑	↑	↑
Triglyceride synthesis	↓				↑
Triglyceride storage	↑				

CLINICAL CHEMISTRY

VITAMINS

Vitamins exert their effects in three main ways: as coenzymes, antioxidants and hormones (Table 6.14).

Vitamins — Organic molecules required for certain metabolic functions that must be supplied in very small amounts (<50 mg/day).

Coenzyme — Non-protein organic molecule that binds to an enzyme to aid in the transfer of small functional groups. When it binds tightly, it is considered to be a *prosthetic* group of an enzyme.

Cofactor — Differs from a coenzyme only because it is usually a metallic ion rather than an organic molecule, e.g. Fe^{2+} in the cytochromes, and Mg^{2+} for enzymes utilizing ATP.

See Tables 6.15 and 6.16.

Table 6.14 Mode of action of vitamins

Coenzymes	Antioxidants	Hormones
Vitamin B_1 (thiamine) (water-soluble)	Vitamin C (water-soluble)	Vitamin A (fat-soluble)
Vitamin B_2 (riboflavin) (water-soluble)	Vitamin E (fat-soluble)	Vitamin D (fat-soluble)
Vitamin B_3 (nicotinic acid) (water-soluble)		
Vitamin B_6 (pyridoxine) (water-soluble)		
Vitamin B_{12} (cobalamin) (water-soluble)		
Biotin (water-soluble)		
Folic acid (water-soluble)		
Pantothenic acid (water-soluble)		
Vitamin K (fat-soluble)		

Table 6.15 Water-soluble vitamins

Vitamin	Source	Function	Deficiency state* and causes	Laboratory diagnosis
Thiamine Vitamin B_1	• Wholemeal flour, cereals (germinal layer), peas, beans and yeast	• Coenzyme: thiamine pyrophosphate (TPP) for decarboxylation of α-ketoacids (pyruvate to acetyl-CoA) and transketolation reactions	1. Glossitis 2. 'Dry' beri-beri: (polyneuritis and weight loss) 3. 'Wet' beri-beri: (high output cardiac failure) 4. Wernicke–Korsakoff syndrome: **Causes:** Occurs in chronic alcoholics and when polished rice is the main food	• ↑ Blood pyruvate and • ↓ Red cell transketolase activity • ↓ Urinary thiamine excretion
Riboflavin Vitamin B_2	• Meat, milk, wholemeal flour, fish and eggs	• Coenzyme of flavoproteins, e.g. flavin adenine dinucleotide (FAD) and flavin mononucleotide (FMN) (act as reversible electron carriers) for oxidation-reduction reactions	1. Angular stomatitis and cheliosis 2. Seborrhoeic dermatitis 3. Vascularized cornea 4. Peripheral neuropathy	• ↓ Plasma glutathione reductase
Niacin, nicotinic acid, nicotinamide Vitamin B_3	• Liver, wholemeal flour, and nuts • Also synthesized from tryptophan in the body	• Coenzyme, e.g. nicotinamide adenine dinucleotide (NAD), and NAD phosphate (NADP) (act as reversible electron carriers) for oxidation-reduction reactions, e.g. glycolysis and oxidative phosphorylation	1. Pellagra (3Ds: diarrhoea, dementia and dermatitis) 2. Neurological disease: (dementia and signs similar to those of subacute combined degeneration of the cord) **Causes:** Alcoholism, malabsorption, Hartnup's disease and isoniazid therapy	• ↑ Urinary excretion of N′-methyl nicotinamide
Pyridoxine Vitamin B_6	• Very widespread	• Coenzyme, e.g. pyridoxal phosphate (PP) for decarboxylation, transamination and deamination of amino acids	1. Glossitis and seborrhoea 2. Peripheral neuropathy and convulsions 3. Hypochromic anaemia **Causes:** Pregnancy, alcoholics, isoniazid or penicillamine therapy administration	• ↑ Urinary excretion of xanthurenate†
Panthothenic acid	• Widespread, but mainly liver, eggs, meat and milk	• Component of coenzyme A for the transport of acetyl and succinyl units	Lethargy and paraesthesia	

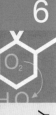

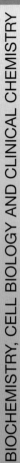

Table 6.15 *(Cont'd)*

Vitamin	Source	Function	Deficiency state* and causes	Laboratory diagnosis
Biotin	• Widespread • Synthesized by intestinal bacteria	• Coenzyme for carboxylation and decarboxylation reactions, e.g. malonyl-coA from acetyl-coA and oxaloacetate from pyruvate	• Seborrhoeic dermatitis, paraesthesia and lethargy • Induced by avidin (a protein in raw egg white), or by antibiotic therapy	
Cyanocobalamin Vitamin B_{12}	• Liver and all foods of animal origin • Normal body stores take 3–5 years for depletion • (Gastric intrinsic factor (IF) facilitates its absorption in the terminal ileum)	1. Coenzyme: (methylcobalamin, 5'-deoxyadenosyl cobalamin) in synthesis of nucleic acids and coenzymes 2. Transfer of methyl groups from N^5-methyltetrahydrofolate to homocysteine, regenerating methionine Homocysteine | *Methylcobalamin* (+ folic acid) ↓ Methionine 3. One-carbon reaction in the conversion of methylmalonyl-coA to succinyl-coA Methylmalonyl-coA | *5'-deoxyadenyl cobalamin* ↓ Succinyl-coA 4. Stimulates erythropoiesis‡	1. Megaloblastic anaemia, leucopenia and thrombocytopenia 2. Peripheral neuropathy: 'glove and stocking' distribution 3. Subacute combined degeneration of the cord 4. Optic atrophy, tobacco amblyopia 5. Depression and psychosis **Causes:** (i) Dietary deficiency (ii) Malabsorption *Stomach* (lack of IF): e.g. pernicious anaemia, partial/total gastrectomy *Gut:* e.g. Crohn's disease, ileal resection, jejunal diverticulae, blind loop syndrome and fish tapeworm	• ↑ AST and ALT • Serum B_{12} • Schilling test: see Table 6.17 • ↑ Methylmalonic acid excretion in urine in deficiency states • ↓ Levels of serum B_{12} in liver disease and myeloproliferative disorders

* Glossitis occurs in all five of the vitamin B deficiency states, in addition to iron deficiency anaemia.

† 24-hour urinary excretion of xanthurenate is measured before and after a loading dose of 2 g of L-tryptophan. Increased levels are excreted in patients with pyridoxine deficiency.

‡ Other substances essential to erythropoiesis include: erythropoietin, vitamins B_1, B_2, B_{12} and C, folic acids, protein, iron and trace elements (Mn, Co), hormones including thyroxine, cortisol, androgen and prolactin.

Table 6.15 (Cont'd)

Vitamin	Source	Function	Deficiency state* and causes	Laboratory diagnosis
Folic acid Contains: 1. Pteridine ring 2. Para-aminobenzoic acid (PABA) 3. Glutamate	• Widespread in small amounts, especially green vegetables, fruits and liver; also, synthesized by gut bacteria	• Coenzyme, e.g. tetrahydrofolic acid for reactions of 1-carbon units (e.g. conversion of homocysteine to methionine and conversion of serine to glycine) and for synthesis of purines and pyrimidines	• Megaloblastic anaemia **Causes:** (i) Dietary deficiency (especially in alcoholics and the elderly) (ii) Malabsorption, e.g. coeliac disease (most common), gastrectomy and Crohn's disease (iii) Excessive utilization, e.g. haematological disease (leukaemia, chronic haemolytic anaemia), malignancy, and inflammatory disease (rheumatoid arthritis, psoriasis) (iv) Drugs, e.g. phenytoin and methotrexate (v) Excessive loss, e.g. chronic dialysis	• ↓ Serum and red cell folate • ↑ Urinary excretion of forminoglutamate (FIGLU)
Vitamin C Ascorbic acid	• Fresh fruit, vegetables and liver • Destroyed by cooking (only primates and guinea pigs can synthesize vitamin C)	• Antioxidant and coenzyme in oxidation reactions. Required for: 1. Collagen synthesis (hydroxylation of proline and lysine residues) 2. Steroid metabolism 3. Electron and cytochrome P450 function 4. Increased gastrointestinal absorption of iron 5. Hydroxylation of tyrosine, tryptophan and proline	• Scurvy	• ↓ Plasma, leucocyte and urinary ascorbate

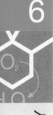

Table 6.16 Fat-soluble vitamins

Vitamin	Source	Function	Deficiency state
Vitamin A* Provitamin = β-carotene Vitamin = retinol	• Liver, dairy produce, fish oils and eggs	• Maintenance of epithelial surfaces and integrity of cartilage • Night vision (11-cis-retinal) 11-cis-retinal + opsin → rhodopsin (visual pigment) + light → trans-retinal + opsin (in dark)	• Night blindness • Xerophthalmia • Follicular hyperkeratosis
Vitamin D Provitamins = ergosterol (plants) and 7-dehydrocholesterol (skin) Vitamins D_2 (ergocalciferol) and D_3 (cholecalciferol) *Synthesis* Provitamins converted to vitamins by UV light Cholecalciferol (vit. D_3) is hydroxylated first in the liver to produce 25-hydroxycholecalciferol (25-HCC) and next in the kidney to generate both 1,25-dihydroxycholecalciferol (1,25-DHCC)† and 24,25-dihydroxycholecalciferol	• Dairy produce, fish liver oils and UV light	• Regulates calcium and phosphate metabolism 1,25-DHCC acts directly on bone, muscle, kidney and intestine • Osteocalcin is a protein secreted by osteoblasts and levels in blood reflect bone metabolic function. Production is induced by binding of 1,25-DHCC to osteocalcin gene. Variations in osteocalcin concentration and levels of bone loss are genetically determined	• Rickets in children and osteomalacia in adults • Tetany and muscle weakness **Causes:** (i) Dietary vitamin D deficiency (ii) Chronic severe liver disease (iii) Malabsorption, e.g. bowel resection, gastric surgery, intestinal bypass operations (iv) Chronic renal failure and renal tubular disease (v) Familial hypophosphataemic rickets and hypophosphatasia

Table 6.16 *(Cont'd)*

Vitamin	Source	Function	Deficiency state
Vitamin E Tocopherols	• Widely distributed in small amounts, especially green vegetables and vegetable oils	• Biological antioxidant	• Areflexia, gait disturbance, gaze paresis and haemolytic anaemia **Causes:** Abetalipoproteinaemia
Vitamin K K_1 = phylloquinone K_2 = menaquinone	• Widely distributed in small amounts, e.g. green vegetables • Synthesized by intestinal bacteria	• Acts as a coenzyme • Essential for activation of clotting factors by the liver (II, VII, IX and X)	• Easy bruising due to impaired clotting • Fat malabsorption **Causes:** (i) Prolonged obstructive jaundice (ii) Prematurity (iii) Gut sterilization (antibiotics) (iv) Drugs, e.g. antibiotics and anticoagulants

* Laboratory diagnosis of deficiency: plasma vitamin A level.
† Production of 1,25-DHCC is stimulated by a low circulating phosphate concentration, a high circulating PTH, oestrogen, prolactin and growth hormone.

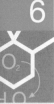

BIOCHEMISTRY, CELL BIOLOGY AND CLINICAL CHEMISTRY

Table 6.17 Urinary B₁₂ excretion in the Schilling test

Oral preparation	Pernicious anaemia	Bacterial overgrowth	Ileal disease
B₁₂	Low	Low	Low
B₁₂ + intrinsic factor	Normal	Low	Low
B₁₂ after antibiotic therapy	Low	Normal	Low

MINERALS

SODIUM

Factors affecting plasma sodium concentration

The intracellular fluid (ICF) Na^+ concentration is less than one-tenth of that in the extracellular fluid (ECF).
1. Aldosterone and the renin–angiotensin system.
2. Changes in glomerular filtration rate and renal blood flow.
3. Atrial natriuretic peptide.

Causes of salt and water abnormalities

See page 196.

Causes of hypo- and hypernatraemia

See pages 197–198.

POTASSIUM

Factors affecting plasma potassium concentration

ICF K^+ concentration is 30-fold that of the ECF. Potassium enters and leaves the ECF compartment via the intestine, kidney and the various other body cells.
1. *Aldosterone*: via effects on the distal tubule (increases renal excretion).
2. *Acid–base balance*: reciprocal relationship between $[K^+]$ and pH. In acidosis ($\uparrow$ ECF $[H^+]$) there is an increase in plasma $[K^+]$, due to reduced entry of K^+ into the cells from the ECF coupled with reduced urinary excretion of the ion. Alkalosis causes a low plasma $[K^+]$ due to a net increase in the entry of potassium into the cells and to an increased urinary loss. K^- loss from the cells causes an intracellular acidosis, because, there is less available for exchange with Na^+, and some is replaced by H^+.
3. *State of hydration*: K^+ is lost from cells in dehydration and returns into cells when dehydration is corrected.
4. *Insulin* promotes entry of K^+ into cells.
5. In *catabolic states*, e.g. major operations, severe infections, starvation and hyperthyroidism, K^+ is lost from cells. In *anabolic states,* K^+ is taken up by cells.

Causes of hypokalaemia

1. *Increased renal loss*
   - Diuretics
   - Renal tubular disorders, i.e. diuretic phase of acute renal failure/chronic pyelonephritis
   - Diabetic ketoacidosis
   - Cushing's syndrome or steroid excess
   - Hyperaldosteronism (primary/secondary).

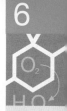

2. *Increased gastrointestinal loss*
   – Diarrhoea, vomiting and intestinal fistulae
   – Laxative abuse
   – Carbenoxolone therapy
   – Chronic mucus-secreting villous adenomas.
3. *Other causes*
   – Insulin therapy
   – Catabolic states
   – Dehydration
   – Intravenous therapy with inadequate K^+ supplements
   – Insulinoma
   – Metabolic or respiratory alkalosis
   – Familial periodic paralysis (abnormal redistribution of potassium between ECF and ICF)
   – Drugs, e.g. carbenicillin, phenothiazines, amphotericin B and degraded tetracycline.

Causes of hyperkalaemia
1. Acute and advanced chronic renal failure
2. Potassium-sparing diuretics
3. Metabolic or respiratory acidosis
4. Haemolysis (e.g. incompatible blood transfusion), tissue necrosis (e.g. major trauma and burns), severe acute starvation (e.g. anorexia nervosa)
5. Adrenal insufficiency (Addison's disease).

IRON

Source
- Liver, meat and cereals. Intake 1.5–2 mg/day.

Absorption
- Iron is absorbed by an active process in the upper small intestine (approximately 10%) and passes rapidly into the plasma. It can cross cell membranes only in the ferrous form.
- Factors increasing absorption: vitamin C, alcohol, gastric acid.
- Factors decreasing absorption: tetracycline, phytates, phosphates, gastric achlorhydria.

Storage
- Within the intestinal cell, some of the iron is combined with apoferritin to form ferritin, which is the principal storage form of iron in tissues. Ferritin is lost in the intestinal tract when the cell desquamates.

Transport
- Iron is carried in the plasma in the Fe^{3+} form, attached to a specific binding protein, transferrin, which is normally about one-third saturated with iron. Transferrin-bound iron is stored as ferritin (apoprotein + Fe^{2+}) and haemosiderin (conglomeration of ferritin molecules) in the bone marrow, liver and spleen, but may pass directly to the developing erythrocyte to form haemoglobin.

Loss
- Most of the loss is via the intestinal tract and the skin (approx. 1 mg per day). In women, the mean daily menstrual loss is about 1 mg and during pregnancy 1.5 mg. Negligible amounts appear in the urine.

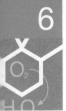

Distribution of iron in the body (Fig. 6.23)

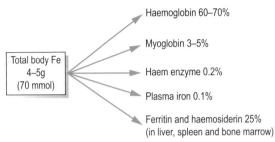

Total body Fe
4–5g
(70 mmol)

Haemoglobin 60–70%

Myoglobin 3–5%

Haem enzyme 0.2%

Plasma iron 0.1%

Ferritin and haemosiderin 25%
(in liver, spleen and bone marrow)

Fig. 6.23 Distribution of iron in the body.

Abnormalities of plasma iron concentration (Table 6.18)

Table 6.18 Plasma iron abnormalities

Disorder	Plasma iron	Transferrin or plasma TIBC*	Plasma ferritin or iron stores
Fe deficiency	↓	↑	↓
Chronic diseases (e.g. infections, malignancy, inflammatory diseases)	↓	↓ or N	↑ (malignancy)
Haemochromatosis	↑	↓ or N	↑
Pregnancy and oral contraceptives	↑	↑	N
Viral hepatitis	↑	↑ (occ)	↑
β-Thalassaemia (major)	↑ or N	N	↑ or N
Sideroblastic anaemia	↑	N	↑

* TIBC, total iron binding capacity; N, normal.
  Other causes of ↑ plasma iron include lead poisoning and haemolytic anaemias.

CALCIUM

Functions
1. Calcification of bones and teeth
2. Regulation of cell metabolism and excitability of nerve and muscle cells
3. 2nd messenger, e.g. calmodulin (see Note) with ATP
4. Cardiac conduction
5. Cofactor in coagulation.

Note: Calmodulin is an intracellular peptide that binds calcium with high affinity. It participates in a variety of different cellular functions requiring calcium, including mitosis, smooth muscle contraction and calcium transport.

Calcium balance

Source
- Present in milk, cheese and eggs.

Distribution in the body
- Most abundant mineral in the body.
- Total body calcium = 32 500 mmol (99% in bone, 1% in teeth as hydroxyapatite, and soft tissues).
- 40–50% of plasma calcium is non-ionized and bound to plasma proteins (mainly albumin).
- 40–50% active and ionized, which is the physiologically important fraction.
- 5–10% complexes with organic anions.

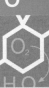

Control of calcium balance

The gastrointestinal tract, kidney and bone control calcium homeostasis through:

1. *Vitamin D* (1,25-DHCC)
   $\uparrow$ Ca^{2+} absorption from the intestine
   $\uparrow$ Ca^{2+} resorption from bone.
2. *Parathyroid hormone* (PTH)
   $\uparrow$ production of 1,25-DHCC by kidney
   $\uparrow$ Ca^{2+} resorption from bone
   $\downarrow$ Ca^{2+} excretion in urine, $\uparrow$ phosphate excretion
   $\uparrow$ Ca^{2+} absorption by intestine.

Causes of hyperparathyroidism
- Primary: parathyroid adenoma or carcinoma.
- Secondary, i.e. (inappropriate physiological increase in parathyroid hormone): hypocalcaemia.
- Tertiary, i.e. (inappropriate autonomous increase in parathyroid hormone): chronic hypocalcaemia, post renal transplant.

Causes of hypoparathyroidism
- DiGeorge's syndrome
- Surgical removal
- Parathyroid infiltration
- Autoimmune.

---

3. *Calcitonin* (minimal clinical significance)
   $\downarrow$ Ca^{2+} resorption from bone, $\uparrow$ renal excretion of phosphate.
4. *Acid–base status*
   If $\uparrow$ [H^+], less calcium is bound to albumin, e.g. in chronic acidosis, plasma [Ca^{2+}] increases.
   If $\downarrow$ [H^+], plasma calcium binds more to albumin and [Ca^{2+}] $\downarrow$.
5. *Others*
   Glucocorticoids, growth hormone and somatomedins, thyroid hormones, oestrogens, insulin, epidermal, fibroblast and platelet-derived growth factor and prostaglandin E_2.

Table 6.19 Biochemical findings in metabolic bone disease

Disease	Ca^{2+}	PO_4^{2-}	Alkaline phosphatase	Urinary hydroxyproline
Osteoporosis	N	N	N	N
Osteomalacia	$\downarrow$	$\downarrow$	$\uparrow$	N
Paget's disease	N	N	$\uparrow$	$\uparrow$
Primary hyperparathyroidism	$\uparrow$	$\downarrow$	N	N
Secondary hyperparathyroidism	$\downarrow$	$\uparrow$	N	N
Tertiary hyperparathyroidism	$\uparrow$	$\downarrow$	N	N

N = normal.

Abnormalities of serum calcium

Causes of hypercalcaemia

1. Primary and tertiary hyperparathyroidism, multiendocrine neoplasia (MEN) and renal transplant

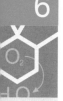

2. Malignancy of lung, breast and kidney (bone metastases), multiple myeloma, lymphoma
3. Sarcoidosis, Paget's disease
4. Endocrine disorders: thyrotoxicosis, acromegaly, adrenal insufficiency
5. Drugs e.g. thiazide diuretics, lithium, hypervitaminosis.

Causes of hypocalcaemia

Table 6.20 Main causes of hypocalcaemia

Disorder	Plasma phosphate	Plasma PTH	Plasma alkaline phosphatase
1. Chronic renal failure	↑ (or N)	↑	↑ (or N)
2. Dietary deficiency of vit. D	↓ (or N)	↑ (or N)	↑
3. Hypoparathyroidism	↑	↓	N
4. Pseudohypoparathyroidism	↑	↑	N
5. Renal tubular defects	↓	N	↑ (or N)
6. Other causes:			

Hypoproteinaemia, hypomagnasaemia, liver disease, respiratory alkalosis, acute pancreatitis, massive transfusion with citrated blood, and drugs, e.g. diuretic therapy, calcitonin, phosphate, diphosphonates, some cytotoxic agents and calcium chelators.

PHOSPHATE

- Major intracellular anion.
- Present in all foods.
- Present with calcium as hydroxyapatite in bones and teeth.

Phosphate balance
- Metabolism follows calcium inversely.
- Acid–base regulation and renal function also affect urinary output of phosphate.

Abnormalities of serum phosphate

Causes of hyperphosphataemia
1. Acute and chronic renal failure
2. Haemolysis
3. Children
4. Hypoparathyroidism and pseudohypoparathyroidism
5. Hypervitaminosis D
6. Catabolic states
7. Metabolic acidosis.

Causes of hypophosphataemia
1. Vitamin D deficiency
2. Hyperparathyroidism
3. Inadequate intake (parenteral nutrition)
4. Renal tubular disease
5. Malabsorption
6. Chronic alcoholism
7. Excessive use of antacids (magnesium and aluminium salts)
8. During recovery from diabetic ketoacidosis.

CHLORIDE

Usually parallels the Na^+ concentration.

Abnormalities of serum chloride levels

Causes of hyperchloraemia
1. Hyperventilation
2. Glomerulonephritis
3. Eclampsia
4. Cystic fibrosis (chloride in sweat is ↑ by five times the reference value).

Causes of hypochloraemia
1. Addison's disease
2. Diabetes
3. Intestinal obstruction and vomiting.

Causes of hyperchloraemic acidosis and hypochloraemic alkalosis
See page 189.

Causes of hypochlorhydria
1. Pernicious anaemia
2. Gastric carcinoma and ulcer
3. Surgery: vagotomy and subtotal gastrectomy
4. Atrophic gastritis
5. Iron deficiency.

MAGNESIUM

- Cofactor for many enzyme reactions and involved in control of muscular contractions.
- Average daily intake (10 mmol) and average daily requirements (8 mmol).
- The majority is distributed in bone and intracellular fluid.

Abnormalities of serum magnesium levels

Causes of hypermagnesaemia
1. Acute renal failure
2. Chronic renal failure
3. Excess intake (parenteral nutrition).

Causes of hypomagnesaemia
1. Malnutrition
2. Malabsorption or severe diarrhoea
3. Alcohol abuse
4. Inadequate intake (parenteral nutrition)
5. Renal tubular acidosis and diabetic ketoacidosis
6. Chronic diuretic therapy or dialysis
7. Acute pancreatitis and hepatic cirrhosis.

TRACE ELEMENTS

See Table 6.21.
Required intake <100 mg/day; necessary for the function of particular compounds.

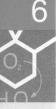

Table 6.21 The trace elements*

Mineral	Source	Function in body	Deficiency state and causes
Iodide	• Iodized salt, seafish, milk and eggs	• Biosynthesis of thyroid hormones	1. Cretinism in children 2. Endemic goitre and hypothyroidism in adults
Magnesium (54% found in bone, rest mainly intracellular)	• Green vegetables and cereal	• Cofactor for many enzymes in metabolism of carbohydrates and fats, e.g. phosphatases and kinases • Cofactor in ATP reactions	1. Paraesthesia, tetany 2. Cardiac arrhythmias (usually with hypocalcaemia) **Causes:** (i) Chronic alcoholism (ii) Malabsorption and fistulae (iii) Diuretic therapy (iv) Chronic dialysis (v) Acute pancreatitis
Copper		• Cofactor for some enzymes and for haem synthesis, e.g. *cytochrome oxidase* • Transported by albumin and bound to caeruloplasmin • Necessary for myelin formation • Metabolism controlled by 3 genes on chromosome 3 (caeruloplasmin), 13 (Wilson's disease) and X chromosome (Menke's syndrome)	1. Anaemia (hypochromic and microcytic) and neutropenia 2. Impaired bone mineralization 3. Wilson's disease: deficiency of caeruloplasmin resulting in low plasma copper levels. Excessive copper deposition occurs in the basal ganglia, liver, renal tubules and eye 4. Menke's syndrome: severe copper deficiency. X-linked recessive. Presents as failure to thrive, cerebral and cerebellar degeneration and death
Zinc	• Herrings, beef, liver, eggs and nuts	• Cofactor for some enzymes, e.g. carbonic anhydrase, alcohol dehydrogenase and carboxypeptidase	1. Confusion, apathy and depression 2. Acrodermatitis enteropathica, skin ulcers and alopecia 3. Diarrhoea 4. Growth and sexual development retarded

*Other trace elements: manganese, cobalt (cofactor of vitamin B_{12}), fluoride (cofactor of hydroxyapatite), chromium, sulphur (present in methionine and cysteine), molybdenum and selenium (cofactor of glutathione peroxidase).

NUTRITIONAL DEFICIENCIES IN SPECIFIC DISEASES/STATES

Nutritional requirements depend on energy requirements

Total daily expenditure (TEE) comprises:

1. Basal metabolic rate (BMR) : the minimal energy expenditure of an individual 12–18 hours after a meal at complete rest. Accounts for 65% of TEE and 90% of REE.
2. Resting energy expenditure (REE) : energy expenditure while resting several hours after a meal or physical activity. Accounts for 75% of TEE.
3. Thermic effect of muscle (TEM) : accounts for 15–20% of TEE.
4. Thermic effect of food : accounts for 10% of TEE.

DAILY DIETARY REQUIREMENTS (adult male)

Carbohydrate 400 g (49%)
Protein 100 g (17%)
Fat 100 g (34%).

- The ratio of the caloric energy yield (kcal/g) of carbohydrates, protein and fats from biological oxidation is respectively **4:4:9**.
- An adult male requires approximately 2500 kcal of energy per day and 6000 kcal for heavy labour.
- These requirements decrease with age, are higher in men than women and are increased by caffeine, thyroxine and catecholamines. Protein requirements increase with disease severity and can rise to 1.5 g/kg/day.

Body mass index

- Body mass index (BMI) is used as a measure of optimal body weight (normal range 18.5–24.9 kg/m^2) (Table 6.22).

Table 6.22 BMI measures

Undernutrition	Overnutrition
Severe: <15.9 kg/m^2	Overweight: 25.0–29.9 kg/m^2
Moderate: 16–16.9 kg/m^2	Obesity: 30.0–39.9 kg/m^2
Mild: 17.0–18.4 kg/m^2	Morbid obesity: >40.0 kg/m^2

Table 6.23 Nutritional deficiencies

Disease/state	Nutritional deficiencies
Post gastrectomy	Iron, B$_{12}$
Coeliac disease	Iron, folic acid
Pancreatic disease	Fat-soluble substances: vitamins A, D, E and K
Crohn's disease	Iron, folic acid, potassium and magnesium, B$_{12}$
Stagnant loop syndrome, alcoholism	Folic acid, thiamine, pyridoxine, protein and calcium
Vegan	B$_{12}$, iron, occ. calcium and phosphorus
Pregnancy and lactation	↑ in requirements for folate, calcium, phosphorus, magnesium, iron, zinc, iodine, vitamins A and C 15% ↑ in calorie and 50% ↑ in protein requirements

PLASMA PROTEINS

CONSTITUENTS AND FUNCTIONS

These are described in Table 6.24.

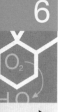

Table 6.24 Plasma proteins

Plasma protein	% of total protein	Constituents	Function
Albumin	50–70%		• Maintains plasma volume and distribution of ECF (40% is intravascular) • Acts as a carrier for bilirubin, non-ionized calcium, free fatty acids, hormones (e.g. thyroxine) and drugs (e.g. salicylates) • Minor role as a buffer
α_1-Globulins	2–6%	Thyroxine-binding globulins High-density lipoproteins (HDL) Orosomucoid Transcortin α_1-Antitrypsin	• Thyroid hormone transport • Lipid transport • Glycoprotein: concentration increases in inflammation • Cortisol-binding globulin • Inhibits proteolytic enzymes (e.g. trypsin and plasmin). High levels in acute illness. Low levels in emphysema and neonatal hepatitis (Three main phenotypes: normal MM, homozygote ZZ and heterozygote MZ)
α_2-Globulins	5–11%	Caeruloplasmin Haptoglobins α_2-Macroglobulin Very low-density lipoproteins (VLDL)	• Copper transport: low levels in Wilson's disease • Binds to haemoglobin released from damaged red cells and prevents loss of iron in the urine • Inhibits proteolytic enzymes, possible transport function • Lipid transport
β-Globulins	7–16%	Transferrin Low-density lipoproteins (LDL) Fibrinogen C3 and C4 complement Plasminogen β_2-Microglobulin	• Iron transport • Lipid transport • Fibrinolysis: deficiency states include congenital afibrinogenaemia and disseminated intravascular coagulation • Sensitive indicator of connective tissue disorders: ↑ in glomerulonephritis and infectious diseases; ↓ in disseminated intravascular coagulation, meningococcal meningitis and leukaemia • Fibrinolysis • Used as an index of renal tubular function (GFR)
γ-Globulins	11–21%	IgA, IgD, IgE, IgG, IgM Antihaemophilia globulin (AHG) Factor VIII α-Fetoprotein C-reactive protein	• See Table 3.9 • Deficiency states include haemophilia, Von Willebrand's disease; and disseminated intravascular coagulation • See page 297 • Concentration increases early in acute inflammation. Parallels the ESR but generally raised first: ↑ in chronic infections, cryoglobulinaemia, Hodgkin's disease, macroglobulinaemia, myeloma and rheumatoid arthritis and Crohn's disease; ↓ in lymphomas, nephrotic syndrome, scleroderma and ulcerative colitis

USE IN DIAGNOSIS (Fig. 6.24)

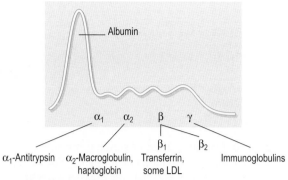

Fig. 6.24 Normal electrophoretic scan.

The patterns of serum proteins on electrophoresis may be used in the diagnosis of disease, e.g.

1. Multiple myeloma: paraprotein band between the α_2 and the γ region; normal or reduced γ-globulin.
2. Nephrotic syndrome: albumin and sometimes γ-globulin lost in urine; $\uparrow$ in α_2-globulin.
3. Liver cirrhosis: $\downarrow$ albumin; $\uparrow$ production of proteins which migrate in the β–γ region.

CHANGES IN PLASMA PROTEIN CONCENTRATIONS

Causes of raised globulins (mainly α_2-globulins)
1. Usually secondary to tissue destruction
2. Malignant disease
3. Chronic inflammatory conditions
4. Chronic infections
5. Nephrotic syndrome.

Causes of raised β-globulins
Hepatitis and acute phase reaction.

Causes of decreased β-globulins
SLE and autoimmune disorders.

Causes of changes in γ-globulins
See page 118.

Proteins decreased in acute inflammation:
- Transferrin
- Albumin
- α-fetoprotein.

C-reactive protein

Marked increase
- Connective tissue disorders (except SLE)
- Malignancy
- Bacterial infection and abscess
- Necrosis (e.g. acute myocardial infarction)
- Crohn's disease
- Trauma.

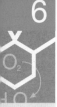
Mild increase
- Viral infection
- Steroids.

Not raised in
- Ulcerative colitis
- SLE
- Leukaemia
- Pregnancy
- Anaemia, polycythaemia, heart failure.

α_1-Antitrypsin (AAT)

- Gene located on chromosome 14. One of a group of serum proteins that inactivates proteolytic enzymes released from inflammatory cells. Failure to inhibit enzyme activity results in progressive alveolar wall destruction and emphysema.
- Normal M allele in 95% of Europeans, associated with normal AAT level. Homozygotes for Z allele have AAT levels less than 20% of normal and are at increased risk of emphysema.

Acute phase reactants are plasma proteins whose concentration alters following trauma (e.g. surgery, myocardial infarction), autoimmune disease (e.g. SLE) or infection:

- C-reactive protein
- Serum amyloid precursor
- α_1-Antitrypsin
- α_1-Antichymotrypsin
- α_1-Acid glycoprotein
- Fibrinogen
- Haptoglobin
- Complement C3, C4
- Caeruloplasmin
- Fibronectin
- Angiotensinogen
- Mannose-binding protein
- Albumin, transferrin.

PLASMA ENZYMES (Tables 6.25 and 6.26)

Table 6.25 Plasma enzymes (see also Table 6.26)

Enzyme	Causes of raised level
Alanine amino transferase (ALT or SGPT) *Sources:* found in the same tissues as AST (see Table 6.26), but ALT present in cytoplasm of hepatocyte only (AST present in cytoplasma and mitochondria of hepatocyte) AST > ALT, if liver cell necrosis severe	Parallels changes in AST, but less affected by trauma or disease of cardiac or skeletal muscle 1. Liver disease, e.g. infectious hepatitis 2. Others: haemolysis, chronic renal failure, dermatomyositis, acute pancreatitis
Alkaline phosphatase (ALP) *Sources:* bone (heat labile), liver (heat stable), intestine, pancreas and placenta (heat stable)	1. Growing children and pregnancy 2. Bone disease, e.g. metastatic bone disease, Paget's disease, osteomalacia or rickets, hyperparathyroidism 3. Liver disease, e.g. obstructive jaundice, cirrhosis, space-occupying lesions 4. Malignancy, e.g. bone or liver tumour *Decreased levels in:* Hypophosphatasia or conditions of reduced bone growth, e.g. cretinism
Leucocyte alkaline phosphatase (LAP)	Polycythaemia rubra vera (PRV), secondary polycythaemia and leukaemoid reactions Pregnancy, oestrogens *Decreased levels in:* Chronic myelocytic leukaemia and paroxysmal nocturnal haemoglobinuria
γ-Glutamyltransferase (γ-GT) *Sources:* liver, kidney, pancreas and prostate gland	1. Liver disease, e.g. alcoholic cholestasis, acute and chronic hepatitis, cirrhosis 2. Enzyme induction by alcohol, barbiturates and phenytoin 3. Acute pancreatitis (rarely) 4. Congestive cardiac failure
Acid phosphatase *Sources:* prostate, platelets, red cells and Gaucher cells	1. Carcinoma of prostate with metastases 2. Benign prostatic hypertrophy 3. After rectal examination or passage of urinary catheter 4. Gaucher's disease 5. Metastatic disease with bony involvement 6. Haemolysis, myeloid leukaemia
Serum amylase *Sources:* pancreas, salivary glands, ovary, lung and prostate gland	1. Acute pancreatitis, obstruction of pancreatic duct (e.g. carcinoma, stricture or stone) 2. Severe diabetic ketoacidosis. 3. Acute abdominal conditions, e.g. perforated peptic ulcer, ruptured ectopic pregnancy 4. Mumps 5. Tumours, e.g. carcinoma of bronchus, colon and ovary 6. Renal failure 7. Drugs, e.g. morphine and codeine
Angiotensin-converting enzyme (ACE) *Source:* capillary endothelial cells of lung	1. Active sarcoidosis 2. Liver disease 3. Leprosy 4. Berylliosis, asbestosis and silicosis 5. May also be elevated in TB, carcinoma of the lung, and primary biliary cirrhosis
Pseudocholinesterase *Source:* liver	*Decreased activity in:* 1. Suxamethonium sensitivity: variants of pseudocholinesterase classified according to dibucaine inhibition number (normal is 75–80; atypical heterozygote 40–70; and for an atypical homozygote 15–30) 2. Organophosphorus poisoning (anticholinesterases) 3. Liver disease (hepatitis, cirrhosis)

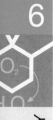

Table 6.26 Enzymes raised after myocardial infarction

Enzyme	Source	First rise (hours)	Peak (hours)	Duration (days)	Other causes of raised levels
Creatine phosphokinase (CPK)*	Skeletal, cardiac, smooth muscle and brain. Not in liver	6	24–48	3–5	Often non-specific: 1. Crush injuries, rhabdomyolysis, surgery, IM injections, severe exercise, generalized seizure 2. Muscular dystrophies and in 60% of carriers, polymyositis, motor neuron disease, myotonic dystrophy 3. Malignant hyperthermia and delirium tremens 4. Hypothyroidism 5. Diabetic ketoacidosis

*CPK has three isoenzymes: MB, myocardium; BB, brain; MM, skeletal muscle.

$$\text{Creatine} \xleftarrow{\quad\text{Creatine kinase}\quad} \text{Creatine phosphate} \rightarrow \text{Creatinine}$$

A constant fraction of the muscle pool, creatine phosphate spontaneously cyclizes to creatinine, which is excreted in the urine.

Enzyme	Source	First rise (hours)	Peak (hours)	Duration (days)	Other causes of raised levels
Aspartate aminotransferase (AST or SGOT)	All tissues including skeletal muscle, liver, heart, pancreas and red cells	6–8	24–48	4–6	1. Liver disease, e.g. cirrhosis (AST > ALT) 2. Haemolytic anaemia 3. Acute systemic infections 4. Skeletal muscle disease, e.g. muscular dystrophies
Lactate dehydrogenase (LDH)†	Widely distributed in skeletal muscle, brain, liver, heart, kidney and red cells	12–24	48–72	7–12	1. Acute myocardial infarction 2. Leukaemia, haemolytic anaemia, polycythaemia rubra vera, pernicious anaemia and megaloblastic anaemia 3. Carcinomatosis, Hodgkin's disease 4. Skeletal muscle disease, e.g. muscular dystrophy 5. Cerebral infarction 6. Renal and hepatic disease (hepatitis, obstructive jaundice) 7. Congestive cardiac failure 8. Pulmonary embolus

†LDH has five isoenzymes, LD1–5, from different tissues. Hydroxybutyrate = isoenzyme 1–2.

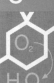

TUMOUR PRODUCTS

Carcinoembryonic antigen (CEA)

- Used mainly for detecting recurrent or metastatic disease and for monitoring therapy in carcinoma of the pancreas, liver, colon, rectum, bronchus and breast.
- Also present in individuals with chronic inflammatory bowel disease.

α-Fetoprotein (AFP)

- Normally synthesized by the fetal liver.
- Present in *plasma* in:
  1. Normal fetus
  2. Elevated maternal AFP may indicate fetal neural tube defect, twin pregnancy or fetal distress
  3. Hepatic carcinoma, germ-cell tumours (not pure seminoma) and testicular teratoma
  4. Viral hepatitis, cirrhosis or liver metastases.
- *Raised amniotic fluid* levels present in:
  1. Neural tube defects, e.g. open spina bifida, anencephaly
  2. Congenital nephrotic syndrome
  3. Oesophageal and duodenal atresia.

CA 125

Raised in:
1. Carcinoma of ovary, breast and liver
2. Pregnancy
3. Cirrhosis
4. Peritonitis.

CA 153

Raised in carcinoma of breast and benign breast disease.

CA 19.9

Raised in colorectal and pancreatic carcinoma and cholestasis.

5-Hydroxyindoleacetic acid (5-HIAA) (Fig. 6.25)

- *Increased urinary levels* occur in the carcinoid syndrome.
- False positives occur with the ingestion of foods high in serotonin e.g. bananas, avocados.

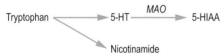

Tryptophan ⟶ 5-HT $\xrightarrow{MAO}$ 5-HIAA
⟶ Nicotinamide

Fig. 6.25 Metabolism of tryptophan.
5HT = 5-hydroxytryptamine (serotonin), 5-HIAA = 5-hydroxyindoleacetic acid, MAO = monoamine oxidase.

Vanillyl mandelic acid level (VMA)

A high urinary level present in:
1. Tumours of sympathetic nervous tissue, e.g. phaeochromocytoma, neuroblastoma
2. Drugs e.g. monoamine oxidase inhibitors (MAOI), phenothiazines, methyl-dopa, tetracyclines and L-dopa
3. Diet e.g. bananas, vanilla, tea, coffee, ice cream, chocolates.

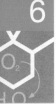

Prostate specific antigen (PSA)

- Raised in prostate cancer and benign prostate hypertrophy.

Prostate cancer	Benign prostate hypertrophy
65% have PSA > 10	1% have PSA > 10
20% have PSA 4–10	8% have PSA 4–10
15% have PSA < 4.	91% have PSA < 4.

5α-reductase inhibitors reduce PSA by 50% after 6 months of treatment.

Human chorionic gonadotrophin (hCG)

- Glycoprotein comprising an α and β subunit.
- β-hCG normally raised in first 2 days of pregnancy and peaks towards end of first trimester.
- *Raised in:*
  1. Choriocarcinoma
  2. Germ-cell tumours, teratomas, seminomas
  3. 20% of breast cancers, especially with metastatic disease, and occasionally with pancreas, ovary and bladder cancers.
- Levels may be helpful in management of germ-cell tumours and trophoblastic disease.

Gastrin, glucagon and VIP

See pages 222–223.

Multiple endocrine neoplasia (MEN) or pluriglandular syndrome

Two or more endocrine glands secrete excessive amounts of hormones. See Table 6.27.

Table 6.27 Multiple endocrine neoplasia	
MEN I	*MEN II*
Parathyroid adenoma	Medullary carcinoma of the thyroid
Pancreatic islet cells (gastrinoma, insulinoma)	Phaechromocytoma
Anterior pituitary gland	Parathyroid carcinoma or adenoma
Adrenal cortex	
Thyroid	

BIOCHEMISTRY OF COAGULATION/FIBRINOLYSIS

COAGULATION CASCADE AND FIBRINOLYTIC PATHWAY (Fig. 6.26)

Platelet activating factor (PAF)

- Phospholipid signalling molecule.
- Produced by endothelial cells, polymorphonuclear leucocytes, eosinophils, macrophages, platelets and mast cells.
- Causes platelet adherence and aggregation, activation of monocytes and macrophages, and production of leucotrienes and cytokines.
- Also plays a role in glycogenolysis in liver, bronchoconstriction, alterations of cardiac rhythm and GFR.
- *Clinical associations:* increased PAF with sepsis, collagen vascular diseases and asthma. Also implicated in pathogenesis of cardiac and cerebrovascular diseases as well as diabetes and renal disease.

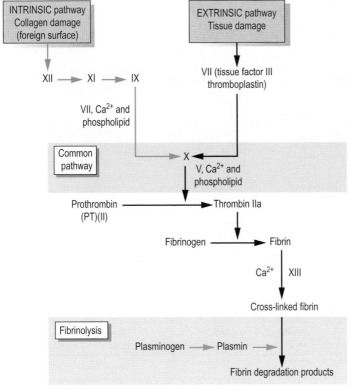

Fig. 6.26 Coagulation cascade and fibrinolytic pathway.

Prothrombin-gene mutation G20210A
- Prothrombotic mutation which increases the risk of cerebral vein thrombosis by tenfold.
- Mutation present in 1–2% of population and in 18% of families with a history of venous thromboembolic disease.
- Most common genetic factor of deep vein thrombosis after factor V (Leiden) gene mutation.

ABNORMALITIES OF COAGULATION

See Tables 6.28 and 6.29.

Other causes of abnormal coagulation
- *Heparin* therapy enhances interaction between thrombin and antithrombin III, and between AT-III and many of the factors in the intrinsic pathway. Prevents activation of factors II, IX, X, XI and probably VII. Therapy may be monitored using APPT and PTT.
- *Vitamin K deficiency* and *warfarin* treatment affects synthesis of factors II, VII, IX and X.
- *Disseminated intravascular coagulation (DIC)* affects factors I, II, V, VIII and XI.
- *Liver disease* affects factors I, II, V, VII, IX and X.

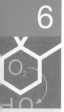
BIOCHEMISTRY, CELL BIOLOGY AND CLINICAL CHEMISTRY

Table 6.28 Abnormalities of coagulation

Causes of abnormal coagulation	Function	Test
Deficiency of factors I, II, V, VII, X	Extrinsic and common pathways	Prothrombin time (PT)
Haemophilia A and B Deficiency of factors I, II, V, VIII, IX, X, XI and XII Not sensitive to factor VII deficiency	Intrinsic and common pathways	Activated partial thromboplastin time (APTT)
Anticoagulants (e.g. heparin), presence of fibrin degradation products (FDPs) or depletion of fibrinogen	Fibrinogen to fibrin conversion	Thrombin time (TT)
Von Willebrand's, uraemia and aspirin* Normal in clotting disorders	Platelet function	Bleeding time
Haemophilia A and B	Final common pathway, intrinsic pathway and platelet function	Clotting time

*Other drugs that prolong bleeding time are phenothiazines, tricyclic antidepressants, dextran, dipyridamole and antihistamines.

Table 6.29 Interpretation of test results

Disorder	Prothrombin time	Partial thromboplastin time	Thrombin time	Platelet count
Liver disease	↑	↑	Usually N	N initially
Warfarin	↑	↑	N	N
Factor VII deficiency	↑	N	N	N
Haemophilia	N	↑	N	N
Christmas disease	N	↑	N	N
Heparin	↑	↑	↑	N
Disseminated intravascular coagulation	↑	↑	↑	↓

APPT and PT normal: platelet or vessel defect.
APPT and PT abnormal: defect in common pathway.
APPT normal and PT abnormal: factor VII deficiency.
APPT abnormal and PT normal: defect in intrinsic system.

INTERPRETATION OF LABORATORY FINDINGS

BLOOD

Effects of delayed transport and haemolysis of blood
↑ levels of plasma potassium, phosphate, total acid phosphatase, lactate dehydrogenase and AST.

Prolonged venous stasis during venesection
↑ levels of plasma total Ca^{2+}, total protein, lipids and T_4.

Taking blood from 'drip' arm
Electrolyte and glucose concentration approximately equal to composition of infused fluid; dilution of all other concentrations.

Use of wrong bottle

1. EDTA or oxalate: $\downarrow$ [Ca^{2+}], $\uparrow$ [Na^+] or [K^+]
2. Failure to use a fluoride tube for a blood glucose specimen results in a high glucose reading (fluoride inhibits erythrocyte glycolysis).

Metabolic effects of pregnancy/oral contraceptive therapy

1. $\uparrow$ Plasma T_4 (due to $\uparrow$ thyroxine-binding globulin), $\uparrow$ plasma cortisol (due to $\uparrow$ cortisol-binding globulin)
2. $\uparrow$ TIBC (due to plasma transferrin), $\uparrow$ plasma iron
3. $\uparrow$ Plasma alkaline phosphatase
4. $\uparrow$ Urinary glucose, and abnormal glucose tolerance tests
5. $\uparrow$ Serum amylase, $\uparrow$ serum cholesterol
6. Low plasma gonadotrophin, $\uparrow$ plasma prolactin.

Drugs that alter thyroid function tests

1. Lithium carbonate ($\downarrow$ in protein binding index (PBI), free T_4 and ^{131}I uptake)
2. Phenytoin ($\downarrow$ in PBI, T_4 and T_3)
3. Salicylates ($\downarrow$ in PBI, T_4 and ^{131}I)
4. Oestrogens and oral contraceptive pill ($\uparrow$ PBI and T_4)
5. Androgens and anabolic steroids ($\downarrow$ T_4 and $\uparrow$ T_3 uptake)
6. Phenylbutazone ($\uparrow$ PBI, T_3 uptake and $\downarrow$ ^{131}I)
7. Propylthiouracil ($\downarrow$ ^{131}I uptake, T_4 and T_3).

Laboratory findings in hypothermia (core temperature <35°C)

1. $\uparrow$ Hb, haematocrit and plasma viscosity
2. Thrombocytopenia and disseminated intravascular coagulation
3. Hyponatraemia, $\uparrow$ blood sugar, creatinine kinase and serum amylase
4. Thyroid function tests unreliable.

CEREBROSPINAL FLUID (CSF)

Composition of CSF (Table 6.30)

Feature	Normal values	Acute purulent meningitis	Aseptic viral meningitis	Tuberculous meningitis
Appearance	Clear	Cloudy	Usually clear	Opalescent
Normal volume	130 ml			
pH	7.3			
Cells/mm³	0–5 lymph.	10–100 000 polymorphs	15–2000 lymph	250–500 lymph
Glucose* (mmol/l)	2.8–4.4	low	normal	very low
Protein (g/l)	0.15–0.35	0.5–5.0	0.2–1.25	0.45–5.00
Albumin:globulin ratio	8:1			
Chloride	20 mmol/l			

Table 6.30 Composition of cerebrospinal fluid in normal and pathological states

Pressure = 10–18 cmH$_2$O (lying on side); 30 cmH$_2$O (standing)

*Normally 60–70% of plasma level.

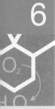
Changes in CSF

Causes of low CSF glucose
1. Hypoglycaemia
2. Infection, e.g. bacterial and fungal meningitis, toxoplasmosis
3. Subarachnoid haemorrhage
4. Leukaemia
5. Sarcoidosis.

Causes of raised CSF protein
1. Intracranial haemorrhage
2. Meningitis (tuberculous, bacterial or fungal)
3. Encephalitis
4. Cerebral tumour
5. Carcinomatous neuropathy
6. Neurofibromatosis (especially acoustic barrier neuroma)
7. Guillain–Barré syndrome

Inflammatory disease:
Globulin:albumin ratio small due to leakage of albumin via the blood–brain barrier

8. Multiple sclerosis
9. Neurosyphilis
10. SLE
11. Cerebral sarcoidosis

Demyelinating disease:
↑ globulin:albumin ratio because of intrathecal synthesis of immunoglobulin

12. Multiple myeloma
13. Lymphoma
14. Benign paraproteinaemia
15. Diabetic neuropathy.

Monoclonal bands of immunoglobulins

URINE BIOCHEMISTRY (Table 6.31)

Table 6.31 Values in urine biochemistry

Feature	Normal values
Volume	400 ml/day–4 l/day
Specific gravity	1.008–1.030
pH	4.5–7.8
Protein	0–90 mg/day
Urobilinogen	up to 6.7 mmol/day
$[Na^+]$	100–250 mmol/day
$[K^+]$	40–120 mmol/day
Cells	Leucocytes and non-squamous epithelial cells, small number of red cells and some hyaline casts
Osmolality	50–1200 mosmol/kg

Urine casts

1. Hyaline casts (most common) arise from tubules. Do not indicate renal dysfunction.
2. Epithelial/granular casts occur when there is acute inflammation or acute oliguric renal failure.
3. White cell casts occur in medullary inflammation, e.g. pyelonephritis.
4. Red cell casts occur in glomerular damage, e.g. SLE and acute glomerulonephritis.

Proteinuria (>1.5 g per day)

1. Glomerular proteinuria commonest; due to increased glomerular permeability.
2. Tubular proteinuria occurs with renal tubular damage from any cause, especially pyelonephritis (mainly α_2- and β-globulin).
3. Also: Bence Jones proteinuria, haemoglobinuria and myoglobinuria.

Positive Clinitest reaction

Colour change from blue to orange in presence of a reducing agent.

Causes

1. Glycosuria, e.g. diabetes mellitus, thyrotoxicosis, postgastrectomy, phaeochromocytoma, gross cerebral injury, severe infection, lag glucose tolerance curve and reduced renal threshold, as in pregnancy.
2. Others
   (i) galactosaemia (galactose)
   (ii) hereditary fructosaemia (fructose)
   (iii) benign fructosuria, pentosuria, and lactosuria
   (iv) alkaptonuria (homogentisic acid).
3. Drugs, e.g. salicylates, isoniazid, L-dopa, vitamin C, tetracyclines.

Myoglobinuria

Causes

1. Crushing injuries
2. Severe muscle damage due to exercise
3. Electrical shock
4. Progressive muscle diseases.

Haemoglobinuria

Causes

1. Incompatible blood transfusion
2. Haemolytic anaemias
3. Burns
4. Paroxysmal cold haemoglobinuria
5. Paroxysmal nocturnal haemoglobinuria.

Elevated urinary calcium

Causes

1. Hyperparathyroidism
2. Bone tumours
3. Hypervitaminosis D
4. Hyperthyroidism
5. Cushing's syndrome.

Decreased urinary calcium

Causes

1. Hypoparathyroidism
2. Vitamin D deficiency
3. Coeliac disease
4. Decreased calcium intake.

Cystinuria

Causes

1. Cystinosis
2. Cystinuria.

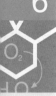

SYNOVIAL FLUID (Table 6.32)

- Aspiration is mainly used to distinguish between infections and crystal arthropathies.
- Normal synovial fluid does not clot because it lacks fibrinogen or other clotting factors. Inflammatory processes allow these to enter, so that if the fluid is allowed to stand a clot will form.
- RA cells: 95% of patients with rheumatoid arthritis have RA cells in their synovial fluid.
- LE cells: 30% of patients with rheumatoid arthritis have ANA in their synovial fluid.
- Crystals: monosodium urate crystals are associated with gout.
- Calcium pyrophosphate crystals are associated with chondrocalcinosis.

Table 6.32 Synovial fluid

	Appearance	Viscosity	White blood cells	Neutrophils
Normal	Clear	High	<200	<25%
Acute inflammation e.g. gout, RA, pseudogout, SLE	Turbid	Decreased	14 000–28 000	50–80%
Sepsis e.g. TB, gonorrhoea, *Staph.*, *Strep.*, Lyme arthritis	Turbid	Decreased	14 000–65 000	60–95%
Non-inflammatory e.g. degenerative joint disease, trauma	Clear	High	<5000	<25%

7

STATISTICS AND EPIDEMIOLOGY

STATISTICS   306
Frequency distributions   306
  Frequency histogram   306
  Cumulative frequency plot   306
Measures of central tendency   307
Measures of dispersion   307
  Sample range   307
  Percentile   307
  Interquartile range   308
  Box and whisker plot   308
  Variance and standard deviation   308
  Coefficient of variation   309
Probability distributions   309
  Normal or Gaussian distribution   309
  Skewed distribution   310
  Log-normal distribution   310
  Binomial distribution   310
  Poisson distribution   310
Sampling   311
  Central limit theorem   311
  Standard error of the mean   312
  Confidence interval   312
  Z score   313
Hypothesis testing and statistical significance   313
  Null hypothesis   313
  Statistical significance   313
  Type I and II errors   315

Tests of significance   315
  Parametric tests   315
  Non-parametric tests   316
  Correlation   317
  Regression   318

EPIDEMIOLOGY   319
Crude rates   319
Adjusted rates   320
Specific rates   320
Principles of study design   321
  Cross-sectional study   321
  Cohort study   322
  Case–control study   322
  Randomized clinical trial   324
Measures of effect   326
Association and causation   331
Diagnostic tests and screening   331
  Validity   332
  Basic requirements of a screening test   334
  Biases in evaluation of screening programmes   334
  Measures used in economic evaluation of healthcare interventions   335

STATISTICS

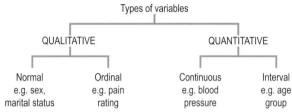

Types of variables

QUALITATIVE

Normal
e.g. sex,
marital status

Ordinal
e.g. pain
rating

QUANTITATIVE

Continuous
e.g. blood
pressure

Interval
e.g. age
group

Fig. 7.1 Types of variables.

FREQUENCY DISTRIBUTIONS

A frequency distribution shows the values which can be taken by a variable and the frequency with which each value is observed, e.g. pie chart, Venn diagram, bar chart and histogram.

FREQUENCY HISTOGRAM (Fig. 7.2)

- With *non-equal* base lines the *area* of each block is proportional to the frequency.
- With *equal* base lines the *height* of each block is proportional to the frequency.

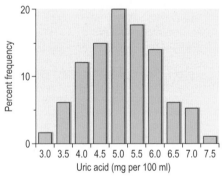

Fig. 7.2 Frequency histogram of serum uric acid distribution in 267 healthy males.

CUMULATIVE FREQUENCY PLOT (Fig. 7.3)

- The frequency of data in each category represents the sum of the data from that category and from the preceding categories.
- Useful in calculating distributions by percentiles, including the median.

Arithmetic scale: equal distances measure equal absolute distances.

Logarithmic scale: equal distances measure equal proportional differences (i.e. percentage change in a variable).

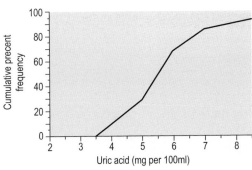

Fig. 7.3 **Cumulative frequency plot.**

MEASURES OF CENTRAL TENDENCY

$$\text{Arithmetic mean} = \frac{\text{Sum of observations}}{\text{Number of observations}}$$

The geometric mean is calculated using first the logarithm of the values, then the arithmetic mean of the logarithm and finally the antilog of the calculated arithmetic mean.
- Used as a substitute for the arithmetic mean when the distribution is skewed, or for describing fractional values, e.g. a series of serum antibody titres. Can only be used for positive values.

The median is the central value of a series of observations arranged in order of magnitude. Unlike the mean, it is not sensitive to extreme values in a series.

The mode is the most frequently observed value in a series of values, i.e. the maximum point in a frequency distribution.

MEASURES OF DISPERSION

(Measures of variation, spread)

1. SAMPLE RANGE

Difference between the highest and lowest values. Disadvantages are that:
1. Range increases as the number of observations increases and extreme values may be unreliable.
2. It provides no information as to the variability of the values between the extremes.

2. PERCENTILE (Fig. 7.4)

- The level of measurement below which a specified proportion of the distribution falls, e.g. the 5th and 95th percentile are the values of a particular measurement below which 5% and 95% of people fall.
- A *quartile* is the division of the distribution using cutpoints at 25%, 50% and 75%. The 'interquartile range' is the difference between the values of the 25th and 75th percentile.

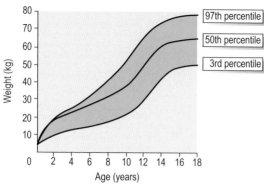

Fig. 7.4 Percentile plot.

3. INTERQUARTILE RANGE (IQR)

- IQR is the interval delimited by the 25th and 75th percentiles (upper and lower quartile), and comprises 50% of the observations available.
- Robust measure that is not influenced by extreme observations.

4. BOX AND WHISKER PLOT (Fig. 7.5)

Graphical method for displaying quantitative variables which have a skewed distribution.

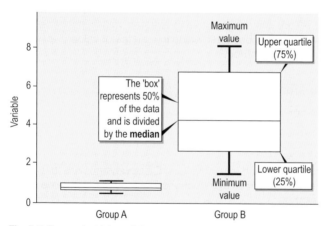

Fig. 7.5 Box and whisker plot.

5. VARIANCE AND STANDARD DEVIATION

Measure of spread of observations about the mean.

$$\text{Variance} = \frac{\text{Sum of (individual observations} - \text{mean)}^2}{\text{Number of observations}}$$

$$\text{Standard deviation (SD)} = \sqrt{\text{Variance}}$$

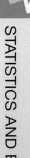

6. COEFFICIENT OF VARIATION

- Ratio of the standard deviation of a series of observations to the mean of the observations. It is without units and expressed as a percentage.

$$\text{Coefficient of variation (\%)} = \left(\frac{\text{SD}}{\text{mean}}\right) \times 100$$

- Used to make comparisons of spread when the means are dissimilar, i.e. standard deviation of 10 around a mean of 40 indicates a greater degree of scatter than a standard deviation of 10 around a mean of 400.

PROBABILITY DISTRIBUTIONS

The probability distribution of a random variable is a table, graph or mathematical expression giving the probabilities with which the random variable takes different values.

1. NORMAL OR GAUSSIAN DISTRIBUTION (Fig. 7.6)

- Theoretical, symmetrical bell-shaped distribution.
- Specified by its mean and standard deviation. The mean, median and mode are equal.
- Approximately 68% of the observations fall within one standard deviation of the mean; 95% of observations fall within two standard deviations from the mean and 99% fall within three standard deviations from the mean.

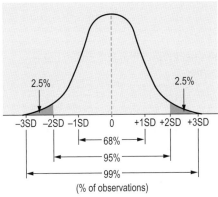

Fig. 7.6 Normal distribution.

Example
1000 men have a mean weight of 160 lb with a standard deviation of 10 lb.
The population weight is normally distributed.
Therefore, 680 (68%) of the men have weights of 160 ± 10 lbs (±1 SD) or between 150 and 170 lbs, and 997 (99.7%) have weights of 160 ± 30 lbs (±3 SD) or between 130 and 190 lbs.

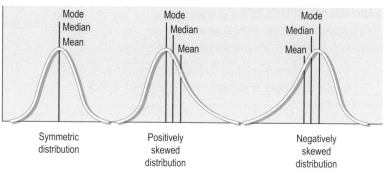

Fig. 7.7 Skewed distribution.

2. SKEWED DISTRIBUTION (Fig. 7.7)

- A distribution that is asymmetric.
- A skewed distribution with a longer tail among the *lower* values is skewed to the *left* or *negatively* skewed.
- A skewed distribution with a longer tail among the *higher* values is skewed to the *right* or *positively* skewed.
- In general, if the curve is skewed, the mean is always towards the long tail, the mode near the short tail, and the median somewhere between the two.

Transformation of data is performed when comparisons are made between two or more samples with unequal variances or when their distributions are non-normal. Logarithmic, square root or square transformations are used most commonly.

3. LOG-NORMAL DISTRIBUTION

This is a skewed distribution when plotted using an arithmetic scale, but is a normal distribution using a logarithmic scale.

4. BINOMIAL DISTRIBUTION

This describes the probability distribution of possible outcomes from a series of data when there are:
1. Only two mutually exclusive outcomes, e.g. success or failure, boy or girl.
2. A known number of independent trials of an event, and the probability of an event or outcome is the same for all trials, e.g. the probability of three male births in a family of six children, where the child's sex is the outcome of the trial.

5. POISSON DISTRIBUTION

This describes the probability of occurrence of rare events in a large population. It represents a limiting case of the binomial distribution, e.g. the probability of occurrence of a specific congenital birth defect in a large number of births.

SAMPLING

Used to estimate unknown characteristics of a population, such as:
1. The mean value of some measurement.
2. The proportion of the population with some characteristic.

Statistical inference is the process of inferring features of the population from observation of a sample.

Sampling error may be due to **systematic** or **random errors**.

Systematic errors (biases)

1. *Selection bias* occurs when comparisons are made between groups of patients that differ with respect to determinants of outcome other than those under study. Methods for controlling for selection bias include:
   (i) Randomization (see p. 324)
   (ii) Restricted study eligibility of patients
   (iii) Matching of patients in one study group to those with similar characteristics in the comparison group
   (iv) Stratification (i.e. comparison of rates within groups of individuals who have the same values for the confounding variable)
   (v) Adjustment, either using simple methods of standardization or the techniques of multiple linear and logistic regression.
2. *Measurement bias* occurs when the methods of measurement are consistently dissimilar among groups of patients, e.g. recall bias occurs when individuals in one group are more likely to remember past events than individuals in another of the study or control groups. Recall bias is especially likely when the study involves serious disease and the characteristics under study are commonly occurring, subjectively remembered events.
3. *Confounding bias* occurs when two factors 'travel together' and the effect of one is confused or distorted by the other.

Random errors

Such errors are determined by heterogeneity of the population and sample size (see p. 315, type I and II errors).

CENTRAL LIMIT THEOREM (Fig. 7.8)

- Means of repeated random samples of a particular size from a population will be normally distributed around the original population mean, regardless of the distribution of the observations in the original population, from which the samples were drawn.
- The mean value of the collection of all possible sample means will equal the mean of the original population.

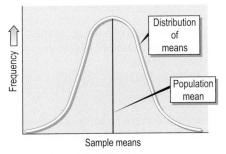

Fig. 7.8 Central limit theorem.

STATISTICS AND EPIDEMIOLOGY

STANDARD ERROR OF THE MEAN (SEM)

- The distribution of the means of these samples has a standard deviation around the population mean. This is called the standard error of the mean and describes the distribution of mean values. It depends on both the standard deviation of the original population and the sample size.

$$\text{Standard error} = \frac{\text{Standard deviation of observations in a sample}}{\sqrt{\text{Sample size}}}$$

- It measures the variability of the sample statistic (mean or proportion) in relation to the true, but unknown, population characteristic, i.e. how accurate is the sample mean as an estimate of the population mean? *(Contrast with the standard deviation which is a measure of the variability of the observations.)*
- Also used when one sample mean is compared to another, and in constructing confidence intervals for a mean or proportion.

Example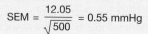

Mean systolic blood pressure of 500 randomly selected males from Glasgow was 130 mmHg and the standard deviation was 12.05 mmHg.

To determine the precision of this mean, i.e. how closely it gives the true mean blood pressure of males in this district:

$$\text{SEM} = \frac{12.05}{\sqrt{500}} = 0.55 \text{ mmHg}$$

This represents an estimate of the standard deviation of means in the sample of 500.

SEM is affected by two main factors:

1. **Sample size (n):** as n increases, SEM decreases: i.e. to halve SEM, the sample size needs to be quadrupled.
2. **Standard deviation** of original population values: as the standard deviation increases, SEM increases: i.e. if original population is uniform (small standard deviation), there will be little variation from sample mean to sample mean, and SEM will be small.

CONFIDENCE INTERVAL (CI)

- The CI is the interval or range about which the 'true' statistic (mean, proportion, correlation coefficient, relative risk) is believed to be found within a given population with a known probability.
- The rationale for calculating CIs is that a single value (or point estimate) in one study sample is likely to be inaccurate. The CI provides additional information about the true population value.
- CIs are also useful in informing the clinical significance of a result, as the lower and upper boundaries may indicate possible treatment effects in negative trials, or the lack of an effect in positive trials.
- Conventional confidence limits are 90%, 95% and 99%.

Sample mean $\pm 2.56 \times$ SE = 99% CI (probability 0.99)

i.e. 99% of *sample means* under normal distribution curve lie within a distance of 2.56 SD from the true population mean, or 99% confident that the interval contains the true population mean. *(Contrast with 99% of observations under any normal distribution curve lie within 2.56 SD from the mean.)*

- It is standard practice to use 95% confidence limits.
Sample mean $\pm 1.96 \times$ SE = 95% CI (probability 0.95)

- A 99% CI will be wider than a 95% CI.
- The width of the CI also depends on the sample size: larger samples provide narrower CIs.
- If the 95% CI contains 0 then the results are not significantly different between the two groups (for relative risk or odds ratio, if the result contains 1 then the results are not significantly different).

Example

Metoprolol trial in acute myocardial infarction: n = 698 patients on metoprolol; percent dying within 90 days on metoprolol = 5.7% with a standard error of 0.88%.
Therefore, the 95% confidence limits for the true percentage dying on metoprolol = $5.7 \pm 1.96 \times 0.88$ = 4.0% and 7.5% (i.e. 95% confident that if the whole population of eligible patients (or if the study were to be repeated) were given metoprolol, the true percentage dying lies somewhere between 4.0% and 7.5%).

Z SCORE

- This is the simplest example of a statistical test. It examines the comparison between a sample mean and a known population mean by calculating the ratio of the difference between means to the standard error.

$$Z = \frac{\text{Sample mean} - \text{Population mean}}{\text{SEM}}$$

- The Z score (or critical ratio) is the number of standard deviations that a value in a normally distributed population lies away from the mean. Thus, in a normally distributed population, 95% of the population lie within 1.96 Z scores of the mean.

HYPOTHESIS TESTING AND STATISTICAL SIGNIFICANCE

NULL HYPOTHESIS

- The null hypothesis underlies all statistical tests. It states that there is no difference between the samples or populations being compared, and that any difference observed is simply the result of random variation.

Null hypothesis (H_0): $P_1 - P_2 = 0$ or $P_1 = P_2$
Alternative hypothesis (H_A): $P_1 - P_2 \neq 0$ or $P_1 \neq P_2$

Where P_1 is the probability of a characteristic in sample or population 1, and P_2 is the probability of the same characteristic in the control sample or comparison population 2.

STATISTICAL SIGNIFICANCE

- The purpose of significance testing is to assess *how strong is the evidence* for a difference between one group and another, or whether random occurrence could reasonably explain the difference.

Significance level (α)

Conventional significance levels are: 5%, 1% and 0.1%. The smaller the value, the less the likelihood of the difference having occurred by chance. A 5%

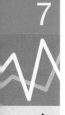

significance level is most often used for statistical comparisons (i.e. a 5% chance of detecting a difference and rejecting the null hypothesis, when the treatments are actually the same, means that one out of 20 times the result would occur by chance). If chosen at the outset of the study, it expresses the risk the investigator is prepared to accept of a type 1 error (see below) occurring.

Critical level (*p* value)
- The strength of the evidence may also be expressed in terms of probabilities (*p* values). Conventional *p* values are 0.05 (5%), 0.01 (1%) and 0.001 (0.1%).
- It is the probability that a given difference is observed in a study sample statistic (mean or proportion) when in reality such a difference does not exist in the population.

Example
A *p* value of 0.04 is interpreted as a 4 in 100 chance of observing a difference of a given magnitude between, for example, the mean cholesterol level of two groups, when in fact in the population the two groups had similar mean cholesterol levels. ✓

- Conventionally a difference is said to be statistically significant if the corresponding *p* value is <0.05.

Confidence intervals (p. 312)
These may also be used to provide an indication of the plausible range of the difference between two proportions. The recommendations of the major scientific journals are that confidence limits should be calculated and shown for all results.

One- and two-tailed tests
- *A two-tailed (-sided) test* is concerned with differences between observations in either direction, (i.e. checks both the upper and lower tails of the normal distribution).
  For example, two alternative treatments, A and B are compared, where either A or B may be better.
- *A one-tailed (-sided) test* is only concerned with differences between observations in one direction, (i.e. only one tail of the normal distribution curve), e.g. whether drug A is better than a placebo. The *p* value for a one-tailed test is generally half that for a two-sided test.

Clinical versus statistical significance
- Statistical significance is not the same as clinical importance. Clinical relevance must be assessed in terms of the magnitude of the difference. A statistically significant difference may not be clinically important i.e. the effect may be too small to warrant changing a treatment policy. Conversely the result may be clinically but not statistically significant. This can be avoided by using a sufficient sample size.
- Clinical significance or importance of a treatment effect is the magnitude of the treatment effect expressed as a relative risk, absolute risk difference, relative risk reduction or numbers needed to treat. Whether an effect is clinically significant requires a clinical of public health judgement as to what is an important effect.

Table 7.1 Type I and II errors

Conclusions from observations	Actual situation	
	Treatment has an effect	Treatment has no effect
Treatment has an effect	True positive $(1 - \alpha)$	False positive (α)
Treatment has no effect	False negative (β)	True negative $(1 - \beta)$

TYPE I AND II ERRORS (Table 7.1)

These concern the incorrect rejection or acceptance of the null hypothesis.
There are two types of errors:
1. **Type I (α) error:** the probability of detecting a significant difference when the parameters, or treatments, are really the same (*significance level α*), i.e. the risk of a false-positive result.
2. **Type II (β) error:** the probability of not detecting a significant difference when there really is a difference, i.e. the risk of a false-negative result. One minus the type II error $(1 - \beta)$ is the *power* of the test to detect a difference.
- **The power of a test** depends on:
1. The significance level
2. The size of the difference you wish to detect
3. The sample size.

Determinants of sample size
1. Magnitude of the difference in outcomes between the two treatment groups.
2. Probability of an α (type I) error, i.e. false-positive result. Usually set at 0.05.
3. Probability of a β (type II) error, i.e. false-negative result. Usually set at 0.20, so there is a 0.8 chance or 80% power to detect a specified degree of difference (effect size) at a defined degree of significance.
4. Proportion of patients experiencing the outcome of interest and the variability of observations. An insufficient number of patients may lead to failure to detect the true difference that may exist (type II error).

TESTS OF SIGNIFICANCE

- Used for comparisons between estimates (sample means or proportions).
- Two types:
    1. *Parametric*
    2. *Non-parametric.*

Selecting a statistical test
Depends on:
1. Type of data and assumptions
2. Study design, e.g. cohort, paired data
3. Number of groups
4. Purpose of analysis.

PARAMETRIC TESTS

Assumptions:
1. The populations from which samples are taken should be normally distributed.
2. The variances of the samples are the same (applies to *t*-test).

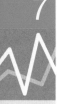

STATISTICS AND EPIDEMIOLOGY

Examples
1. *t*-tests
2. Pearson's correlation.

Student's *t*-test
- Based on the *t* distribution and is used for comparing a single small sample with a population or to compare the difference in means between two small samples.
- The *t*-test is inappropriate if more than two means are compared.
- As the sample size increases, the *t* distribution closely resembles the normal distribution, and at infinite degrees of freedom, the *t* and normal distribution are identical.

$$\text{Calculated } t \text{ value} = \frac{\text{Observed difference in means}}{\text{Standard error of the difference in means}}$$

- Calculated *t* value is compared with a critical *t* value from tables at a predetermined significance level and appropriate degrees of freedom. The larger the value of *t* (+ or −), the smaller the value of *p*, and the stronger the evidence that the null hypothesis is untrue.

Degrees of freedom (df) are the number of independently varying quantities, i.e. the number of variables in a series or distribution that can be freely assigned values when the sum of the values is fixed. Used in preference to sample size.

(a) Using paired data
The paired *t*-test compares the means of two small paired observations, either on the same individual or on matched individuals, e.g. comparison of the effects of two drugs on a particular patient, at different points in time.

$$t = \frac{\bar{x}}{\sqrt{\dfrac{s^2}{n}}}$$

where s = SD
$\bar{x}$ is the mean difference between the pairs, and n is the number of pairs.
(df = n − 1.)

(b) Using unpaired data
The unpaired *t*-test compares the means of two small, independent samples, e.g. two separate groups of patients.

$$t = \frac{\bar{x}_1 - \bar{x}_2}{s\sqrt{\left(\dfrac{1}{n_1} + \dfrac{1}{n_2}\right)}}$$

where s = pooled SD
n_1 and n_2 = number of patients in treatment groups
$\bar{x}_1$ and $\bar{x}_2$ are the means from samples 1 and 2.
(df = (n₁ − 1) + (n₂ − 1).)

NON-PARAMETRIC TESTS

- Make no assumptions about the underlying distribution of the sample.
- Used when data is qualitative, i.e. measured by ordinal (rank) scale, or not normally distributed.
- Not as powerful as parametric tests when data is normally distributed.

Examples
1. Chi-square (χ^2) test.
2. Fisher's exact probability test: used to determine the exact probability that an observed distribution is due to chance, when the expected frequencies in any one cell of a contingency table are less than 5.
3. Wilcoxon rank sum test: used for unpaired data.
4. Mann–Whitney U test: gives equivalent results to the Wilcoxon rank sum test.
5. Wilcoxon signed rank test: used for matched or paired data.
6. Kruskal–Wallis test:
Data transformations (e.g. to a log scale) are an alternative to using non-parametric methods.

Chi-square test
- Used to determine the extent to which an observed series of proportions (or frequencies) differs from an expected series of proportions (or frequencies), or that two or more proportions (or frequencies) differ from one another, based on the χ^2 probability distribution.
- Can only be used on count data, and the categories of data used must be mutually exclusive and discrete.

$$\chi^2 = \frac{\text{Sum of (observed – expected)}^2}{\text{Expected}}$$

- Calculated χ^2 value is compared with a critical value of χ^2 from tables at a predetermined significance level and appropriate degrees of freedom. The larger the value of χ^2, the smaller the probability p, and so the stronger the evidence that the null hypothesis is untrue.

Yates' correction factor
The χ^2 test is based on a normal approximation of the binomial distribution, and therefore a correction for continuity, called the Yates' correction factor, is often included in the χ^2 test equation. The Yates' correction factor is used with small samples, and decreases the χ^2 value, so that the null hypothesis is less often rejected.

CORRELATION

Describes the strength of the linear relationship between variables and is denoted by the *correlation coefficient (r)* or *Pearson's product moment correlation coefficient* (a parametric test) (Table 7.2).
- Its value can range from –1 to +1.
- A correlation coefficient may be strong but statistically non-significant because of sample size. The statistical significance of the correlation coefficient is based on the associated p value.
- Assumes that one or both variables are normally distributed (i.e. parametric correlation).

Table 7.2 Correlation

Correlation coefficient (r)	Degree of association
0.8 to 1.0	Strong
0.5 to 0.8	Moderate
0.2 to 0.5	Weak
0 to 0.2	Negligible

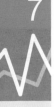

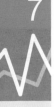

STATISTICS AND EPIDEMIOLOGY

- *Scattergrams* show the relationship between X and Y, e.g. height and weight (Fig. 7.9).
- Spearman's and Kendall's rank correlation coefficients are the non-parametric alternatives to Pearson's correlation coefficient.

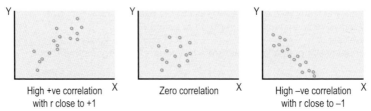

Fig. 7.9 Scattergrams.

REGRESSION

- Describes the relationship between two variables, and how one value varies depending on the value of another, e.g. the incidence of myocardial infarction and number of cigarettes smoked per day.
- Mainly used when there is one measured dependent variable and one or more independent variables.
- A regression line is a line that minimizes the sum of the squares of the vertical distances to the line of each data point, i.e. 'least squares regression' (Fig. 7.10).
- Used when the main purpose is to develop a predictive model, i.e. to predict Y for a given value of X, using the equation: $Y = a + bx$.
- As with the correlation coefficient (r), a slope of 0 represents no relationship between the variables. But a regression coefficient can vary between $-\infty$ and $+\infty$, and is expressed in the same units as outcome variable.
- Two regression techniques: *multiple linear regression* and *logistic regression*.

1. *Multiple linear regression* predicts a single dependent or response variable using a number of independent variables, e.g. blood pressure predicted by weight, age, smoking and family history can only be used for normally distributed responses, and not for binary outcomes, e.g. disease/no disease.
2. *Logistic regression* is used to predict the probability of a binary outcome occurring, e.g. breast cancer/no cancer using several predictor or explanatory variables, e.g. age, family history. It is often used to assess odds ratios in case–control studies and allows for the correction of multiple potential confounding factors.

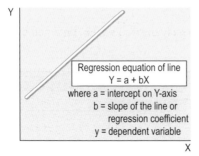

Regression equation of line
$Y = a + bX$
where a = intercept on Y-axis
b = slope of the line or
regression coefficient
y = dependent variable

318   Fig. 7.10 Regression line.

EPIDEMIOLOGY

CRUDE RATES

- These are summary rates for a given population, i.e. not standardized for age, sex or other variables, e.g. crude birth and death rate.
- They cannot be used to compare events in different populations because these rates will vary depending on the age–sex composition of the total population.

Incidence rate

Number of new cases of a disease in a given period
Total population at risk during the same period of time

Change in incidence indicates a change in the balance of aetiological factors.

Attack rate

Incidence rate calculated in an epidemic situation, using a particular population observed for a limited period of time.
Normally expressed as a percentage.

Prevalence rate (point)

Total number of cases in a population at one particular time
Total population at risk at the time

Point prevalence refers to a particular point in time.
Period prevalence refers to a given time interval.
Prevalence rates are influenced both by the incidence of the disease and the duration of the illness:
Prevalence = Incidence × average duration of illness.
Used mainly to measure the amount of illness and therefore the health needs of a community.

Mortality rate

$$\frac{\text{Number of deaths during one year}}{\text{Total population at mid-year}} \times 1000$$
= Deaths per 1000

Case fatality rate

$$\frac{\text{Number of deaths due to a disease in a specified period of time}}{\text{Number of cases of the disease in the same period of time}} \times 100$$

i.e. the risk of dying if the disease is contracted.
Normally expressed as a percentage.

Proportionate mortality rate (PMR)

$$\frac{\text{Number of deaths from a given cause in a specified period of time}}{\text{Total number of deaths in the same period of time}} \times 100$$

Used to determine the relative importance of a specific cause of death in relation to all causes of death in a population, e.g. the three leading causes of deaths in the US in 1980 were heart disease (PMR = 38.2%); cancer (PMR = 20.9%) and stroke (PMR = 8.6%).

319

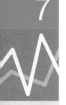

STATISTICS AND EPIDEMIOLOGY

It is not a rate and therefore does not measure the probability of dying from a particular cause. Usually expressed as a percentage.

Person-time at risk
Can be used as the denominator in calculation of rates:
Sum of the individual lengths of time each subject is under observation, and can be estimated as number at risk of the event, e.g. death × average length of study period usually expressed in years, i.e. (PYAR) but also in months:

Example
Patient   *Duration of follow-up*
1   2 years
2   3 years 1 month
3   1 year 3 months
4   4 years
PYAR = 10 years and 4 months, i.e. 10.333 years.
If 2 deaths are observed during study period:
Mortality rate = 2 per 10.333 PYAR
            = 0.19 per PYAR
            = 19 per 100 PYAR

ADJUSTED RATES

- These equalize the differences in the populations at risk so that the rates are comparable. Age-adjusted rates are most frequently used.
- The direct and indirect methods of standardization are two statistical methods employed to compute adjusted rates.

Standardized mortality ratio (SMR)
Ratio of observed deaths in a particular population to the number that would be expected if a standard mortality rate for that population applied, i.e. age/sex standardized rate. It is calculated using the indirect method of standardization. Usually expressed as a percentage.
If the SMR > 100, then more events are occurring in the population than expected.

SPECIFIC RATES

- These relate only to a specific part of the population, e.g. age, sex, race, occupation, cause-specific death rates, and therefore can be used to compare events in different populations.

Still birth rate

$$\frac{\text{Number of still births (See Note)}}{\text{Total births (live and still) in the same period of time}} \times 1000$$

Perinatal mortality rate (PMR)

$$\frac{\text{Number of still births and early neonatal deaths (<7 days old) in a period of time}}{\text{Total number of births (live and still) in the same period of time}} \times 1000$$

Infant mortality rate (IMR)

$$\frac{\text{Number of deaths under 1 year of age in a period of time}}{\text{Number of live births in same period}} \times 1000$$

IMR consists of two segments: the neonatal mortality rate (deaths <28 days old) and the postneonatal mortality rate (deaths 28 days to 11 months). Neonatal and perinatal mortality are generally affected by causes of death related to maternal health, while the postneonatal mortality is more closely linked to environmental factors.

Note: Still birth is defined as delivery of a fetus that shows no signs of life after a presumed 28-week gestation.

PRINCIPLES OF STUDY DESIGN (Fig. 7.11 and Table 7.3)

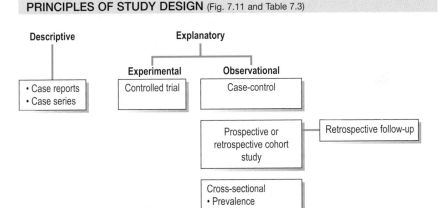

Fig. 7.11 The terminology of study designs.

Table 7.3 Matching the strongest research designs to clinical questions	
Question	*Design*
Diagnosis	Prevalence/Cross-sectional
Prevalence	Prevalence/Cross-sectional
Incidence	Cohort
Risk	Cohort / Case–control
Prognosis	Cohort
Treatment	Clinical trial
Causation	Cohort / Case–control

CROSS-SECTIONAL STUDY

- A survey of the frequency of a disease or risk factor in a defined population at a given time.
- Provides information in a population at a particular point in time and may generate hypotheses about associations between risk factors and disease.
- It cannot evaluate hypotheses about causation, as it does not take into account how the timing of exposure to a risk factor relates to the development of disease.

COHORT STUDY

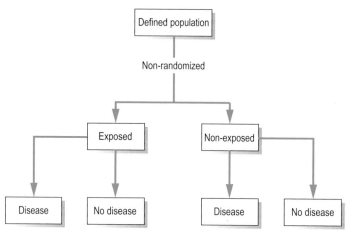

Fig. 7.12 Prospective (cohort) studies.

- A cohort study (Table 7.4 and Fig. 7.12) is an observational study of a group of subjects with a specific disease or characteristic who are followed up over a period of time to detect complications or new events. This group may be compared with a control group. If this type of study requires follow-up over several years, it may be prone to loss of subjects.
- Persons exposed (a + b) to the suspected cause and those not exposed (c + d) are followed prospectively over time, to determine the rate of specific diseases or events.

- Incidence rate of outcome in the exposed group $= \dfrac{a}{a + b}$

- Incidence rate of outcome in the non-exposed group $= \dfrac{c}{c + d}$

Table 7.4 Simple 2 × 2 table used in cohort and case–control studies

		Disease		Total
		Present	*Absent*	
Exposure	Present	a	b	a + b
	Absent	c	d	c + d
Total		a + c	b + d	n

CASE–CONTROL STUDY

- A case–control study (Fig. 7.13) is a type of observational study in which the investigator selects cases with the disease, and appropriate controls without the disease, and obtains data regarding past exposure to possible aetiological factors in both groups. The investigator then compares the rate of exposure of the two groups. The validity of this type of study depends on the appropriate selection of control subjects.

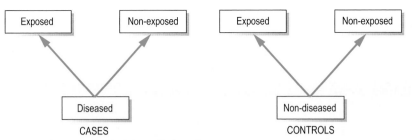

Fig. 7.13 Case–control (retrospective) study.

- Persons with a disease (a + c) and those without (b + d) are identified, and then compared regarding specific characteristics to determine their possible association with the disease.

- Exposure rate among cases = $\dfrac{a}{a + c}$

- Exposure rate among controls = $\dfrac{b}{b + d}$

Table 7.5 Comparison of case–control and cohort studies

Case–control	Cohort
1. Suitable for rare diseases	1. Suitable for common diseases
2. Short study time and cheaper to perform	2. Prolonged study time with potential for increasing drop-out rates and therefore more costly
3. Smaller number of subjects required	3. Large number of subjects usually required
4. Bias may occur in the selection of cases and controls and in ascertaining exposure	4. Less selection bias occurs
5. Because data collected retrospectively, some data may not be available or of poorer quality	5. Prospective data collection may be more accurate
6. No volunteer subjects needed	6. Subjects usually volunteer
7. Cannot determine true incidence or relative risk. Results expressed as odds ratios	7. Incidence, relative risk and attributable risk can be determined
8. Estimate of time from exposure to development of disease not possible	8. Estimate of time from exposure to development of disease possible

Table 7.6 Methods of controlling for selection bias

Strategy	Comment
Randomization	Assigns patients to groups in a way that gives each patient an equal chance of falling into one or the other group
Restriction	Limits the range of characteristics of patients in the study
Matching	For each patient in one group, selects one or more patients with the same characteristics (except for the one under study) for a comparison group
Stratification	Compares rates within subgroups (strata) with otherwise similar probability of the outcome
Adjustment	
Simple	Mathematically adjusts crude rates for one or a few characteristics so that equal weight is given to strata of similar risk
Multiple	Adjusts for differences in a large number of factors related to outcome, using mathematical modelling techniques

STATISTICS AND EPIDEMIOLOGY

RANDOMIZED CLINICAL TRIAL (RCT) (Table 7.7 and Fig. 7.14)

- Experimental design used to assess the differences between two or more groups receiving different interventions or treatments.

Table 7.7 The five stages of drug development in clinical trials		
Phase	Main aims	Study subjects
Preclinical	Pharmacology Toxicology	In vitro In laboratory animals
Phase 1	Clinical pharmacology and toxicology Drug metabolism Drug/treatment safety	Healthy individuals and/or patients
Phase 2	Initial treatment studies Drug treatment efficacy	Small numbers of patients
Phase 3	Large randomized controlled trials Comparing new to standard treatments Drug/treatment safety and efficacy	Large numbers of patients
Phase 4	Post-marketing surveillance Long-term safety and rare events	All patients prescribed the drug

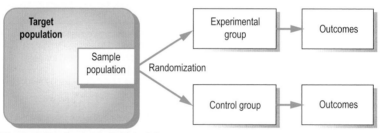

Fig. 7.14 Randomized clinical trial.

Clinical trial terminology

Effectiveness   The extent to which a treatment produces a beneficial effect when implemented under the *usual* clinical conditions for a particular group of patients.

Efficacy   The extent to which a treatment produces a beneficial effect when assessed under the *ideal* conditions of an investigation.

Randomization   Method of assignment of subjects to either the experimental or control treatments, whereby each patient has an equal chance of appearing in any one treatment group.
- Protects against selection bias in the assignment process.
- Allows the control of other clinical variables which may affect the outcomes under investigation, and so minimizes the effects of systematic error (bias).
- Ensures the two groups are similar for baseline characteristics so outcomes can be attributed to therapy, and not to dissimilar groups.

Placebo
A pharmacologically inert dummy, identical in appearance to the treatment(s), should normally be used for the control group, when there is no conventional treatment available.
- It dissociates the effects of treatment from the suggestive element imposed by the receipt of treatment.

Double-blinding (masking) technique
Neither the subject/patient nor the investigator/doctor knows to which group the subject is assigned
- Most desirable in trials where the endpoints used are subjective, i.e. improved/unchanged/worse. Especially in trials of pain and depression.
- Single-blinded implies that only the patient/subject is unaware of which treatment he or she is assigned to.

Analysis by 'intention to treat'
Outcome among all those allocated to treatment after randomization is compared to all those allocated to control, irrespective of whether patients actually received or completed allocated treatment(s) or had missing data or poor compliance. This avoids introducing bias into the assessment of treatment.

Interim analysis
Analyses that are carried out before the end of the trial in order to assess whether the accumulating data are beginning to demonstrate a beneficial effect of one treatment over the other with sufficient certainty. This can avoid further patients being randomized to the inferior treatment.

Cross-over or 'within-patient' trial (Fig. 7.15)
A comparison of the effects of two or more treatments in the same patient, when the treatments are applied at different points in time over the course of the illness. Important that therapies have a 'carry over' period and a sufficiently long 'wash out' period between them to avoid the effect of the trial therapies influencing the outcome of the comparison therapy.
- Suitable for the assessment of short-term effects of treatment in relatively stable, chronic conditions.

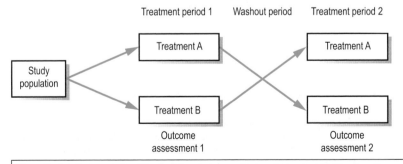

The patient undergoes pairs of treatment periods organized so that one period involves the use of the experimental treatment, and another period the use of another. Treatment periods are repeated until the doctor and patient are convinced that the treatments are definitely different or not different.

Fig. 7.15 Cross-over trial.

| **Meta-analysis** | Mathematical analysis performed on data from two or more different but similar studies, usually clinical trials, for the purpose of drawing a global conclusion concerning the usefulness of a drug or procedure, the contribution of a risk factor to a disease, or the role of a condition in the aetiology of a disease. The main problems relate to pooling results from heterogeneous studies (Fig. 7.16). |

- The results of a meta-analysis are usually expressed as odds ratios or relative risks.

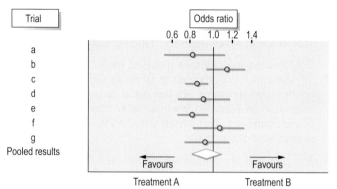

Fig. 7.16 A theoretical plot showing the results of a meta-analysis comparing Treatments A and B.

The individual trials are listed on the left hand side and their results are represented by the dark circles and horizontal lines. The diamond represents the pooled results of all included studies.

MEASURES OF EFFECT (Table 7.8)

Table 7.8 Measures of effect

	Disease develops	Disease does not develop	Total	Incidence rates of disease
Exposed (or treatment A)	a	b	a + b	$\dfrac{a}{a+b}$ = Incidence in exposed
Not exposed (or control treatment B)	c	d	c + d	$\dfrac{c}{c+d}$ = Incidence in non-exposed

Absolute risk (AL)	Rate of occurrence of a disease, i.e. incidence in exposed population or treatment A in an RCT.

Relative risk (RL)	$\dfrac{\text{Incidence rate among exposed or treatment A in an RCT}}{\text{Incidence rate among non-exposed or treatment B in an RCT}}$ $\dfrac{a/(a+b)}{c/(c+d)} = \dfrac{ad}{bc}$

(When the incidence of disease is *low*, this simplifies to ad/bc.)

- Thus, relative risk measures strength of association between a factor and outcome. The stronger the association between the exposure and the disease, the higher the relative risk (Table 7.9).
- Can be used to quantify the risk of an event between control and experimental groups in an RCT.

Table 7.9 Interpreting relative risk of a disease

If RR = 1	Risk in exposed = Risk in unexposed (no association)
If RR > 1	Risk in exposed > Risk in unexposed (positive association; ? causal)
If RR < 1	Risk in exposed < Risk in unexposed (negative association; ? protective)

Attributable risk Incidence rate among exposed – the incidence rate among non-exposed;
i.e. measures the amount of risk that can be attributed to a particular factor.

Population attributable risk The excess incidence of disease in a community that is associated with a risk factor. It is a product of the attributable risk and the prevalence of the risk factor in the population.

Population attributable fraction The fraction of disease in a population that is attributable to exposure to a particular risk factor and therefore that may be prevented (in principle) by removal of the exposure. It is obtained by dividing the population attributable risk by the total incidence of disease in a population.

Example

Death rate from lung cancer in smokers (i.e. absolute risk) = 0.80/1000/year.
Death rate from lung cancer in non-smokers = 0.05/1000/year.
Prevalence of smoking = 50%
Total death rate from lung cancer = 0.50/1000/year
Therefore:

Relative risk = $\dfrac{0.80/1000}{0.05/1000}$ = 16.0

Attributable risk = 0.80/1000/year – 0.05/1000/year
= 0.75/1000/year

Population attributable risk = 0.75/1000/year × 0.50
= 0.375/1000/year

Population attributable fraction = $\dfrac{0.375/1000}{0.50/1000}$ = 0.75

Absolute risk reduction (ARR) Incidence rate in control treatment group – incidence rate in experimental treatment group.
This is more clinically relevant than the relative risk reduction (RRR) because the RRR 'factors out' the baseline risk (see below), so that small differences in risk can seem significant compared to a small baseline risk.

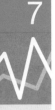

STATISTICS AND EPIDEMIOLOGY

Relative risk reduction (RRR)

An alternative way of expressing the RR. Calculated as:

$$RRR = (1 - RR) \times 100\%$$

i.e. the population or % of the baseline risk which was reduced by a given intervention:

> **Example**
> The RR for effect of aspirin versus no aspirin on vascular death = 0.80
>
> RRR = 1 − 0.80 × 100% = 20%
>
> So aspirin reduced the risk of death by 20%.

Number needed to treat (NNT)

Another measure of the impact of an intervention. It states how many patients need to be treated with the intervention to prevent one event which would otherwise occur. It is calculated as:

$$NNT = \frac{1}{RRR}$$

Because it is based on the absolute risk difference, it is possible for a treatment of only moderate efficacy to have a small NNT, and to have a considerable impact when used to treat a common disease:

> **Example**
> If 3 deaths are prevented per 100 patients with acute myocardial infarction then NNT = 1/0.3 × 100 = 33.
> In the event of the treatment having important side-effects, then the 'number needed to harm' (NNH) should also be calculated.

> **Example: Summary of measures of effect**
> 2000 patients with mild hypertension are randomly allocated to treatment or placebo. 4 patients in the placebo group have had a CVA at the end of the year and only 2 in the treated group have suffered a CVA:
>
> Absolute risk, treated group   = 2/1000
>
> Absolute risk, untreated group = 4/1000
>
> Relative risk (RR)   = 0.5
>
> Absolute risk reduction (ARR)   = 2/1000
>
> Number needed to treat (NNR) = 500

Odds ratio
(Table 7.10)

With a case–control study, it is not possible to obtain a relative risk by dividing the incidence of disease among those exposed by the incidence of disease among those not exposed. An alternative approach uses the odds ratio, which is conceptually and mathematically similar to the relative risk.
The odds is itself the ratio of two probabilities:

$$= \frac{\text{Probability of an event}}{1 - \text{probability of an event}}$$

Table 7.10 Odds ratio

	Cases (with disease)	Controls (without disease)
History of exposure	a	b
No history of exposure	c	d

Odds that a case is exposed $= \dfrac{a/(a + c)}{c/(a + c)} = \dfrac{a}{c}$

Odds that a control is exposed $= \dfrac{b/(b + d)}{d/(b + d)} = \dfrac{b}{d}$

The ratio of the odds $= \dfrac{a/c}{b/d} = \dfrac{ad}{bc}$

Odds ratio and relative risk
The odds ratio is approximately equal to the relative risk only when the incidence of disease is *low*.

Life-table (Kaplan–Meier) or survival analysis (Fig. 7.17)	A method of estimating the survival (or failure) events of a cohort over time, when some individuals are followed for longer periods of time than others and the status of some patients at the end of follow-up is not known. The chance of surviving to any point in time is estimated from the cumulative probability of surviving each of the time intervals that preceded it (syn: Kaplan–Meier life tables).

- Mainly used for comparing the survival experience of two or more groups, or predicting length of survival based on a number of given prognostic factors.
- The Kaplan–Meier method differs from the life-table method, in which the 'time' variable is grouped.
Comparison of survival curves: The survival curves of two or more separate groups can be compared statistically using the log-rank test.

Constructing a survival curve (Fig. 7.17)
- With the life table method, the chance of surviving to any point of time is estimated from the cumulative probability of surviving each of the time intervals that preceded it.
- For many of the time intervals no one dies, and the probability of surviving is 1. At other times, one or more patients die and the probabilities of surviving the time interval are then calculated as:

$$\frac{\text{no. of deaths in time interval}}{\text{no. at risk of dying at start of time interval}}$$

- Patients who have already died, dropped out or who have not yet been followed up to that time point are not at risk of dying, and are therefore not used to estimate survival at that time.
- When patients are lost from the study at any point in time, for any reason, e.g. loss to follow-up, drop-outs, these are called 'censored'.

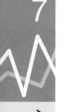

STATISTICS AND EPIDEMIOLOGY

- The cumulative probability of surviving all the time intervals is then used to construct the survival curve, and the overall probability of surviving up to a particular time point is calculated from the cumulative probability of surviving all the time intervals up to this point.

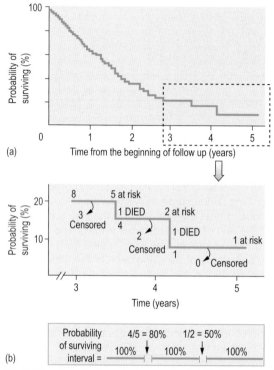

Fig. 7.17 a, A typical survival curve; b, detail of one part of the curve.
Adapted from Fletcher RH, Fletcher SW, Wagner WH 1996 Clinical epidemiology: the essentials, 3rd edn. Williams and Wilkins.

Evidence-based medicine (EBM)	EBM is the 'conscientious, explicit and judicious use of current best evidence in making decisions about individual patients'. This involves 'integrating individual clinical expertise with the best available external clinical evidence from systematic research'.
The hazard ratio (HR)	Measure of relative risk used in survival studies. An HR = 1 suggests the hazard risk of the event is the same in the two comparison groups. An HR >1 suggests one group is more likely to experience the event.

ASSOCIATION AND CAUSATION

- An association may be artefactual (because of bias in the study), non-causal or causal.

> **Five criteria adopted as a test of causation**
> 1. Consistency of the association, i.e. dose–response.
> 2. Strength of the association, i.e. size of relative risk.
> 3. Specificity of the association, i.e. degree to which one particular exposure produces one particular disease.
> 4. Temporal relationship of the association, i.e. exposure to factor must precede the development of the disease.
> 5. Biological plausibility of the association.

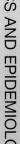

Cause–effect studies

Types of studies which examine cause–effect relationships and their relative strength of evidence are shown in Table 7.11.

Table 7.11 Study design and strength of evidence

Strong ↑ ↓ Weak	Clinical trial Cohort study Case–control study Cross-sectional Aggregate risk or ecological studies Case series Case report

Ecological (or aggregate) survey

A study based on *aggregated* data for a population at a point in time. Used to investigate the relationship of an exposure to a known or presumed risk factor for a particular outcome, e.g. comparing rate of cardiac mortality in 18 developed countries with wine consumption in these countries.

Ecological fallacy

The type of error that can occur when the existence of a group association is used to imply the existence of a relationship that does not exist at the individual level.

DIAGNOSTIC TESTS AND SCREENING (Table 7.12)

Table 7.12 2 × 2 table notation for expressing the results of a diagnostic test

		Disease or result of gold standard test		Totals
		Present	*Absent*	
Diagnostic test result or screening	Positive	a	b (false +ve)	a+b
	Negative	c (false –ve)	d	c+d
	Totals	a+c	b+d	a+b+c+d

VALIDITY

Sensitivity	= a/(a+c)
Specificity	= d/(b+d)
Prevalence in the study	= (a+c)/(a+b+c+d)
Positive predictive value (of the test)	= a/a(a+b)
Negative predictive value (of the test)	= d/(c+d)

The ability of a screening test to provide an indication of which individuals have the disease and which do not.

Five components:

1. **Sensitivity** (%) is the test's ability to correctly identify those individuals who truly have the disease.

$$\frac{\text{Persons with the disease detected by the screening test}}{\text{Total number of persons tested with the disease}} \times 100$$

$$= \frac{a}{a + c} \times 100$$

- A high sensitivity implies few false negatives (Fig. 7.18) which is important for very rare or lethal diseases, e.g. phenylketonuria.

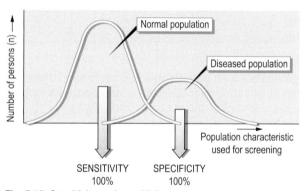

Fig. 7.18 Sensitivity and specificity.

2. **Specificity** (%) is the test's ability to correctly identify those individuals who do not have the disease.

$$\frac{\text{Persons without the disease who are negative to the screening test}}{\text{Total number of persons tested without the disease}} \times 100$$

$$= \frac{d}{b + d} \times 100$$

A high specificity implies few false positives, which is important for common diseases, e.g. diabetes.

3. **Predictive value** (%) is the test's ability to identify those individuals who truly have the disease (true positives) amongst all those individuals whose screening tests are positive.

$$\frac{\text{True positive (a)}}{\text{True positive (a) + false positive (b)}} \times 100$$

- The predictive value of a positive test increases with increasing disease prevalence.
- Lowering the screening cut-off level *increases* the sensitivity and number of false positives and *decreases* the specificity and number of false negatives.

Receiver operator curve (ROC)

- One way to express the relationship between sensitivity and specificity is to construct a receiver operating characteristic (ROC) curve. This may be used to describe the accuracy of a test over a range of cut-off points. The overall accuracy of the test can be described as the area under the curve (Fig. 7.19).

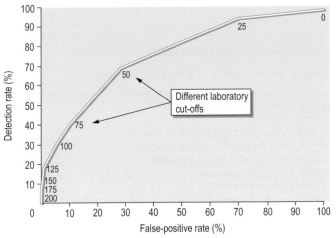

Fig. 7.19 ROC curve.

- Plot of sensitivity or detection rate is false-positive rate (100 – specificity %) for selected cut-offs.
- This allows the performance of different cut-offs to be compared. The choice of cut-off is a trade off between the false positive and negative rates.
- A good cut-off should be close to the top left-hand of the graph, i.e. high detection rate, low false positive rate.

Example

1000 participants in a screening programme
Disease prevalence 2%, i.e. 20 with the disease
Sensitivity of screening test = 95%
Specificity of screening test = 90%

Sensitivity: $\dfrac{95}{100} = \dfrac{a}{a + c}$

$a + c = 20$; so a (true positive) = 19, c (false negative) = 1

Specificity: $\dfrac{90}{100} = \dfrac{d}{b + d}$

$b + d = 980$; so b (false positive) = 98, d (true negative) = 882

Positive predictive value $= \dfrac{a}{a + b} = \dfrac{19}{19 + 98} = 16.24\%$

STATISTICS AND EPIDEMIOLOGY

SpPIN:	When a test has a high **sp**ecificity, a **p**ositive result rules **in** the diagnosis.	
SnNOUT:	When a test has a high **s**ensitivity a **n**egative result rules **out** the diagnosis.	

4. **The likelihood ratio** for a particular value of a diagnostic test is defined as: the probability of that test result in the presence of a disease, divided by the probability of the result in people without the disease.

Likelihood ratios express how many times more (or less) likely a test result is to be found in diseased as compared to non-diseased people.

5. **Reproducibility:** the variability of repeated measurements under different conditions.

BASIC REQUIREMENTS OF A SCREENING TEST

Modified Wilson criteria for screening of a disease (see box)

Mnemonic spells **IATROGENIC**
1. Condition should be **I**mportant.
2. An **A**cceptable treatment should be available for disease.
3. Diagnostic and **T**reatment facilities should be available.
4. A **R**ecognizable early symptomatic stage is required.
5. **O**pinions on who to treat must be agreed.
6. The safety of the test is **G**uaranteed.
7. The test **E**xamination must be acceptable to the patient.
8. The untreated **N**atural history of the disease must be known.
9. The test should be **I**nexpensive.
10. Screening must be **C**ontinuous.

- Also test parameters should be high (i.e. high sensitivity and specification), valid (i.e. measures relevant outcome not just surrogate markers), and reproducible.

BIASES IN EVALUATION OF SCREENING PROGRAMMES

Length–time bias	Bias which results from the preferential diagnosis of disease in patients with long preclinical stage of disease. Because of the positive association between duration of preclinical and clinical stages of disease, early detection through screening may appear to lead to longer survival.
Lead time bias	The spurious finding that patients diagnosed at an earlier stage of disease appear to have a longer survival compared to those diagnosed after developing symptoms. If patients are not all enrolled at similar well-defined points in the course of their disease, differences in outcome over time may just reflect differences in duration of illness.

MEASURES USED IN ECONOMIC EVALUATION OF HEALTHCARE INTERVENTIONS

Cost–benefit analysis
Comparison of the costs and outcomes of *different interventions* when these interventions have *different effects*, or similar effects of different magnitude, e.g. compare ratio of cost of intervention to cost savings through reduction in a particular outcome from intervention for a cervical cancer screening programme versus an influenza immunization programme.

Cost–effectiveness analysis
Comparison of the costs and outcomes of *different interventions* when the interventions are thought to have the *same outcome*, but a different magnitude of effect, e.g. kidney transplantation versus dialysis for patients with renal failure.

Cost–utility analysis
Comparison of the costs and outcomes of *different interventions* when these have *different effects*, or *similar effects of different magnitude*. This type of analysis allows individual values to be taken into account, as the impact of some interventions may vary. Outcomes are translated into utility value, usually quality-adjusted life-years or QALYs, which are then used to compare the costs of different interventions.

8

CLINICAL PHARMACOLOGY

GLOSSARY 338

DRUG INTERACTIONS 342
Major mechanisms of drug interactions
    342
  Drug absorption 342
  Plasma protein binding 342
  Metabolism 342
  Excretion 346
  Pharmacological interactions 346

**ADVERSE EFFECTS AND
    INTERACTIONS OF DRUGS** 346
Antihypertensive drugs 347
Antiarrhythmic drugs 352
Anticoagulants, thrombolytic and
  fibrinolytic drugs 355
Antirheumatic drugs 359
Lipid-lowering drugs 361
Peptic ulcer disease drugs 363
Antidepressant, anxiolytic, antipsychotic
  and antimania drugs 364
Anticonvulsant drugs 371
Antiparkinsonian drugs 373
Drugs used in Alzheimer's disease
  374
Drugs used for erectile dysfunction 374
Alcohol and other drugs with CNS effects
  375
Corticosteroids 377
Oral contraceptives 378
Oral hypoglycaemic drugs 379
Insulin 381
Drugs used in gout 381
Drugs used in hyperthyroidism 381
Antibacterial drugs 382
Antituberculous drugs 385
Antifungal drugs 386

Antiprotozoal drugs 387
Antiviral and antiretroviral drugs 388
Immunosuppressant drugs 393
  Cytotoxic drugs 393
  Other anticancer or transplantation
    drugs 394
  Immunotherapy 396

**ADVERSE EFFECTS IN SPECIAL RISK
    GROUPS** 396
Drugs in pregnancy 396
Drugs excreted in breast milk 398
Drugs in the elderly 398
Drugs in liver disease 399
Drugs in renal disease 399

ANTIDOTES USED IN OVERDOSE 400

**SUMMARY OF DRUG-INDUCED
    DISEASE** 401
Cardiovascular system 401
Respiratory system 402
Renal system 403
Gastrointestinal system 404
  Intrahepatic cholestasis ± hepatitis 405
  Cholestasis alone 405
  Hepatotoxins 405
Endocrine system 405
Metabolic 406
Blood diseases 407
Neuropsychiatric 409
Sexual dysfunction 410
  Decreased libido and erectile
    dysfunction 410
  Failure of ejaculation 411
Otological 411
Eye 411
Dermatological 411

CLINICAL PHARMACOLOGY

8

GLOSSARY

Pharmacokinetics	Study of the time course of drug absorption, distribution, metabolism and excretion.
Pharmacodynamics	Study of the biochemical and physiological effects of drugs and their mechanisms of action.
Plasma half-life	The time taken for drug plasma concentration to fall by 50% (for first-order reactions only). Symbol, $t_{1/2}$. Half-life is the main determinant of dose frequency. A drug achieves 50% of its steady-state concentration after one half-life, 75% after two half-lives, 88% after three, 94% after four and 99% after five.
Steady state	Occurs when the amount of drug administered during the dosage interval equals the amount of drug eliminated during a dosage interval. Dependent on $t_{1/2}$.

A loading dose or increased frequency of initial doses is used to achieve a steady state more rapidly, e.g. digoxin, phenytoin (Fig. 8.1). The actual steady state concentration is directly proportional to the size of the dose, and indirectly proportional to the volume of distribution and the eliminator constant.

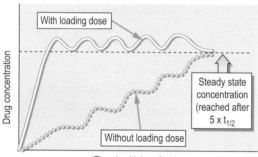

Fig. 8.1 Steady state.

Clearance	The volume of plasma cleared of drug in unit time. Expressed in ml/min or l/hour.
Bioavailability	Extent to which a drug is absorbed systemically. It depends on formulation, gut motility, disease states and first-pass effect.
First-pass effect	Metabolic breakdown of certain drugs before entering the systemic circulation on initial passage through either the liver (e.g. propranolol, GTN, lidocaine, pethidine and oestrogens), the intestinal mucosa (e.g. L-dopa, chlorpromazine, ethanol) or lungs (e.g. isoprenaline). This results in some drugs being unavailable if given by certain oral routes (Table 8.1).

Table 8.1 Drugs with extensive first-pass-metabolism

Cardiac drugs	CNS drugs	Analgesics	Others
Propranolol, metoprolol	Chlorpromazine	Aspirin	Oral contraceptive
Verapamil, nifedipine	Nortriptyline	Paracetamol	Salbutamol
Prazosin	L-dopa	Morphine	
GTN, isosorbide dinitrate	Clormethiazole	Pethidine	
Lidocaine			

Volume of distribution (Vd)
The theoretical fluid volume which would contain the total body content of a drug at a concentration equal to the plasma concentration. Expressed in m/s/kg. Drugs that are highly lipophilic and extensively tissue-bound have a large volume of distribution, e.g. nortriptyline, chloroquine. Drugs that are poorly lipophilic and highly plasma protein-bound have a low volume or distribution, e.g. warfarin, aspirin, gentamicin, theophylline. A knowledge of Vd can be used to determine the size of a loading dose, if an immediate response to treatment is required.

Area under the curve (Fig. 8.2)
Area under a concentration versus time curve for a drug. Calculated from the time of dosing to the last data point by summation of the trapezoids. The unit of measurement is g/l/hour.

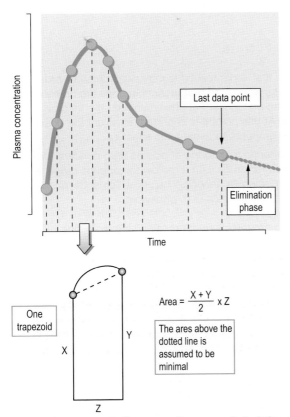

$$\text{Area} = \frac{X + Y}{2} \times Z$$

The ares above the dotted line is assumed to be minimal

Fig. 8.2 Drug concentration versus time curve. Calculation of area under the curve.

Drug elimination

First-order (linear) elimination (Fig. 8.3). Most common type for both drug absorption and elimination. The rate of reaction is directly proportional to the amount of drug available, i.e. constant fraction of drug absorbed or eliminated in unit time. Time taken to reach steady state (i.e. when rate of drug administration = rate of drug elimination) = 5 half-lives.

Zero-order elimination or saturation kinetics (Fig. 8.3). Proceeds at a constant rate and is independent of the amount of drug available. This usually occurs when a high concentration of the drug is present or when the normal elimination mechanism of a drug is saturated, e.g. inhalational anaesthetics or IV infusions.

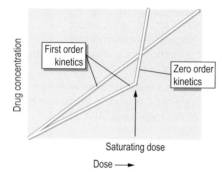

Fig. 8.3 First-order elimination.

Some first-order reactions may switch to zero-order kinetics when high drug concentrations are present, e.g. hepatic metabolism of phenytoin near the therapeutic level. At this point it is important to adjust the dose in small amounts to avoid toxic effects.

Therapeutic monitoring of plasma drug concentrations is used for drugs with a narrow therapeutic range (e.g. lithium, digoxin, theophylline), or which show dose-dependent kinetics (e.g. phenytoin).
1. Digoxin
2. Antiarrythmics, e.g. procainamide, quinidine
3. Anticonvulsants, e.g. phenobarbital, phenytoin, valproate and carbamazepine
4. Antibiotics, e.g. aminoglycosides
5. Others, e.g. theophylline, lithium.

Therapeutic index (TI) (Fig. 8.4)

Margin of safety of a drug. Ratio of the lethal or toxic dose (LD) and the therapeutically effective dose (ED). In animal experiments, the therapeutic index is often taken as the dose at which 50% of the population respond.

$$\text{Therapeutic index} = \frac{LD_{50}}{ED_{50}}$$

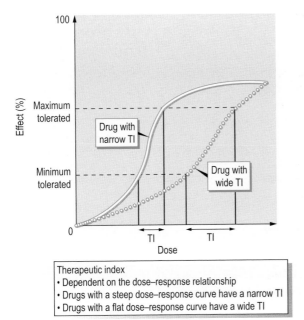

Therapeutic index
• Dependent on the dose–response relationship
• Drugs with a steep dose–response curve have a narrow TI
• Drugs with a flat dose–response curve have a wide TI

Fig. 8.4 Dose–response relationship for drug with narrow and wide therapeutic indices.

• Drugs with a broad therapeutic window or index are penicillins, β_2 agonists and thiazide diuretics.
• Drugs with a narrow therapeutic window are digoxin, theophylline, lithium, phenytoin (i.e. require therapeutic drug monitoring).

Dose–response curves	Graphs of drug concentration plotted as a function of the response. *Competitive antagonism* In the presence of different concentrations of an antagonist the dose–response curves show parallel displacement but with the same maximal effect, i.e. antagonism can be overcome by raising the concentration of the agonist drug, e.g. β-blockers. *Non-competitive antagonism* The maximal effect declines with higher concentrations of the antagonist, e.g. omeprazole.
Drug potency	Relative concentrations of two or more drugs that elicit the same effect (Fig. 8.5).
Drug efficacy	Maximal effect that a particular drug may elicit (Fig. 8.5).

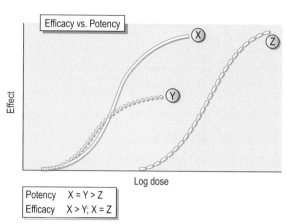

Fig. 8.5 Drug efficacy versus potency.

DRUG INTERACTIONS

MAJOR MECHANISMS OF DRUG INTERACTIONS

DRUG ABSORPTION

- Drugs causing decreased absorption, e.g. anticholinergic agents ($\downarrow$ gastric emptying); cholestyramine (ion exchange resin binder); iron and other chelating agents.
- Drugs causing increased absorption ($\uparrow$ gastric emptying), e.g. metoclopramide.

PLASMA PROTEIN BINDING (Table 8.2)

- Drug displacement affects drugs that are highly protein-bound, e.g. clofibrate, salicylates, sulphonamides, phenylbutazone, tolbutamide, phenytoin, warfarin.

Table 8.2 Plasma protein binding

Bound drugs	Displacing drug	Effect
Bilirubin	Sulphonamides Vitamin K Salicylates	Kernicterus
Tolbutamide	Salicylates Phenylbutazone Sulphonamides	Hypoglycaemia
Warfarin	Salicylates Clofibrate Phenylbutazone Phenytoin	Haemorrhage

METABOLISM

- Main site of drug metabolism is in the liver, but also to a lesser extent in other organs, e.g. gut and kidney.
- Two phases of metabolism (Fig. 8.6).

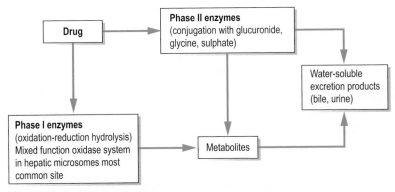

Fig. 8.6 Phase I and II enzymes.

Mixed function oxidase system (MFOS)

Dependent on $NADPH_2$, cytochrome P450 and cytochrome P450 reductase, which catalyse the incorporation of molecular oxygen.

Cytochrome P450 enzymes (Table 8.3)

- Present in large quantities in endoplasmic reticulum of liver, but also lung, kidney and intestinal wall.
- There are three families of the P450 cytochromes that are important for the oxidative metabolism of certain drugs.
- Each P450 enzyme has a unique but overlapping range of drug substrates, and several are under polymorphic genetic control; their frequency differs across ethnic groups.
- There are many potential drug interactions with cytochrome P450 which require dose adjustments (Table 8.3)

Table 8.3 Examples of drugs and isoforms of cytochrome P450 with potential for metabolic interactions

Family	Isoform	Major drugs affected by inhibition	Inhibitory drug
CYP1	CYP1A2	Theophylline Clozapine Haloperidol Propranolol	Fluvoxamine Cimetidine
CYP2	CYP2D6	Codeine Amitriptyline Flecainide Propranolol Thioridazine	Amiodarone Fluoxetine Cimetidine Quinidine Paroxetine
CYP3*	CYP3A4	Ciclosporin Amiodarone Astemizole Carbamazepine Diazepam Fentanyl Simvastatin	Cimetidine Erythromycin Fluconazole Indinavir Omeprazole Sertraline

* The CYP3A subfamily is the major constitutive form in the liver, but it is also expressed in significant amounts in other tissues, e.g. gastrointestinal tract. Lower activity is associated with an increased risk of adverse drug reactions, and higher activity with inhibitory interactions. Grapefruit juice downregulates CYP4503A4 in the intestinal wall, which can lead to increased bioavailablity and toxic effects of drugs broken down by this enzyme, e.g. terfenadine, ciclosporin, verapamil, midazolam and saquinavir.

Factors affecting metabolism

1. Enzyme *inducers*, e.g. barbiturates, carbamazepine, griseofulvin, phenytoin, omeprazole, alcohol, cigarette smoking, spironolactone and rifampicin.
2. Enzyme *inhibitors*, e.g. allopurinol, cimetidine, ciprofloxacin, erythromycin, isoniazid, chloramphenicol, ketoconazole, quinidine, phenylbutazone and grapefruit juice.
3. Age, sex and disease states.
4. Genetic constitution: genetic factors influence both *drug response* and *drug metabolism* (see Tables 8.4 and 8.5).

Genetic variation and drug response (Table 8.4)

Table 8.4 Genetic variation associated with drug sensitivity		
Pharmacogenetic trait	*Adverse effects*	*Drugs to avoid*
G6PDH deficiency in erythrocytes (X-linked recessive) Mainly in Africans, some Mediterranean races, Iraqi Jews, Chinese and South-East Asians	Haemolysis (see below and Fig. 8.7)	'Oxidant' drugs **Analgesics:** Aspirin, phenacetin **Antibacterials:** Chloramphenicol, sulphonamides, nitrofurantoin, dapsone, co-trimoxazole **Antimalarials:** Chloroquine, primaquine, quinine, mepacrine **Others:** Quinidine, probenecid
Methaemoglobin-reductase deficiency (autosomal recessive)	Methaemoglobinaemia	As above plus nitrates, nitrites, local anaesthetics
Malignant hyperpyrexia (autosomal recessive)	Hyperpyrexia with muscular rigidity	Suxamethonium
Acute intermittent porphyria (autosomal dominant)*	(See p. 271) Pyrexia Abdominal pain Constipation Confusion Peripheral neuropathy Tachycardia ↑BP	**CNS drugs:** Alcohol, barbiturates **Antibacterials:** Rifampicin, sulphonamides, griseofulvin, chloroquine, oral contraceptives **Others:** Phenytoin, sulphonylureas, methyldopa

*Drugs considered safe: *Analgesics*, e.g. salicylates, morphine and related opiates; *Antibiotics*, e.g. penicillins, tetracyclines, chloramphenicol; *CNS drugs*, e.g. phenothiazines, diazepam; *Antihypertensives*, e.g. propranolol; *Others*, e.g. digoxin, nitrous oxide, succinylcholine and atropine.

G6PDH deficiency and haemolysis
G6PD maintains low levels of methaemoglobin in red cells. If the methaemoglobin level increases, haemolysis occurs (Fig. 8.7).

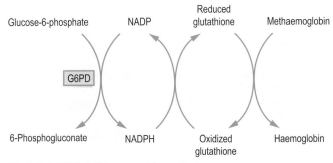

Fig. 8.7 G6PDH deficiency and haemolysis.

Genetic variation and drug metabolism (Table 8.5)

Table 8.5 Genetic variation in drug metabolism

Pharmacogenetic trait	Adverse effects	Drugs to avoid or take in reduced dose
Acetylation (fast acetylation = autosomal dominant) (Prevalence of rapid acetylation: Canadian Eskimos, 100%; Japanese 88%; UK, 38%; Egyptians, 18%)	Lupus-like syndrome (see below) or neuropathy in slow acetylators; fast acetylators show a diminished response Features of a drug induced SLE (see below)	Hydralazine Isoniazid Procainamide Dapsone Nitrazepam Sulphonamides Sulfasalazine
Suxamethonium sensitivity due to an abnormal plasma pseudocholinesterase (autosomal recessive) (1 in 2500 in UK, but absent in Japanese and Eskimos, rare in Africans)	Prolonged muscle paralysis and apnoea	Suxamethonium
Phenacetin-induced methaemoglobinaemia (autosomal recessive)	Methaemoglobinaemia	Phenacetin
G6PD deficiency (N. Europeans 0%, S. Europeans up to 25%, Afro-Caribbeans 10%)	Haemolysis	Antimalarials Sulphonamides Aspirin Phenacetin
Hypolactasia (Europeans <20%, Asians 100%)		

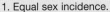

Features of a drug-induced SLE syndrome
1. Equal sex incidence.
2. Most commonly affects persons of HLA type DR4 (i.e. slow acetylators).
3. Dose-related and usually reversible.
4. Renal and CNS disease unlikely.
5. Positive antinuclear antibody.
6. Complement usually unaffected.

EXCRETION

- Changes in urine pH, e.g. alkalinization of urine increases the elimination of phenobarbital and aspirin in overdose; amphetamine overdose is treated by urine acidification.
- Competition for active renal tubular excretion, e.g. probenecid and penicillin; digoxin and quinidine.
- Drugs which undergo an enterohepatic circulation (EHC) include thyroxine, oestrogens, diethylstilbestrol and rifampicin.
- Dubin–Johnson's syndrome: failure of excretion of bilirubin glucuronide into bile; inherited as autosomal recessive.

PHARMACOLOGICAL INTERACTIONS

For example, at drug receptor site (see Tables 8.6–8.38).

ADVERSE EFFECTS AND INTERACTIONS OF DRUGS

Table 8.6 Classification of adverse drug reactions

Type A (commonest 75%)	Type B
Dose dependent	Non-dose dependent
Predictable	Unpredictable
Insidious onset	Usually acute onset
Low mortality	High mortality
May be attenuated by dose reduction	Not attenuated by dose reduction
Commoner in renal and liver disease	Related to hypersensitivity reactions and hereditary enzyme deficiencies

Table 8.7 Receptor types classified according to agonist sensitivity

Receptor	Subtype	Agonist	Antagonist
Cholinergic	Muscarinic	Acetylcholine	Atropine
	Nicotinic	Acetylcholine	Tubocurare
Adrenergic	α_1	Noradrenaline (norepinephrine)	Prazosin
	α_2	Noradrenaline, clonidine	
	β_1	Adrenaline (epinephrine), dobutamine	Atenolol
	β_2	Adrenaline, salbutamol	Propranolol
Histaminergic	H_1	Histamine	Chlorpheniramine
	H_2	Histamine	Ranitidine
Dopaminergic	D_1	Apomorphine	
	D_2	Bromocriptine	{ Metoclopramide, Domperidone
	D_2	Apomorphine	Phenothiazines
Opioid	χ	Dynorphin	
	δ	Enkephalins	
	ϵ	β-Endorphin	Naloxone
	γ	β-Endorphin, morphine	Naloxone
GABA	GABA A		
	GABA B		

Important drug adverse effects and interactions are summarized in Tables 8.8–8.38.

Table 8.8 Antihypertensives

Class/drug	Adverse effects	Interacting drug(s)	Interacting effect
All antihypertensives		Corticosteroids Oral contraceptives NSAIDs	– Antagonism of hypotensive effect (due to fluid retention)
Centrally acting			
	1. Depression and drowsiness 2. Dry mouth 3. Nasal stuffiness 4. Fluid retention		
Methyldopa	*Specific side-effects:* 1. Fever 2. Diarrhoea 3. Failure of ejaculation 4. Positive Coombs' test (20%) 5. Haemolytic anaemia 6. Hepatitis 7. Pancreatitis 8. Gynaecomastia	Tricyclic antidepressants Phenothiazines	– Antagonism of hypotensive effect
Clonidine	*Specific side-effects:* 1. Constipation 2. Rebound hypertension on sudden withdrawal	Tricyclic antidepressants	– Antagonism of hypotensive effect – Exacerbates the rebound hypertension in clonidine withdrawal
Moxonidine	1. Similar sedative properties to clonidine but no rebound hypertension	Other antihypertensive agents Benzodiazepines	– Potentiation of antihypertensive effect – Potentiation of sedation

Table 8.8 (Cont'd)

Class/drug	Adverse effects	Interacting drug(s)	Interacting effect

β-Blockers
Mechanism of action:
Reduce the ability of the
sympathetic nervous system
to raise blood pressure
Non-selective ($β_1$-/$β_2$)
  Propranolol
Selective ($β_1$)
  Atenolol
  Metoprolol
  Bisoprolol
  Betaxolol
  Nadolol
  Carvedilol
Intrinsic sympathomimetic
activity ($β_1$ partial agonist)
  Pindolol
Antiarrhythmic properties
  Sotalol
Dual antihypertensive
action ($β_1$-/$α_1$)
  Labetolol
	1. Precipitate cardiac failure
	2. Exacerbate Raynaud's and peripheral
	   vascular disease
	3. Bradycardia and heart block
	4. Hypoglycaemia
	5. β-Blockers inhibit
	   hypoglycaemia-related tachycardia
	6. Bronchospasm esp. in asthmatics
	7. Lethargy, depression, and sleep disturbance
	8. Oculocutaneous syndrome (Practolol)
	9. Male sexual dysfunction,
	10. GI disturbance, liver damage (Labetalol)
		Verapamil (high dose, IV)
		Disopyramide
		Oral hypoglycaemics
		Insulin
			– Profound hypotension
			– Heart failure
			– Prolonged hypoglycaemic action
			– Increased hypoglycaemic action of insulin

Vasodilators *Mechanism of action:* Relax vascular smooth muscle and reduce peripheral resistance	1. Headache 2. Flushing 3. Nasal congestion 4. Postural hypotension 5. Tachycardia 6. Fluid retention		

Table 8.8 (Cont'd)

Class/drug	Adverse effects	Interacting drug(s)	Interacting effect
Vasodilators (Cont'd)			
Hydralazine	*Specific side-effects:* 1. SLE syndrome (+ve ANF), esp. with slow acetylators or high dose (> 200 mg/day) 2. Bone marrow depression 3. Peripheral neuropathy		
Prazosin, doxazosin Minoxidil	1. First-dose dizziness or syncope 2. Hypertrichosis 3. Pulmonary hypertension (with long-term treatment)		
Nitrates/nitrites[†]	1. Flushing with severe headache 2. Severe hypotension		
Nicorandil (nitrate and potassium channel activator); new class of antianginal drug	1. Headaches 2. Dizziness, nausea 3. Palpitations 4. Flushing	Avoid in patients with hypovolaemia, acute MI and left ventricular dysfunction	
Angiotensin-converting enzyme inhibitors (ACE) *First generation* Captopril Enalapril Lisinopril *Second generation* Fosinopril Perindropril Quinapril Ramipril Trandolapril	1. First-dose hypotension (esp. in renal failure or with diuretics) 2. Hyperkalaemia 3. Rashes. Angio-oedema 4. Proteinuria/haematuria 5. Loss of taste 6. Leucopenia, esp. with pre-existing immune complex disease 7. Persistent dry cough	Potassium-sparing diuretics NSAIDs	− Hyperkalaemia − Antagonism of antihypertensive effect − Contraindicated in pregnancy − Patients with low renin concentrations and Afro-Caribbeans may respond less well

Table 8.8 (Cont'd)

Class/drug	Adverse effects	Interacting drug(s)	Interacting effect
Angiotensin II antagonists *Mechanism of action:* Reduce peripheral resistance and blood volume, with no effect on heart rate Losartan Valsartan (Angiotensin II binds to the AT$_1$ receptor which is coupled to a G protein and causes vasoconstriction and aldosterone release. Losartan blocks this effect)	Similar adverse effect profile to ACE inhibitors but without cough, because does not inhibit the breakdown of bradykinin. 1. Hypotension, esp. in patients with intravascular volume depletion 2. Hyperkalaemia 3. Angio-oedema		
Calcium antagonists *Dihydropyridines* Nifedipine Nicardipine Amlodipine	1. Vasodilator side-effects (headache and facial flushing, palpitations) 2. Ankle swelling 3. Hypotension	β-Blockers	↑ Cardiodepressant effect
Verapamil	1. Bradycardia, hypotension, AV conduction defects 2. Constipation		
Diltiazem	1. Bradycardia, hypotension, AV conduction defects 2. Skin rash		

†*Action:* Nitrates are converted to nitrous oxide (NO), which combines with sulphydryl groups to form nitrosothiols. These activate the enzyme guanyl cyclase to produce the second messenger cyclic group, which causes smooth muscle relaxation and vasodilatation.

Table 8.8 (Cont'd)

Class/drug	Adverse effects	Interacting drug(s)	Interacting effect
Diuretics			
Thiazides	1. Hypokalaemia	Digoxin ⎱	– Potentiation of side-effects of thiazides
Mechanism of action:	2. Hypomagnesaemia	Lithium ⎰	
Increase Na⁺ excretion and	3. Hyperuricaemia		
reduce blood volume	4. Hyperglycaemia		
	5. Acute urinary retention		
	6. Precipitates hepatic encephalopathy		
	7. Pancreatitis		
	8. Inhibits Ca²⁺ excretion‡ (Used for treatment of idiopathic hypercalciuria)		
	9. Rashes		
	10. Thrombocytopenia		
	11. Impotence (20%)		
Loop diuretics	(As above)	Gentamicin ⎱	– ↑ Risk of nephrotoxicity and ototoxicity
	Specific side-effects:	Cephalosporins ⎰	
	1. Deafness (esp. in renal failure)		
	2. Thrombocytopenia		
	3. ↑ Ca²⁺ excretion		
	4. ↓ Uric acid secretion		
Potassium-retaining diuretics	1. Hyperkalaemia		
	2. Gynaecomastia		

Effect of antihypertensive drugs on serum lipids and lipoproteins

Thiazide diuretics – ↑ total cholesterol, LDL and triglycerides
β-Blockers – ↑ triglycerides and ↓ HDL
Prazosin, clonidine and methyldopa – ↓ cholesterol and LDL
Angiotensin-converting enzyme inhibitors and calcium blockers – no apparent effect on lipid levels

Positive inotropes that improve cardiac contractility

- Cardiac glycosides, e.g. digoxin
- β-Agonists e.g. dopamine and dobutamine
- Phosphodiesterase inhibitors, e.g. enoximone and milrinone.

Mechanism: Phosphodiesterase is responsible for the degradation of cAMP. Inhibiting this enzyme raises cAMP levels, and thus produces an increase in myocardial contractility and cardiac output and vasodilatation.

ANTIARRHYTHMIC DRUGS (Tables 8.9 and 8.10)

See conducting system of the heart (p. 209).

Table 8.9 Antiarrhythmic drugs: classification of drug actions

Class	Drugs	Electrophysiological actions
I Fast sodium channel inhibitors	Ia Quinidine, procainamide, disopyramide	Blocks conduction, increases ERP
	Ib Lidocaine, phenytoin, mexiletine, tocainide	Blocks conduction, decreases ERP
	Ic Flecainide, encainide	Blocks conduction, no effect on ERP
II Antisympathetic agents	β-Blockers	Decreases sinus node automaticity
III Prolongation of action potential duration	Amiodarone, bretylium, sotalol	No effects on conduction, delays repolarization
IV Slow calcium channel antagonists	Verapamil, diltiazem	Slows conduction velocity in the atrioventricular node
Not classified	Digoxin, adenine nucleotides	—

ERP = effective refractory period.

Table 8.10 Antiarrhythmic drugs: adverse effects and interactions

Drug	Adverse effects	Interacting drug(s)	Interacting effect

Digoxin
Mechanism: At a cellular level, digoxin blocks the exchange of intracellular Na$^+$ for extracellular K$^+$ by inhibiting Na$^+$/K$^+$-ATPase in the cell membrane. This increases intracellular Na$^+$ and encourages its exchange for Ca^{2+}, raising intracellular Ca^{2+} and causing a positive inotropic effect.
	1. Confusion and insomnia
	2. Colour vision defects (yellow/green)
	3. Xanthopsia
	4. Anorexia, nausea and vomiting
	5. Arrhythmias esp.
	  (i) Ventricular extrasystoles and bigeminy
	  (ii) Atrial tachycardia with AV block
	6. Gynaecomastia
		Hypokalaemia due to potassium-depleting diuretics, corticosteroids, carbenoloxone, and amphotericin B
		Verapamil
		β-Blockers
		Hypercalcaemia
		Quinidine
		Amiodarone
		Also in the elderly, renal failure, hypoxia, severe heart and pulmonary disease
			– Digoxin toxicity enhanced

Verapamil	1. Dizziness and constipation 2. Hypotension and AV block 3. Cardiac failure and peripheral oedema	β-Blockers Digoxin	– ↑ AV block – ↑ Digoxin levels
Quinidine	1. 'Cinchonism' 2. Cardiac failure 3. Hypotension, AV block 4. Hypersensitivity	Antihypertensive agents Digoxin Amiodarone Warfarin	– Potentiation of hypotensive effects – ↑ Digoxin toxicity – ↑ Quinidine levels – ↑ Anticoagulant effect
Disopyramide	1. Anticholinergic effects 2. Myocardial depressant	Antihypertensive agents	– Potentiation of hypotensive effect
Procainamide	1. Ventricular arrhythmias 2. SLE syndrome 3. Agranulocytosis 4. Hypersensitivity		

CLINICAL PHARMACOLOGY

CLINICAL PHARMACOLOGY

Table 8.10 (Cont'd)

Drug	Adverse effects	Interacting drug(s)	Interacting effect
Lignocaine (lidocaine)	1. Hypotension 2. Convulsions 3. Myocardial depression	Phenytoin	– Cardiac depression
Amiodarone	1. Photosensitivity 2. Thyroid dysfunction 3. Fibrosing alveolitis 4. Corneal deposits (do not interfere with sight and reverse on stopping drug) 5. Flattened T wave 6. Tremor, peripheral neuropathy 7. Proarrhythmic effect	Digoxin and warfarin Class I A and C antiarrhythmics β-Blockers, verapamil	– ↑ Risk of digoxin and warfarin toxicity – Proarrhythmic effect – ↑ AV block
Adenosine (adenosine receptor agonist used for treatment of supraventricular tachycardias)	1. Short-lived vasodilator effects (flushing, dyspnoea, chest pain, hypotension). Cardiac transplant patients are particularly susceptible 2. Bronchoconstriction in asthmatics 3. Transient heart block	Theophylline Dipyridamole	– ↓ Effect of adenosine – ↑ Effect of adenosine

ANTICOAGULANTS, THROMBOLYTIC AND FIBRINOLYTIC DRUGS (Tables 8.11–8.13)

Table 8.11 Oral anticoagulants

All produce *increased anticoagulant effect in*: alcoholism, liver disease, renal failure, cardiac failure, thyrotoxicosis, fever and hypoalbuminaemia.

Drug	Adverse effects	Interacting drug(s)	Interacting effect
Warfarin	1. Alopecia 2. Haemmorrhagic skin necrosis		**↑ anticoagulant effect**
		NSAIDs Oral hypoglycaemics Metronidazole Co-trimoxazole	– Due to displacement of warfarin from protein binding
		Ampicillin Cephalosporins Erythromycin Clofibrate Salicylates	
		Chloramphenicol Alcohol (acute) Phenylbutazone Cimetidine Amiodarone	– Due to liver enzyme inhibition
		Salicylates (high dose)	
		Broad-spectrum antibiotics (neomycin)	– Due to ↓ clotting factor synthesis – Due to ↓ vit. K synthesis
		Also: age, biliary disease, congestive heart failure, hyperthyroidism	
			↓ anticoagulant effect
		Barbiturates Phenytoin Rifampicin Carbamazepine Griseofulvin Oral contraceptives	– Due to enzyme induction (sudden ↑ effect when interacting drug is stopped)
		Vitamin K	– Due to increased clotting factor synthesis inhibition
		Cholestyramine	– Due to reduced absorption
		Also: hypothyroidism, nephrotic syndrome	

CLINICAL PHARMACOLOGY

Table 8.11 (Cont'd)

Drug	Adverse effects	Interacting drug(s)	Interacting effect
Aspirin Mechanism: Inhibition of cyclo-oxygenase (Fig. 8.8)	1. GI disturbance and haemorrhage 2. 'Salicylism' (deafness, tinnitus and vomiting) 3. Hypersensitivity (asthma, urticaria and angio-oedema) 4. Gout (urate retention with low doses (1–2 g/day), uricosuric with high doses) 5. Analgesic nephropathy 6. Aggravation of bleeding disorders (hypoprothrombinaemic) 7. Reye's syndrome in children	GI irritants Oral hypoglycaemics Warfarin, NSAIDs Steroids	– ↑ Peptic ulceration – ↑ Hypoglycaemic effect – ↑ Anticoagulant effect – ↓ Aspirin effect
ADP agonists Dipyridamole Ticlodipine Clopidogrel Mechanism: block adenosine receptors, adenosine initiates platelet aggregation	1. Bleeding 2. Neutropenia, agranulocytosis (ticlodipine) 3. GI disturbance 4. Rash		
Glycoprotein IIa/IIIb receptor antagonists Tirofiban Abciximab (monoclonal antibody) Mechanism: block receptor essential for final activation of platelet aggregation	1. Haemorrhage 2. Nausea, vomiting 3. Hypotension		

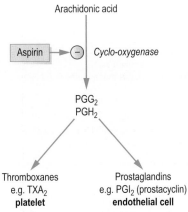

Fig. 8.8 Mechanism of action of aspirin.

Table 8.12 Intravenous thrombolytic agents	
Drug	*Adverse effect*
Heparin Dalteparin Low molecular weight heparins are purified derivatives that have more consistent activity, require less monitoring and have a longer duration of action than unfractionated heparins	1. Local bleeding 2. Hypersensitivity (rare) 3. Thrombocytopenia 4. Osteoporosis 5. Hair loss Reversal with protamine monitored by measuring APTT (activated partial thromboplastin time). Dose is adjusted until the APTT is 2–3 times longer than normal
Streptokinase *Mechanism:* see Fig. 8.9 *Contraindications:* Recent haemorrhage (e.g. from a peptic ulcer), trauma, surgery, bleeding diatheses, aortic dissection, coma, history of cerebrovascular disease, post cardiac massage, severe uncontrolled hypertension, recent treatment with streptokinase.	1. Bleeding 2. Allergic reactions 3. Nausea and vomiting
Tissue-type plasminogen activators (tPAs) Alteplase Reteplase *Mechanism:* see Fig. 8.9	As for streptokinase but less likely to cause bleeding and allergic reactions.

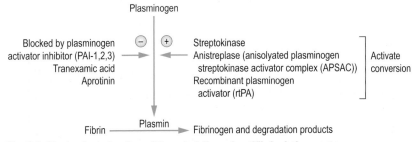

Fig. 8.9 Mechanism of action of thrombolytic and antifibrinolytic agents.

Table 8.13 Antifibrinolytic agents

Drug	Adverse effects
Tranexamic acid *Mechanism:* see Fig. 8.9 *Indications:* gastrointestinal haemorrhage and conditions with risk of haemorrhage, e.g. haemophilia, menorrhagia and dental extraction	1. Nausea and vomiting 2. Diarrhoea 3. Thromboembolic events (rare)
Aprotinin *Mechanism:* see Fig. 8.9 *Indications:* to reduce blood loss after open heart surgery *Contraindications:* thromboembolic disease	1. Allergy 2. Localized thrombophlebitis

ANTIRHEUMATIC DRUGS (Table 8.14)

Table 8.14 Disease modifying antirheumatic drugs (DMARDs)

Drug	Adverse effects	Interacting drug(s)	Interacting effects
Aspirin (see p. 356)			
Non-steroidal anti-inflammatory drugs (NSAIDs) *Actions:* – Anti-inflammatory – Anti-pyretic – Analgesic – Antiplatelet *Mechanisms:* NSAIDs inhibit cyclo-oxygenase (COX) which has 2 isoenzymes: – COX-1 has housekeeping functions, including gastric cytoprotection – COX-2 is a gene product of inflammatory cells, and inhibition has anti-inflammatory effects Most NSAIDs are non-selective (e.g. ibuprofen, naproxen, indomethacin) New specific COX-2 inhibitors have been developed, e.g. rofecoxib	1. Gastrointestinal: indigestion, peptic ulceration, bleeding. (COX-2 inhibitors less prone) 2. Sodium and water retention 3. Renal impairment reduces GFR, and chronic exposure can cause papillary necrosis 4. Asthma 5. Hepatitis and blood dyscrasias (indomethacin) 6. Recent evidence suggests an increased risk of cardiovascular events with COX-2 inhibitors	Diuretics Lithium Aminoglycosides, penicillins, cephalosporins	– NSAIDs cause salt retention and ↓ potency of diuretics – ↓ Clearance of lithium – May precipitate acute renal failure

Table 8.14 (Cont'd)

Drug	Adverse effects	Interacting drug(s)	Interacting effects
Gold	1. Skin reactions, e.g. dermatitis and mucosal lesions 2. Nephritis, proteinuria 3. Blood dyscrasias		
Penicillamine	Approx. 40% of patients: 1. Nausea, loss of taste, rashes 2. Thrombocytopenia 3. Neutropenia 4. Proteinuria/nephrotic syndrome 5. Autoimmune conditions, e.g. AIHA		
Sulfasalazine	1. Severe skin reaction 2. Blood dyscrasias		
Antimalarials e.g. chloroquine (see p. 387),			
Glucocorticoids (see p. 377)			
Cytotoxic drugs e.g. methotrexate, azathioprine, ciclosporin (see p. 395), infliximab (monoclonal antibody against tumour necrosis factor used in rheumatoid and Crohn's disease)			
Drugs used in treatment of osteoporosis 1. Calcium (vitamin D) 2. Hormone replacement therapy 3. Bisphosphonates: etidronate (inhibits osteoclasts and osteoblasts), alendronate (inhibits osteoblasts)	1. Gastrointestinal upsets 2. Oesophageal ulceration (alendronate only) 3. Hypocalcaemia		

LIPID-LOWERING DRUGS (Tables 8.15 and 8.16)

Table 8.15 Lipid-lowering drugs: summary of actions

Drug	Major mechanisms (Fig. 8.10)	LDL	HDL	Triglycerides
HMG-CoA reductase inhibitors	Competitive inhibition of cholesterol biosynthetic enzyme induces LDL expression and enhanced LDL clearance	↓↓	↑	→
Fibrates	Enhance VLDL catabolism (Apo C) and increase HDL cholesterol content (Apo AI/II)	↓	↑	↓
Bile acid sequestrant resins	Increase intestinal clearance of cholesterol	↓	→	→
Others Nicotinic acid (niacin) Probucol	Decrease fatty acid flux from adipose tissue. Decrease VLDL production	↓ ↓	↑ ↓	↓ →

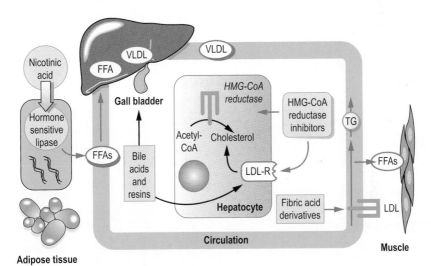

Adipose tissue

Fig. 8.10 Sites of action of lipid-lowering drugs.

Table 8.16 Lipid-lowering drugs

Drug	Adverse effects	Interacting drug(s)	Interacting effect
HMGCoA reductase inhibitors ('statins')			
Simvastatin	1. Myopathy, elevation of CPK, hepatic transaminase elevation 2. Skin reactions	Warfarin Fibrates Ciclosporin, erythromycin, diltiazem	– Extensively bound to albumin – Potentiation of myopathy – CYP3A4 interactions
Pravastatin Fluvastatin Atorvastatin Lovastatin	1. Myalgia 1. Headache		
Fibrates			
Bezafibrate Gemfibrozil Fenofibrate	1. Myopathy 2. GI upset 3. Headaches 4. Fatigue 5. Skin reactions 6. Possible increased risk of cholelithiasis	Statins	– Potentiation of myopathy
Resins			
Colestyramine Colestipol	1. GI upset 2. Dyspepsia, flatulence 3. Mild triglyceride elevation 4. Fat malabsorption (rare)	Vitamin K Folic acid Digoxin (↑ Interactions if other drugs administered 1 hour before or up to 4 hours after resin)	– Interfere with absorption
Nicotinic acid	1. Cutaneous flushing, pruritus, rash 2. Hepatotoxicity 3. Impaired glucose tolerance 4. Hyperuricaemia 5. Acanthosis nigricans 6. Exacerbation of peptic ulcer		

PEPTIC ULCER DISEASE DRUGS (Table 8.17)

Table 8.17 Drugs used in peptic ulcer disease

Drug	Adverse effects	Interacting drug(s)	Interacting effect
H₂-receptor antagonists Cimetidine Ranitidine Famotidine	1. Confusion 2. Drowsiness 3. Gynaecomastia (rarely) 4. Galactorrhoea 5. Loss of libido (antiandrogenic effect with cimetidine)	Diazepam Theophylline β-Blockers Phenytoin Quinidine Tricyclic antidepressants Warfarin	↑ effect of interacting drugs (cimetidine inhibits cytochrome P450 metabolism)
Proton pump inhibitors (Fig. 8.11)	1. Hypergastrinaemia 2. Increase the risk of Campylobacter infections tenfold in persons over 45 years old		
Omeprazole	1. Mild and infrequent diarrhoea	Diazepam	Omeprazole reduces the clearance and prolongs elimination
Lansoprazole	1. Skin rash 2. Headache	Phenytoin Warfarin	

Cimetidine and omeprazole, but not famotidine, inhibit cytochrome P450 enzymes.
Helicobacter pylori eradication. Proton pump inhibitor (e.g. omeprazole) and two antibiotics (amoxicillin, clarithromycin and metronidazole) for 1 week.

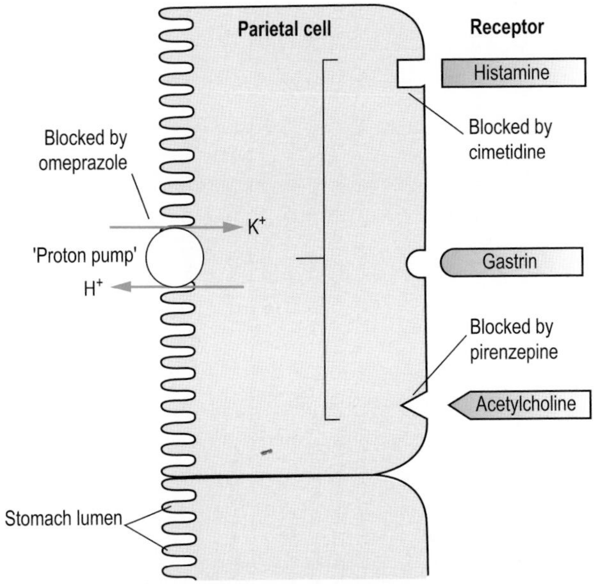

Fig. 8.11 Site and mechanism of action of H₂ receptor antagonists and proton pump inhibitors.

ANTIDEPRESSANT, ANXIOLYTIC, ANTIPSYCHOTIC AND ANTIMANIA DRUGS (Tables 8.18–8.20)

Table 8.18 Antidepressants

Drug	Adverse effects	Interacting drug(s)	Interacting effect
Tricyclic antidepressants *Older tricyclics* e.g. amitryptyline, imipramine, dothiepin *Tetracyclics* e.g. mianserin *5HT-uptake blocks (SSRI)* *Mixed* e.g. trazodone, lofepramine *Selective* e.g. fluoxetine *Monoamine oxidase inhibitors* e.g. phenelzine *Thioxanthines* e.g. flupenthixol *Mechanism:* Block reuptake into the presynaptic neuron of NA and 5HT, and so increases their availability to postsynaptic membrane	1. Postural hypotension 2. Arrhythmias and conduction defects (quinidine-like), e.g. prolonged PR, QRS, PR intervals, T wave flattening, ST depression 3. Anticholinergic effects 4. Confusion in the elderly 5. Lowering of seizure threshold 6. Weight gain 7. Hepatotoxicity and blood dyscrasias (idiosyncratic) Newer agents have less cardiotoxic and anticholinergic effects. Selective 5HT inhibitors are not sedating, but can cause nausea, tremor, sexual dysfunction and dizziness	Phenothiazines Anticholinergic agents Antihistamines Antiparkinsonian drugs MAOI Ethanol, sedatives	– ↑ Anticholinergic effects – (See below) – ↑ CNS effects of interacting drugs
Monoamine oxidase inhibitors (MAOI) (Fig. 8.12) *Hydrazine group* e.g. iproniazid, phenelzine *Non-hydrazine groups* e.g. tranylcypromine, pargyline	As for tricyclics 1. Jaundice 2. Anticholinergic effects	(a) **Tyramine-containing foodstuffs** Mature cheese (cream and cottage cheeses safe), yeast extracts, red wine and beer, chicken liver, broad beans, coffee (b) **Indirect sympathomimetic amines** Tricyclic antidepressants Amphetamines Pethidine Barbiturates L-Dopa	(i) Hypertensive crisis (risk of subarachnoid haemorrhage) (ii) CNS excitation, hyperpyrexia (iii) Prolongs action of interacting drugs

Table 8.18 (Cont'd)

Drug	Adverse effects	Interacting drug(s)	Interacting effect
Monoamine oxidase inhibitors (cont'd) *Reversible inhibitors of MAO (RIMAs)* Moclobemide	1. Mild agitation		
Selective serotonin reuptake inhibitors (SSRIs) (Fig. 8.12) *Mechanism:* Cause selective inhibition of 5HT reuptake by postsynaptic nerve terminals, e.g. fluoxetine, sertraline	1. Nausea, vomiting, dry mouth 2. Seizures, agitation 3. Weight loss and sexual dysfunction 4. Hyponatraemia 5. Vasculitic rash (rare) Do not have sedative, hypotensive or anticholinergic effects of tricyclics, and have less effect on cardiac conduction. Also better tolerated in overdose	Lithium	
Serotonin-noradrenaline reuptake inhibitors (SNRIs) Venlafaxine	1. Sedation 2. Mania		

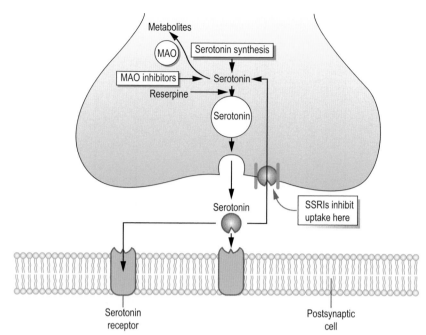

Fig. 8.12 Site of action of MAOIs and SSRIs.

Table 8.19 Anxiolytic drugs

Drug	Adverse effects	Interacting drug	Interacting effect
Benzodiazepines *Longer-acting* Diazepam ($t_{1/2}$ = 14–70 h) Chlordiazepoxide Nitrazepam ($t_{1/2}$ = 15–30 h) Flurazepam Clonazepam	1. Drowsiness and agitation (esp. in the elderly) 2. Incontinence, nightmares and confusion 3. Excessive salivation 4. Thrombophlebitis with IV injections 5. Respiratory depression, hypotension 6. Withdrawal can be associated with rebound, increased agitation, hallucinations and seizures	Other sedative drugs	– Do not interfere with metabolism of other drugs or with warfarin – Additive CNS depression
Shorter-acting Oxazepam ($t_{1/2}$ = 3–25 h) Lorazepam ($t_{1/2}$ = 8–24 h) Temazepam ($t_{1/2}$ = 3–25 h)			
Ultra-short-acting Midazolam		Cimetidine	– Inhibits metabolism of midazolam
Mechanism: Gamma-aminobutyric acid (GABA) is a major inhibiting neurotransmitter that works by inhibiting postsynaptic chloride channels. Benzodiazepines potentiate GABA and receptors for these drugs are found close to GABA receptors and chloride channels			
Clormethiazole **Chloral hydrate**	1. Nasal, conjunctival and bronchial discomfort 2. Respiratory and CVS depression	Cimetidine	– Prolongs half-life
Non-benzodiazepine hypnotics Zopiclone *Mechanism:* Act on GABA receptors	Short duration of action and little/no hangover effect		
5-Hydroxytryptamine IA agonists Buspirone Sumatriptan	1. Headache 2. Dizziness 3. Nervousness		

Table 8.20 Antipsychotic and antimania drugs

Drug	Adverse effects	Interacting drugs	Interacting effect
Lithium carbonate	1. Metallic taste 2. Anorexia and diarrhoea 3. Polyuria and polydypsia 4. Nephrogenic diabetes insipidus 5. Tremor 6. Muscle weakness 7. Goitre and hypothyroidism 8. Leucocytosis 9. ECG and EEG changes 10. Worsens psoriasis 11. May be teratogenic *Toxicity:* 1. Slurred speech 2. Coarse tremor 3. Ataxia 4. Confusion and fits	Thiazide diuretics Phenothiazines NSAID Carbamazepine Phenytoin Methyldopa	– ↑ lithium toxicity

Phenothiazines
Chlorpromazine
Promazine
Thioridazine
Prochlorperazine
Perphenazine
Fluphenazine
Mechanism: Act by blocking dopamine D_2 receptors, mainly in mesolimbic system (Fig. 8.13)
	1. Extrapyramidal effects (blockade of D_2 receptors)
	  (i) Parkinsonism
	  (ii) Dystonic reactions (also with haloperidol)
	  (iii) Akathesia
	  (iv) Tardive dyskinesia (up to 40% of patients; caused by dopamine receptor upregulation)
	2. Neuroleptic malignant syndrome (potentially fatal hypertension, muscle rigidity and autonomic dysfunction) (idiosyncratic)
	3. Glucose intolerance
	4. Anticholinergic effects (dry mouth, blurred vision, constipation, urinary retention, ejaculatory failure)
	5. Cardiac arrhythmias and postural hypotension (anti-adrenergic effects)
		Alcohol
		Narcotic analgesics
			– ↑ CNS effects of interacting drugs

Table 8.20 (Cont'd)

Drug	Adverse effects	Interacting drugs	Interacting effect

Phenothiazines (cont'd)	6. Gynaecomastia, galactorrhoea, hyperprolactinaemia, infertility
	7. Corneal and lens opacities
	8. Retinal pigmentation
	9. Lowering of seizure threshold
	10. Hypothermia in the elderly
	11. Hypersensitivity reactions not related to dose
	   — Cholestatic jaundice
	   — Skin pigmentation and photosensitivity
	   — Agranulocytosis, leucopenia and eosinophilia		

Non-phenothiazine neuroleptics Haloperidol (butyrophenone) Pimozide (diphenylbutypiperidine) Flupenthixol (thioxanthine) Sulpiride (resubstituted benzamide) Clozapine (dibenzepine)	Less likely to cause sedation or extrapyramidal side effects		
Atypical neuroleptics (act on D_2 receptors) Risperidone Sulpiride Pimozide *Mechanism:* Dopamine/5HT blockers	Cause fewer extrapyramidal side-effects 1. Sleep disturbance 2. Anxiety 3. Rhinitis 4. Sudden death (rare) in patients with pre-existing cardiac disease 5. Fewer extrapyramidal side-effects		
Olanzapine	1. Cardiac arrhythmias 2. Agranulocytosis		
Clozapine	1. Agranulocytosis 2. Weight gain 3. Convulsions		

CLINICAL PHARMACOLOGY

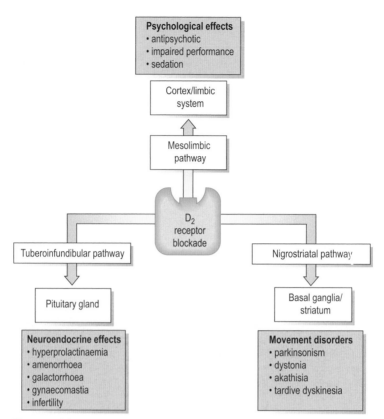

Fig. 8.13 Adverse effects of D$_2$ dopamine receptor blockade.

ANTICONVULSANT DRUGS (Table 8.21)

Table 8.21 Anticonvulsants

Drug	Adverse effects	Interacting drug(s)	Interacting effect
All anticonvulsants		Phenothiazines Tricyclic antidepressants	– ↓ Anticonvulsant effect (i.e. lowering of convulsive threshold)
Phenytoin *Mechanism*: Maintains deactivation of voltage-sensitive sodium channels, and so blocks repetitive firing of neurons	1. Nystagmus, dizziness, ataxia 2. Drowsiness *Long-term effects:* 3. Gum hyperplasia 4. Folate deficiency and megaloblastic anaemia 5. Hypocalcaemia and osteomalacia 6. Hypersensitivity reactions (idiosyncratic) 7. Rashes, SLE syndrome (idiosyncratic) 8. Lymphadenopathy 9. Slurred speech	Disulfuram Warfarin Corticosteroids Carbamazepine Alcohol Oral contraceptive pill Chloramphenicol Isoniazid Warfarin Cimetidine Oestrogens	– ↓ Effect of phenytoin and Interacting drugs (due to enzyme induction) – ↓ Effect of phenytoin (due to drug displacement)
Barbiturates Phenobarbital *Mechanism*: Potentiates the effects of GABA and antagonizes effects of excitatory transmitter glutamate	1. Tolerance and dependence 2. Sedation 3. ↓ REM sleep 4. Confusion in elderly 5. Precipitates porphyria in susceptible individuals 6. Respiratory depression 7. Rashes	Alcohol Narcotic analgesics Antihistamines Antidepressants Warfarin Corticosteroids Phenothiazines Aminophylline Phenytoin Oral contraceptives	– ↑ Effect of interacting drugs, i.e. ↑ CNS depression – ↓ Effect of interacting drugs (due to liver enzyme induction)

Table 8.21 (Cont'd)

Drug	Adverse effects	Interacting drug(s)	Interacting effect
Sodium valproate *Mechanism:* Increases CNS levels of GABA with potentiation of changes in Na⁺/K⁺ conductance	*Concentration-dependent:* 1. Anorexia nervosa and vomiting 2. Tremor 3. Hair loss or curling 4. Peripheral oedema 5. Weight gain *Idiosyncratic:* 6. Hepatoxicity, pancreatitis and thrombocytopenia (rare) 7. Spina bifida in babies exposed in utero (1%)		– Minor inhibitor of drug metabolism – Can ↑ concentrations of other anticonvulsant drugs
Carbamazepine *Action:* Blocks Na⁺ channels postsynaptically and so reduces response to excitatory neurotransmitter binding	1. Hyponatraemia 2. Aplastic anaemia, agranulocytosis, rashes, hepatic dysfunction (idiosyncratic reactions) 3. Teratogenicity (spina bifida) 4. Concentration-related diplopia, ataxia and sedation	Erythromycin Lithium Isoniazid Warfarin Oral contraceptive pill	– ↑ Effect of interacting drugs – ↓ Warfarin effect – ↓ Contraceptive effect
Vigabatrin *Mechanism:* Inhibits enzymatic breakdown of GABA and so increases levels	1. Sedation 2. Weight gain 3. Confusion, psychosis (rare) 4. Visual field defects (may persist after stopping treatment) Less cognitive impairment or sedation		
Lamotrigine *Mechanism:* Inhibits release of excitatory neurotransmitter, e.g. glutamate	1. Skin rash 3% 2. Severe skin reactions, angio-oedema and multiorgan failure 3. Hepatic dysfunction 4. Agitation in elderly	Sodium valproate	– Inhibits lamotrigine metabolism, so use at a lower starting dose
Gabapentin *Mechanism:* Alters GABA metabolism	1. Sedation 2. Ataxia		

ANTIPARKINSONIAN DRUGS (Table 8.22)

Drugs are used to restore nigrostriatal dopaminergic activity or to inhibit striatal cholinergic overactivity.

Table 8.22 Antiparkinsonian drugs

Drug	Adverse effects	Interacting drug(s)	Interacting effect
Anticholinergic drugs Benzhexol Benztropine Orphenadrine Procyclidine	1. Confusion 2. Anticholinergic side-effects	Tricyclic antidepressants Phenothiazines Antihistamines MAOI	– ↑ Anticholinergic effects
L-Dopa *Mechanism:* Metabolized by decarboxylation to dopamine centrally, which causes adverse effects. Therefore used with a decarboxylase inhibitor (e.g. carbidopa or benserazide) that does not cross blood–brain barrier or a selective MAOI (e.g. selegiline) or a catechol-O-methyltransferase (COMT) inhibitor (e.g. entacapone)	1. Nausea and vomiting 2. Postural hypotension 3. Cardiac arrhythmias 4. Dystonic reactions ('on–off' responses) 5. Psychosis, confusion 6. Positive Coombs' test 1. Peripheral effects of L-Dopa can be prevented by combining with domperidone, a peripheral dopamine antagonist 2. Bromocriptine (a dopamine agonist) and amantadine (increases dopamine release) are also used to treat Parkinson's disease	Vitamin B$_6$ Phenothiazines Haloperidol Methyldopa Metoclopramide MAOI	– ↓ L-Dopa effect
Selegiline and entacapone *Mechanism:* Dopamine is metabolized in CNS by 2 pathways: MAO-B is inhibited by selegiline COMT is inhibited by entacapone Selegiline is used with L-dopa to restore clinical response or in patients with 'on–off' symptoms	1. Gastrointestinal upset 2. Confusion		

DRUGS USED IN ALZHEIMER'S DISEASE (Table 8.23)

Table 8.23 Treatment of Alzheimer's disease

Drug	Adverse effects
Cholinesterase inhibitors Tacrine (Significantly better than placebo at increasing (by about 10%) short-term memory, language abilities and selective attention.) Velnacrine Donepezil	1. GI disturbance 2. Polyuria, bladder outflow obstruction 3. Cardiac conduction abnormalities 4. Headaches, fatigue, agitation 5. Increase in CPK
Enhance release of acetylcholine (ACh) Hydergine	
ACh precursor Lecithin	

DRUGS USED FOR ERECTILE DYSFUNCTION (Table 8.24)

Table 8.24

Drug	Adverse effects	Interacting drugs and effects	

Sildenafil
Mechanism: Erectile response mediated by release of nitric oxide (NO) from nerves supplying vessels in corpora cavernosa. This increases intracellular cGMP levels which cause vasodilatation. Effects terminated by phosphodiesterase type 5 enzyme, which is inhibited selectively by sildenafil, which enhances vasodilatory actions of NO
 	
Contraindicated:
1. Severe hepatic impairment
2. BP <90/50 mmHg
3. Recent stroke or myocardial infarction
	1. Headache, flushing, dyspepsia, nasal congestion
	2. Green/blue tinging of vision (3%)
		CYP3A4 inhibitors e.g. cimetidine, erythromycin, azole antifungals, protease inhibitors
		Hepatic or renal disease
		Nitrates
			– ↑ blood
			  levels
			  of
			  sildenafil

ALCOHOL AND OTHER DRUGS WITH CNS EFFECTS (Table 8.25)

Table 8.25 Alcohol (see also Fig. 8.14)

Adverse effects	Interacting drug(s)	Interacting effect
GI 1. Peptic ulceration; malabsorption 2. Fatty liver 3. Cirrhosis and recurrent pancreatitis	Metronidazole Sulphonylureas (esp. chlorpropamide) Chloramphenicol	– Antabuse reaction. Flushing, abdominal colic, vomiting, dizziness and tachycardia (due to inhibition of aldehyde dehydrogenase)
CVS 1. Arrhythmia esp. atrial fibrillation 2. Congestive cardiomyopathy	Warfarin Phenytoin Tolbutamide	– ↑Effects of interacting drugs with acute alcohol (due to enzyme inhibition)
Haematology 1. Macrocytosis	Phenformin	– ↑ Risk of lactic acidosis
Neuropsychiatric 1. Wernicke's and Korsakoff's syndrome 2. Peripheral neuropathy 3. Cerebellar degeneration 4. Retrobulbar neuropathy 5. Psychoses, hallucinations	Hypnotics Sedatives Narcotic analgesics Antihistamines	– ↑ Sedative effects (potentiation of central depression)
Metabolic effects 1. Hypoglycaemia (↓ gluconeogenesis) 2. Hypertriglyceridaemia and hyperuricaemia 3. ↓ Albumin and transferrin synthesis 4. ↑ Catecholamine release 5. ↑ Lipoprotein synthesis 6. Accumulation of fatty acids, ketoacidosis 7. Diuresis and electrolyte disturbance 8. Haemochromatosis and porphyria cutanea tarda 9. Deficiency of protein, calcium and water-soluble vitamins especially thiamine, folate and pyridoxine	Ethanol can prevent the lethal effects of the ingestion of ethylene glycol (antifreeze). In the presence of ethanol, ethanol and ethylene glycol compete for alcohol dehydrogenase.	

Ethanol → Acetaldehyde → Acetate

NAD$^+$ NADH   NAD$^+$ NADH

Alcohol dehydrogenase

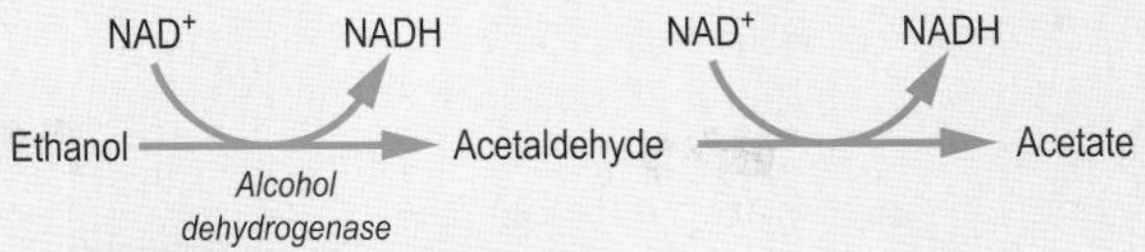

Fig. 8.14 Ethanol metabolism.

Table 8.25 (Cont'd) **Other drugs with CNS effects**

Adverse effects	Interacting drug(s)	Interacting effect
Ecstasy (3,4-methylenedioxymethamphetamine MDMA)		
Class A drug		
Deaths associated with disseminated intravascular coagulation, rhabdomyolysis, acute renal failure, hyperpyrexia, convulsion, cardiac arrhythmias, cerebral infarction		
Amphetamines		
Associated with psychiatric disorders: psychoses, hallucinations and depersonalization, depression, panic attacks and anxiety		

CORTICOSTEROIDS (Tables 8.26 and 8.27)

Table 8.26 Relative properties of various corticosteroids compared to cortisol

Steroid	Glucocorticoid activity	Mineralocorticoid activity
Cortisol	1.0	1.0
Cortisone	0.7	1.0
Aldosterone	0.3	3000
Fludrocortisone	10	125
Prednisolone	4	1
Dexamethasone	25	0

Table 8.27 Cortisol

Adverse effects	Interacting drug(s)	Interacting effect
General 1. Weight gain 2. Redistribution of body fat (moon face and truncal adiposity) 3. Skin atrophy, striae, purpura, acne, pigmentation and hirsutism 4. Cataracts, glaucoma	Barbiturates Phenytoin Rifampicin Warfarin	− ↓ Corticosteroid effect (due to enzyme induction) − ↑ Anticoagulant effect
CVS/metabolic 1. Sodium retention and potassium loss 2. Thirst and polyuria 3. Hypertension 4. Hyperglycaemia 5. Adrenal atrophy and insufficiency (hypotension during anaesthesia and infection)		
Musculoskeletal 1. Muscle weakness and wasting 2. Osteoporosis 3. Growth retardation in children 4. Aseptic bone necrosis		
GI 1. Reactivation of peptic ulcer		
Haematological 1. Polycythaemia		
Immunological 1. Increased susceptibility to and masking of infection 2. Reactivation of latent TB 3. Delayed wound healing		
Psychiatric 1. Mental disturbances, e.g. euphoria, depression and psychoses		

ORAL CONTRACEPTIVES (Table 8.28)

Table 8.28 Oral contraceptives

Adverse effects (generally reflect the role of oestrogens)	Interacting drug(s)	Interacting effect
Oestrogens (ethinyloestradiol, norethisterone), progestogens		
General		
1. Nausea	Phenytoin	
2. Headache	Carbamazepine	
3. Fluid retention and weight gain	Phenobarbitone	– ↓contraceptive
4. Hypertension (5–10% have a significant BP rise)	Rifampicin	effect (due to enzyme induction)
5. Depression	Isoniazid	
6. Loss of libido	Benzodiazepines	
7. Urinary tract infection	Griseofulvin	
8. Genital candidiasis		
9. Jaundice (rare)		
10. Persisting amenorrhoea after stopping pill		
11. Venous thrombosis and embolism (Risk trebled by OC to 15/100 000 women years. More common with higher oestrogen doses. Caused by decrease in antithrombin production and increase in fibrinogen in liver.)		
12. Thrombotic and haemorrhagic stroke		
13. Myocardial infarction (More common with higher oestrogen dose; in older women (> 35 years) and smokers. Due to alteration of clotting factors and increased platelet aggregation.)		

Metabolic
1. Precipitate porphyria in susceptible individuals
2. Impaired glucose tolerance
3. Increase in cholesterol and triglycerides
4. Increase in gall bladder disease
5. ↑ TBG: altered thyroid function tests
6. Increase in hepatic adenoma (rare)
7. Cholestatic jaundice
8. Combined pill protects against endometrial and ovarian malignancy, but associated with an increased risk of cervical and breast cancer

Progestogen-only pill (Norethisterone, medroxyprogesterone)
1. Menstrual irregularities
2. Nausea and vomiting
3. Breast discomfort
4. Breakthrough bleeding
5. Weight gain and oedema

Hormone replacement therapy (Estradiol)
1. Increase in risk of endometrial cancer
2. Increase in risk of breast cancer by 10–30%
3. Increase in risk of thromboembolism
4. Other oestrogen effects as above
Contraindications fewer than with OCP: thromboembolic disease, liver disease

---

Contraindications

Absolute: liver disease, cerebrovascular disease, venous thrombosis, undiagnosed vaginal bleeding, hyperlipidaemia, hormone-dependent tumours of the breast, uterus, kidney and malignant melanoma.

Relative: hypertension, gall bladder disease, cardiac failure and nephrogenic oedema.

Use with caution: diabetes mellitus, smoker, older patient (>35 years), hypertension, migraine sufferers.

ORAL HYPOGLYCAEMIC DRUGS (Table 8.29)

Table 8.29 Oral hypoglycaemics

Drug	Adverse effects	Interacting drug(s)	Interacting effect
All *Mechanism:* Stimulates release of endogenous insulin from pancreas		Alcohol MAOI β-Blockers (inhibits hypoglycaemia-induced tachycardia) NSAID Aspirin (large doses) Warfarin Chloramphenicol	− ↑ Hypoglycaemic effect (due to inhibition of metabolism)
		Corticosteroids Thiazide diuretics Phenothiazines Oral contraceptives Phenytoin Barbiturates Salicylates Lithium Rifampicin	− ↓ Hypoglycaemic effect (due to enzyme induction)
Sulphonylureas Chlorpropamide Tolbutamide ($t_{1/2}$ 3–6 h) Glibenclamide (up to 24 h) Glipizide Gliclazide (6–12 h) *Mechanism:* Stimulates insulin release from pancreas	1. Hypoglycaemia 2. Alcohol intolerance 3. Jaundice (esp. chlorpropamide) 4. Hyponatraemia 5. Weight gain	As above	

Table 8.29 (Cont'd)

Drug	Adverse effects	Interacting drug(s)	Interacting effect
Biguanides Metformin *Mechanism*: Increases peripheral utilization of glucose and decreases absorption of glucose from gastrointestinal tract	1. Lactic acidosis 2. Nausea, anorexia and diabetes 3. Malabsorption of vit. B_{12} Contraindicated in renal or hepatic failure	Alcohol	– ↑ Risk of lactic acidosis
Glitazones Rosiglitazone Pioglitazone *Mechanism*: Increases cell sensitivity to insulin	1. Hepatitis 2. Weight gain 3. GI disturbance 4. Fluid retention and heart failure		
α-Glucosidase inhibitors Acarbose *Mechanism*: Inhibits intestinal α-glucosidases, and so delays absorption of starch and sucrose	1. Flatulence and diarrhoea		

INSULIN (see p. 235)

Insulin preparations

1. Short acting (e.g. soluble insulins). Peak effect at 1–2 hours when given s.c. and duration of action is 4–8 hours.
2. Intermediate acting (e.g. amorphous insulin zinc suspensions). Peak effect is at 3–6 hours, and duration of action is about 12–24 hours.
3. Long acting (crystalline insulin zinc suspension). Peak action is 5–12 hours and duration of effect is 16–30 hours.
4. New very short acting (insulin lispro and insulin aspart) and very long acting insulin analogues (insulin glargine).

DRUGS USED IN GOUT (Table 8.30)

Table 8.30 Drugs used in gout

Drug	Adverse effects	Interacting drug(s)	Interacting effect
Prophylaxis against recurrent attacks			
Allopurinol *Mechanism:* Reduces uric acid synthesis by blocking xanthine oxidase	1. Hypersensitivity reaction 2. May precipitate acute gout	Azathioprine Cyclophosphamide	– ↑ Toxicity of cytotoxic drugs (due to inhibition of metabolism by xanthine oxidase)
Probenecid *Mechanism:* Blocks reuptake of uric acid by proximal renal tubule	1. Rashes 2. Nephrotic syndrome 3. May precipitate acute gout and renal colic	Aspirin (<2 g daily)	– ↓ Uricosuric effect
Acute attacks			
Colchinine *Mechanism:* Binds to microtubule protein and inhibits leucocyte migration	1. GI toxicity (nausea, vomiting and diarrhoea in 80%) 2. Bone marrow suppression and renal failure (rare)		

Uricosuric drugs: Probenecid, sulphinpyrazone, salicylate in high doses (i.e. 5–6 g/day). Should not be used during an acute attack of gout. NSAIDs or colchicine should be given for first 3 months as treatment may precipitate an acute attack.

Drugs causing gout: Thiazide diuretics, loop diuretics, pyrazinamide, ethambutol, salicylate in low doses, alcohol, cytotoxic agents, drugs causing haemolysis.

DRUGS USED IN HYPERTHYROIDISM (Table 8.31)

Table 8.31 Drugs used for hyperthyroidism

Drug	Adverse effects
Thiouracils Carbimazole Methimazole	Common, dose dependent: 1. Allergy with fever, rash and arthralgia 2. Neutropenia Contraindicated in pregnancy and breast feeding

ANTIBACTERIAL DRUGS (Table 8.32)

Table 8.32 Antibacterial drugs (for mechanisms of action see p. 58)

Drug	Adverse effects	Interacting drugs	Interacting effect

Penicillins
Benzylpenicillin
Ampicillin
Amoxicillin
Active against β-lactamase-producing-
bacteria
  Flucloxacillin
  Amoxycillin + clavulanate
Active against Pseudomonas aeroginosa
  Carbenicillin
  Ticarcillin
  Piperacillin
	1. Skin hypersensitivity, fever (including
	   Stevens–Johnson syndrome) and anaphylaxis
	2. Neurotoxicity, e.g. convulsions (esp. in renal failure and
	   with intrathecal administration)
	3. Hyperkalaemia
	4. Interstitial nephritis
	5. Sodium overload
	6. Haemolytic anaemia, thrombocytopenia		

Tetracyclines	1. Diarrhoea 2. Photosensitivity 3. Candidal infections 4. ↑ Urea in patients with impaired renal function 5. Staining of teeth during tooth development	Antacids Oral Fe preparations	– ↓ Tetracycline absorption (due to chelation)

Cephalosporins
First generation
  Cefadroxil (oral)
  Cephradine
  Cephalexin
Second generation
  Cefuroxime (oral)
  Cephamandole
  Cefaclor
Third generation
  Cefixime (oral)
  Cefotaxime
  Ceftazidime
	1. Hypersensitivity
	2. Cross-sensitivity with penicillins (10%)
	3. Nephrotoxic (large doses)
		Furosemide
		Alcohol
			– ↑ Risk of nephrotoxicity
			– Disulfiram-like reaction

Table 8.32 (Cont'd)

Drug	Adverse effects	Interacting drugs	Interacting effect
Chloramphenicol	1. Dose-related bone marrow depression 2. Non-dose-related aplastic anaemia (rare) 3. Haemolysis in G6PDH deficiency 'Grey baby syndrome'	Warfarin Sulphonylureas Phenytoin Barbiturates	– ↑ Effect of interacting drugs (due to liver enzyme inhibition)
Aminoglycosides Gentamicin Amikacin Tobramycin Streptomycin	1. Ototoxicity ⎫ dose related 2. Nephrotoxicity ⎭ 3. Malabsorption syndrome (oral neomycin) 4. Aggravation of myasthenia gravis	Furosemide Cephalosporins Amphotericin B	– ↑ Risk of ototoxicity and of nephrotoxicity
Quinolones Ciprofloxacin Ofloxacin	1. GI disturbance 2. Arthritis 3. Lowers seizure threshold	Theophylline	– ↑ Side-effects of theophylline due to ↓ elimination
Nitrofurantoin	1. Nausea and vomiting 2. Rashes and fever 3. Peripheral neuropathy (esp. in renal failure) 4. Hypersensitivity reactions, e.g. pneumonitis 5. Haemolysis in G6PDH deficiency 6. Pulmonary complications with chronic therapy		
Metronidazole	1. GI disturbance 2. Metallic taste 3. Peripheral neuropathy and seizures	Alcohol Warfarin	– 'Antabuse reaction' – ↑ Anticoagulant effect (due to enzyme inhibition)
Macrolides Erythromycin Clarithromycin Azithromycin	1. GI disturbance 2. Liver damage and jaundice		

Table 8.32 (Cont'd)

Drug	Adverse effects	Interacting drugs	Interacting effect
Sulphonamides	1. Rashes and photosensitivity 2. Stevens–Johnson syndrome 3. Fever 4. Hepatitis 5. Erythema nodosum 6. Kernicterus in the newborn 7. Blood dyscrasias: haemolytic anaemia/aplastic anaemia 8. Nephrotoxicity due to crystalluria	Warfarin Phenytoin Sulphonylureas	– ↑ effect of interacting drugs
Glycopeptides Vancomycin Teicoplanin	Ototoxicity and nephrotoxicity at high plasma levels 1. Thrombophlebitis, 'Red man syndrome' 1. Nausea, anaphylaxis		

ANTITUBERCULOUS DRUGS (Table 8.33)

Table 8.33 Antituberculous drugs

Drug	Adverse effects	Interacting drug(s)	Interacting effect
Isoniazid	1. Peripheral neuropathy (corrected by pyridoxine, 50 mg/day) 2. Pellagra-like syndrome 3. Hepatotoxicity and transient rise in aminotransferases 4. +ve ANA and SLE syndrome in slow acetylators 5. Agranulocytosis, haemolytic anaemia	Phenytoin Carbamazepine	– ↑ Effects of interacting drugs (due to liver enzyme inhibition)
Ethambutol	1. Retrobulbar neuritis and yellow/green colour vision defects 2. Transient rise in aminotransferases		
Rifampicin	1. Hepatitis, transient rise in aminotransferases 2. Nephritis 3. Immune thrombocytopenia 4. Colours urine and sputum pink	Warfarin Oral contraceptives Diazepam Barbiturates β-Blockers Digoxin Oral hypoglycaemics Protease inhibitors (indinavir)	– ↑ Effect of interacting drugs (due to liver enzyme induction) – ↑ Levels of rifampicin and ↓ Levels of indinavir (rifampicin enhances metabolism)
Pyrazinamide	1. Hepatitis 2. Interstitial nephritis 3. Hyperuricaemia		
Second line drugs Capreomycin Cycloserine New macrolides (Clarithromycin, azithromycin) Quinolones (Ciprofloxacin) Ansamycin	Ototoxicity and nephrotoxicity CNS toxicity 1. Thrombocytopenia and leucopenia 2. GI disturbance	Ketoconazole	– Levels of ansamycin and ketoconazole reduced

ANTIFUNGAL DRUGS (Table 8.34)

Table 8.34 Antifungal drugs

Drug	Adverse effects	Interacting drug(s)	Interacting effect
Griseofulvin	1. Porphyria in susceptible individuals 2. Photosensitivity, hypersensitivity 3. Hepatitis 4. Headaches	Phenobarbital Warfarin	– ↑ Antifungal effect (due to enzyme induction) – ↓ Anticoagulant effect (due to enzyme induction)
Amphotericin B	1. Nausea, vomiting, fever, chills 2. Hypersensitivity reactions 3. Nephrotoxicity with long-term use Creatinine clearance must be monitored 4. Normochromic anaemia 5. Hypokalaemia 6. Phlebitis at injection sites	Corticosteroids	– Enhanced potassium loss
Imidazoles Ketoconazole	1. Nausea, vomiting 2. Hepatitis 3. Rashes 4. Gynaecomastia	Ciclosporin Warfarin Rifampicin Terfenadine Astemizole Cisapride	– ↑ Serum levels of ciclosporin – ↑ Anticoagulant effect – ↓ Levels of rifampicin and/or ketoconazole – High risk of arrhythmia (torsade de pointes)
Miconazole	1. Reversible liver dysfunction 2. Nausea and vomiting	Warfarin, phenytoin Oral hypoglycaemics	– ↑ Effect of interacting drugs (due to protein-binding displacement)
Triazoles Fluconazole Itraconazole Voriconazole	1. GI disturbance 2. Rash 3. Nausea, headache 4. Liver damage (fluconazole)	Rifampicin Warfarin Phenytoin Tacrolimus Ciclosporin Rifabutin	– ↓ Fluconazole levels – ↑ Warfarin effect – ↑ Plasma levels – ↑ Rifabutin levels
Flucytosine	1. Marrow depression 2. Accumulation in renal failure		
Echinocardins Caspofungin	1. Increase in liver transaminases Less nephrotoxicity	Ciclosporin	– ↑ Caspofungin levels

ANTIPROTOZOAL DRUGS (Tables 8.35 and 8.36)

Table 8.35 Antimalarial drugs

Drug	Acts against	Adverse effects
4-Aminoquinolones Chloroquine	Blood schizonticide	1. Nausea, vomiting and headaches 2. Retinal and corneal damage 3. Photosensitivity 4. Myopathy 5. Exacerbation of cutaneous porphyria and psoriasis 6. Increase in epilepsy and neuropsychiatric illness
8-Aminoquinolones Primaquine	Tissue schizonticide Hypnozonticide Gametocytocide Sporonticide	1. Haemolytic anaemia in G6PD deficiency 2. Nausea and vomiting 3. Bone marrow suppression
Arylamino alcohols Quinine	Blood schizonticide	1. Tinnitus, headache, blurring of vision 2. Hypoglycaemia 3. Overdosage 'cinchonism', profound hypotension due to peripheral vasodilatation and myocardial depression Safe in pregnancy
Mefloquine	Blood schizonticide	1. Neuropsychiatric disturbance, acute psychosis 2. GI disturbance 3. Postural hypotension Contraindicated in renal and severe hepatic impairment, past psychiatric history, epilepsy, cardiac conduction defects, lactation and pregnancy
Halofantrine	Blood schizonticide	1. Nausea, abdominal pain, diarrhoea 2. Prolongation of QT interval, serious arrhythmias
Antifolates *Type I (compete with p-aminobenzoic acid (PABA) free enzyme in parasites)* Sulfadoxine	Blood schizonticide	1. Folic acid deficiency 2. Skin rashes, Stevens–Johnson syndrome
Dapsone *Type II* *(inhibits dihydrofolate)*	Blood schizonticide	
Proguanil	Blood and tissue schizonticide Sporonticide	1. Aphthous mouth ulceration 2. Alopecia
Pyrimethamine	Blood and tissue schizonticide Sporonticide	1. Folic acid deficiency 2. Bone marrow suppression (in high doses) 3. Stevens–Johnson syndrome
Antibiotics Tetracycline Doxycycline	Blood schizonticide	1. GI disturbance 2. Photosensitivity
Qinghaosu Artemisin	Blood schizonticide Gametocytocide	Relatively safe to date

Doxycycline and primaquine are contraindicated in pregnancy.
Mefloquine is contraindicated in first trimester.
Quinine, chloroquine and proguanil are all safe in pregnancy.

Table 8.36 Drugs for treatment of trypanosomiasis and leishmaniasis

Drug	Adverse effects
Suramin	1. Fatal collapse 2. Heavy albuminuria 3. Stomal ulceration 4. Exfoliative dermatitis 5. Severe diarrhoea and fever
Pentamidine	1. Hypotension 2. Hypoglycaemia 3. IDDM 4. Reversible renal failure
Melarsoprol	1. Encephalopathy 2. Myocardial damage 3. Renal failure 4. Hepatotoxicity
Eflornithine	1. Usually mild and reversible
Pentavalent antimony	Well tolerated

ANTIVIRAL AND ANTIRETROVIRAL DRUGS (Tables 8.37–8.39)

Table 8.37 Antiviral drugs

Drug	Adverse effects
Amantadine, rimantadine (Influenza A)	1. Renal failure 2. Seizures at high dose
Interferon-alpha (Chronic hepatitis B and C)	1. Flu-like syndrome with fever, fatigue, myalgia, chills, headache and arthralgia. Attenuated by antipyretic analgesics 2. Bone marrow suppression 3. Neurotoxicity (anxiety, dizziness and depression) 4. Nausea, vomiting and diarrhoea 5. Hypo- and hypertension 6. Cough, dyspnoea and nasal congestion 7. Proteinuria 8. Hyper- and hypothyroidism
Foscarnet* (CMV, aciclovir-resistant HSV infection, VZV)	1. Nephrotoxicity 2. Hypokalaemia 3. Hypo- and hypercalcaemia
Nucleoside analogues Aciclovir, famciclovir, valaciclovir (HSV and VZV infections)	1. High therapeutic index 2. Neurotoxicity (<4%) with seizures and hallucinations
Ganciclovir (CMV pneumonitis and retinitis)	1. Bone marrow suppression, neutropenia 2. Avoid all potentially nephrotoxic drugs, e.g. aminoglycosides, amphotericin B_1, foscarnet, NSAIDs, radiographic contrast dye
Cidofovir (CMV infections)	1. Dose-dependent nephrotoxicity. Can be prevented by coadministration of probenicid 2. Teratogenic
Fomivirsen	1. Iritis, vitritis, raised intraocular pressure
Ribavarin (aerosol)	1. Reticulocytosis 2. Respiratory depression
Neuraminidase inhibitors Zanamivir (inhaled) Oseltamivir (oral)	1. GI disturbance

*Does not require intracellular metabolism, and directly inhibits herpes virus DNA polymerase. Requires IV administration.

Table 8.38 Antiretroviral agents

Drug	Major adverse effects	Interacting drug(s)	Interacting effect
Nucleoside reverse transcriptase inhibitors (NRTIs) *Mechanism*: Activated intracellularly by phosphorylation by cellular kinases; triphosphate form competitively inhibits reverse transcriptase; incorporation into DNA causes chain termination	Hepatic steatosis and lactic acidosis due to inhibition of mitochondrial DNA polymerase and subsequent mitochondrial dysfunction		
Zidovudine (ZDV)	1. Anaemia 2. Neutropenia (2–30%) 3. Myopathy 4. Anorexia 5. Nausea (4–25%) 6. Fatigue 7. Headache (12–18%) 8. Malaise 9. Myalgia 10. Insomnia 11. Lipoatrophy	Ganciclovir Probenicid d4T	– ↑ Risk of haematological toxicity – ↑ ZDV levels – Antagonism
Didanosine (ddl)	1. Pancreatitis (5–9%)* 2. Peripheral neuropathy* (5–12%) 3. Hyperamylasaemia 4. Diarrhoea (15–25%) 5. Increase in serum urate levels 6. Transaminase elevation 7. Lipoatrophy	Avoid drugs that may cause pancreatitis or peripheral neuropathy (e.g. ddC, d4T, isoniazid) Drugs requiring gastric acidity should be given 2 hours before or after ddl, e.g. tetracyclines, dapsone, ketoconazole and itraconazole	
Dideoxycytidine (ddC)	1. Peripheral neuropathy (17–31%) 2. Pancreatitis* 3. Vomiting 4. Rash 5. Stomatitis (10–20%) 6. Lipoatrophy	Avoid drugs that cause peripheral neuropathy	

Table 8.38 (Cont'd)

Drug	Major adverse effects	Interacting drug(s)	Interacting effect
Nucleoside reverse transcriptase inhibitors (NRTIs) (Cont'd)			
Stavudine (d4T)	1. Peripheral neuropathy (15–21%) 2. Transaminase elevation 3. Anaemia 4. Lipoatrophy	Avoid drugs that cause peripheral neuropathy	
Lamivudine (3TC)	1. Headache 2. Nausea 3. Abdominal pain 4. Insomnia		
Abacavir	1. Hypersensitivity syndrome (4%). Rechallenge has been associated with fatal cardiovascular collapse 2. Rash		
Tenofovir	1. Renal dysfunction	Avoid other nephrotoxic drugs	
Non-nucleoside reverse transcriptase inhibitors (NNRTIs) *Mechanism:* Inhibit HIV replication by binding to a pocket of reverse transcriptase which leads to inactivation. Do not require intracellular phosphorylation for their antiviral activity. The presence of a single RT mutation at position 103 confers crossresistance to all NNRTIs			
Nevirapine	1. Rash (20%) Stevens–Johnson (rare) 2. Hepatitis	Rifampicin Clarithromycin	– ↓ Nevirapine levels – ↑ Clarithromycin levels (prolonged QT interval)
Efavirenz	1. Rash (5–10%) 2. Dizziness, headache 3. Insomnia, abnormal dreams Contraindicated in pregnancy	Rifampicin	– ↓ Efavirenz levels

Table 8.38 (Cont'd)

Drug	Major adverse effects	Interacting drug(s)	Interacting effect
Fusion inhibitors Fuzeon (T20)	Injection site reactions		
Protease inhibitors (PI) *Mechanism:* interferes with post-translational processing of HIV-1 precursor proteins	Lipodystrophy (fat wasting or accumulation), hyperlipidaemia, diabetes mellitus	All eliminated via hepatic cytochome P450, and all are P450 inhibitors (ritonavir > indinavir > lopinavir > nelfinavir > amprenavir > saquinavir)	
Saquinavir (Soft gel and a hard gel capsule combined with ritonavir)	1. Dose-related GI intolerance 2. Elevated liver function tests (2–6%)	Rifampicin Rifabutin Phenobarbital	– ↓ Saquinavir levels by 80% – ↓ Saquinavir levels by 40%
		Phenytoin Dexamethasone Carbamazepine	– ↓ Saquinavir levels
		Ketoconazole Itraconazole Fluconazole Ritonavir	– ↑ Saquinavir levels (inhibition of cytochrome p450) – ↑ Saquinavir levels
		Terfenadine Astemizole Cisapride	– Saquinavir ↑ drug levels

Table 8.38 (Cont'd)

Drug	Major adverse effects	Interacting drug(s)	Interacting effect
Protease inhibitors (PI) (cont'd)			
Indinavir	1. Asymptomatic hyperbilirubinaemia (10%) 2. Nephrolithiasis 3. GI intolerance 4. Hair, skin and nail changes	Ketoconazole Rifampicin Rifabutin	– ↑ Indinavir levels – ↓ Indinavir levels – ↑ Rifampicin and rifabutin levels
Ritonavir	1. GI intolerance 2. Circumoral paraesthesia 3. ↑ cholesterol levels (by 30–40%), and triglyceride levels by 200–300% 4. Altered taste 5. Elevated liver function tests 5%	Astemizole Amiodarone Cisapride Diazepam Midazolam Piroxicam Rifabutin	– Contraindicated because ritonavir is potent inhibitor of P450 system
Nelfinavir	1. Diarrhoea		
Lopinavir	1. GI disturbance 2. Hyperlipidaemia		
Amprenavir	1. Rash		
Atazanavir	1. Hyperbilirubinaemia		

Table 8.39 Examples of drugs metabolized by cytochrome P450 enzymes, with clinically important adverse interactions when administered concomitantly with antiretroviral protease inhibitor drugs, and alternative drugs

Drug class	Representative drug	Alternative drug
Non-sedating antihistamines	Terfenadine, astemizole	Loratidine, cetirizine, fexofenadine
Antiarrhythmics*	Amiodarone, quinidine, flecainide	(Monitor effects closely)
Antihyperlipidaemics	Lovastatin, simvastatin	Atorvastatin, pravastatin
Gastrointestinal motility agents	Cisapride	Metoclopramide
Psychoactive agents*	Bupropion, clozapine, pimozide	SSRIs, haloperidol, respiridone
Benzodiazepines	Midazolam, triazolam, diazepam	Lorazepam, oxazepam

*Principal risk is with concurrent ritonavir use.

IMMUNOSUPPRESSANT DRUGS

CYTOTOXIC DRUGS (Fig. 8.15)

- Most drugs affect DNA synthesis. They are classified according to their site of action on DNA synthesis in the cell cycle.
- Some drugs are phase specific, i.e. only effective at killing cells during specific parts of the cell cycle. Other drugs are cycle specific, i.e. cytotoxic towards cycling cells throughout the cell cycle (e.g. alkyating agents).

Adverse effects

- Antiproliferative effects, e.g. marrow suppression, ulceration of GI tract, and, especially with cyclophosphamide, infertility, hair loss, cystitis.
- Steroid effects, e.g. cushingoid appearance, hypertension, diabetes, peptic ulceration, stunted growth, osteoporosis, avascular bone necrosis, cataracts, myopathy.
- Infection: viral, e.g. CMV, HSV, VZV; fungal, e.g. aspergillus, candida, pneumocystis; bacterial, e.g. tuberculosis, listeria, nocardia.

Late complications

- Malignancy, e.g. lymphomas, skin tumours
- Myelodysplasia, testicular and ovarian failure, secondary cancers
- Teratogenesis.

Resistance to cytotoxic drugs

- Can be inherent to the cancer cell line or acquired during therapy.
- Mechanisms of genetic resistance: abnormal transport, decreased cellular retention, increased cellular activation (binding/metabolism), altered target protein, enhanced repair of DNA, altered processing.

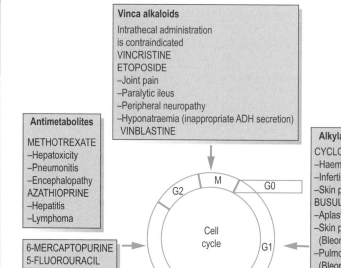

Fig. 8.15 Cell cycle and phase specificity of cytotoxic agents and main adverse effects.
G0 = latent phase, G1 = resting phase, G2 = premitotic phase, S = synthesis of DNA, M = mitosis and division.

Principles of cytotoxic cancer therapy
- Drugs kill a constant fraction, not a constant number, of cells.
- Cells may have discrete periods of vulnerability to cytotoxic drugs.
- Cytotoxic drugs slow the progression of cells through the cell cycle.
- Cytotoxic drugs are not selectively toxic toward cancer cells.
- Cytotoxicity is proportional to total drug exposure.

OTHER ANTICANCER OR TRANSPLANTATION DRUGS

Paclitaxel (Taxol)
- Cytotoxic against many tumours, e.g. ovarian and breast.
- Promotes polymerization of tubulin and disrupts cell division.
- *Adverse effects:*
    1. Neutropenia after 8–10 days
    2. Hypersensitivity
    3. Peripheral neuropathy
    4. Bradycardia, 2nd/3rd degree heart block
    5. Alopecia
    6. Mild vomiting.

Mycophenolate mofetil (MMF)

- Inhibitor of de novo purine synthesis during cell division. Affects T and B cell proliferation.
- Associated with less bone marrow toxicity and gastrointestinal problems.

Ciclosporin

- Main immunosuppressant action is against T cells and the production of cytokines, e.g. IFN-γ.
- After entry into the T cell, ciclosporin binds to its cytoplasmic binding protein, cyclophilin. Inhibition of calcineurin by the ciclosporin–cyclophilin complex inhibits the production of IL-2 by T cells.
- *Adverse effects:*
  1. Nephrotoxicity (almost always occurs and may be permanent or reversible)
  2. Hyperkalaemia, hyperuricaemia, hypophosphataemia
  3. Hyperlipidaemia
  4. Tremor
  5. Hirsutism
  6. Hypertension (in 50%)
  7. Diabetes mellitus
  8. Hepatotoxicity
  9. Haemolytic-uraemic syndrome
  10. Increased incidence of lymphoma.

Absence of bone marrow problems.

Tacrolimus (FK506) and rapamycin

- Bind to the FK binding protein. Tacrolimus also inhibits the production of IL-2 and other cytokines. Rapamycin blocks T-cell proliferation through inhibition of IL-2-dependent pathways but does not affect cytokine expression.
- Similar mechanism of action to ciclosporin.

Adverse effects:
1. Nephrotoxicity
2. New onset IDDM
3. Less hyperlipidaemia, hirsutism and gum hyperplasia than ciclosporin.

Tamoxifen

- Oestrogen-receptor antagonist on breast tissue, and is used in treatment of oestrogen-dependent cancer.
- May prevent development of breast cancer in high-risk patients. Reduces total cholesterol and coronary artery disease and preserves bone density in postmenopausal women.
- *Adverse effects*: hot flushes, nausea and vomiting, hypercalcaemia and ocular changes, i.e. retinopathy and ↓ visual acuity. May increase endometrial cancer and thromboembolic events.

Raloxifene

- Another selective oestrogen modulator, but does not stimulate endometrium.

Antilymphocyte globulin

- *Adverse effects*: serum sickness, fever.

IMMUNOTHERAPY

Colony-stimulating factors (CSF)

E.g. granulocyte-CSF (G-CSF), granulocyte macrophage-colony-stimulating factor (GM-CSF).

• Stimulate haematopoiesis. Produced by recombinant DNA technology.
Adverse effects: bone pain and liver dysfunction with G-CSF, and rashes, fever and myalgia with GM-CSF. Vasculitis, deep vein thrombosis and pulmonary embolus have been reported with high-dose GM-CSF.

ADVERSE EFFECTS IN SPECIAL RISK GROUPS

DRUGS IN PREGNANCY

Adverse effects may occur at any time but especially during the first trimester.

1st trimester (Table 8.40)

Period of greatest risk is considered to be 3rd–11th week of pregnancy ('teratogenesis').

Table 8.40 Drugs to be avoided in pregnancy: 1st trimester	
Teratogenic drugs	*Adverse effects on fetus*
Cytotoxic drugs e.g. methotrexate, cyclophosphamide	Fetal malformations
Thalidomide	Phocomelia, congenital heart disease and stenosis
Androgens	Virilization and other congenital defects
Danazol	
Diethylstilbestrol	Adenocarcinoma of vagina, uterine malformations
Warfarin	Fetal warfarin syndrome*
Alcohol	Fetal alcohol syndrome[†]
Radioactive iodine	Fetal thyroid damage
ACE inhibitors	Abnormalities of the skull, renal failure, hypotension
Chloroquine	Chorioretinitis, deafness
Lithium	Cardiac defects (Ebstein's anomaly)
Phenytoin	Cardiac defects, cleft palate, digital hypoplasia
Retinoids	Ear and eye defects, hydrocephalus
Streptomycin	Deafness
Tetracycline	Dental enamel hypoplasia
Sodium valproate	Neural tube defects, characteristic facies, spina bifida
Carbamazepine	Craniofacial and limb abnormalities
Fluoroquinolones	Cartilage damage
Others: live vaccines, oral contraceptives, metformin, quinine, amphetamines	

*Hypoplastic nose, upper airway difficulties, optic atrophy, mental handicap.
[†]Mental handicap, microcephaly, congenital heart disease, renal anomaly, growth retardation, cleft palate, characteristic facies.

2nd and 3rd trimesters (Table 8.41)

Drugs with important adverse effects on fetal growth and development.

Table 8.41 Drugs to be avoided in pregnancy: 2nd and 3rd trimesters	
Drug	Adverse effects
Aminoglycosides	Ototoxicity
Tetracyclines	Impaired fetal bone growth, teeth discoloration
Chloramphenicol	Peripheral vascular collapse ('grey baby syndrome')
Sulphonamides	Kernicterus, methaemoglobinaemia
Quinine, chloroquine	Retinopathy, congenital deafness, corneal opacities
Quinolones	May damage cartilage development
Isoniazid, rifampicin	Risk of hepatitis
Antithyroid drugs	Neonatal hypothyroidism and goitre
Aspirin	Haemorrhagic disease of the newborn
NSAIDs (Prostaglandin-synthetase inhibitors)	Kernicterus, premature closure of ductus arteriosus
Thiazide diuretics, β-blockers	Neonatal thrombocytopenia Fetal bradycardia
High concentrations of O_2 (>35%)	Retrolental fibroplasia and blindness
Opiates, barbiturates, diazepam	Respiratory depression, drowsiness
Lithium	Congenital heart disease (Ebstein's complex)
Sodium valproate	Neural tube defect (1–2%), hypospadias, microstomia, developmental delay
Corticosteroids	Growth inhibition
Cytotoxic drugs	Inhibition of intellectual development

Drugs in the pregnant mother

1. *Absorption*: Gastrointestinal motility is slowed, which increases absorption of poorly soluble drugs, e.g. digoxin.
2. *Distribution*: Plasma volume and extracellular fluid increase up to 50%. This reduces the plasma concentration of drugs with a small volume of distribution for a given dose. Albumin falls by almost 20%. This means increased free drug for a given concentration for acidic drugs (phenytoin, valproate), and decreased free drug for basic drugs (propranolol, chlorpromazine).
3. *Elimination*: Increased renal plasma flow, but renal elimination unaltered. Liver metabolism induced by progesterone in pregnancy.
4. *Use of drugs with specific diseases:*

> **Epilepsy**: Carbamazepine least likely to cause deformities. Need to perform frequent phenytoin levels during pregnancy.
>
> **Hyperthyroidism**: Use lowest possible dose of carbimazole.
>
> **Malaria**: Doxycycline and primaquine are contraindicated in pregnancy. Mefloquine is contraindicated in first trimester. Quinine, chloroquine and proguanil are all safe in pregnancy.
>
> **Anticoagulation**: Heparin is the drug of choice for anticoagulation at any time during pregnancy, as it does not cross the placenta.

DRUGS EXCRETED IN BREAST MILK

Drugs to be avoided when breast feeding

1. Antibiotics, e.g. aminoglycosides, sulphonamides, ciprofloxacin, tetracycline, metronidazole, chloramphenicol.
2. Anti-TB drugs, e.g. isoniazid.
3. CNS drugs, e.g. narcotic analgesics, benzodiazepines, chlorpromazine.
4. Antithyroid drugs, e.g. carbimazole, radioactive iodine.
5. Anticonvulsant drugs, e.g. phenytoin, phenobarbital.
6. Sulphonylureas.
7. Anticoagulant drugs, e.g. phenindiones (warfarin and heparin are acceptable). Aspirin is associated with a theoretical risk of Reye's syndrome.
8. Cytotoxic drugs and high dose corticosteroids.

Lactation is suppressed by: thiazide diuretics, furosemide, bromocriptine, oestrogens and progestogens (high doses).

Drugs safe in breast feeding

1. Antibiotics: Penicillins, cephalosporins.
2. Theophylline, salbutamol by inhaler, prednisolone.
3. Anticonvulsants: sodium valproate, carbamazepine, phenytoin.
4. Antihypertensives: Beta-blockers, methyldopa, hydralazine (but higher-doses may affect fetus and cause adrenal suppression).
5. Anticoagulants: Warfarin, heparin.
6. Psychotropic drugs: Haloperidol, chlorpromazine.
7. Antidepressants: Tricyclic antidepressants.

DRUGS IN THE ELDERLY (Table 8.42)

Effects of age on drug metabolism

- Concentration of albumin decreases with age, resulting in reduced drug-binding capacity and an increase in the free fraction of drug.
- Lean body mass decreases with age and so volume of distribution may change.
- Expression of cytochrome P450 enzyme changes with age, with a reduced ability to oxidize drugs, mainly in elderly males.

Table 8.42 Drugs to be avoided in the elderly	
Drugs to be used with caution	Adverse effects
Benzodiazepines (especially if long $t_{1/2}$)	Prolonged CNS depression
Barbiturates	Confusional states, hypothermia
Phenothiazines	Hypotension, parkinsonism, extrapyramidal reactions, hypothermia
Antiparkinsonian drugs, (e.g. benzhexol, L-dopa) Anticholinergic drugs and Tricyclic antidepressants	↑ Anticholinergic effects, hallucinations and disorientation
Antihypertensive agents	More prone to postural hypotension
Diuretics	Hypokalaemia, hypomagnesaemia, incontinence
Digoxin	Toxic effects more common
Anticoagulants	↑ Risk of haemorrhage

DRUGS IN LIVER DISEASE (Table 8.43)

Table 8.43 Drugs to be avoided in liver disease	
Drugs to be used with caution	Adverse effects
Drugs whose main route of metabolism is via the liver, e.g. phenytoin, warfarin, narcotic analgesics, theophylline, corticosteroids, barbiturates, phenothiazines and antimicrobials (clindamycin, rifampicin, isoniazid, ethambutol, erythromycin)	↑ Risk of toxic effects
Drugs causing fluid retention, e.g. NSAIDs, corticosteroids	Exacerbate fluid retention
Sedative drugs	May precipitate hepatic encephalopathy
Hepatotoxic drugs	Dose-dependent and hypersensitivity reactions more likely
Diuretics (especially non-potassium sparing)	May precipitate hepatic encephalopathy

DRUGS IN RENAL DISEASE

Drugs accumulate in renal failure if excreted mainly or entirely by the kidney.

Drugs to be avoided

1. Antimicrobials, e.g. tetracyclines (except doxycycline and minocycline that inhibit protein synthesis and induce a catabolic effect that may aggravate renal failure); nitrofurantoin (increased risk of peripheral neuropathy), amphotericin B.
2. Potassium-sparing diuretics, potassium supplements.
3. Opioid analgesics, e.g. meperidine, may produce prolonged CNS effects.
4. Aspirin and NSAIDs.
5. Psychotropic drugs, e.g. lithium.
6. Uricosuric agents, e.g. probenecid and sulfinpyrazone, are ineffective.

Drugs requiring dose adjustment in renal failure

1. Antimicrobials, e.g. penicillin G, ampicillin, aminoglycosides, cephalosporins, sulphonamides, vancomycin, metronidazole.
2. Cardiovascular drugs, e.g. methyldopa, digoxin (reduced excretion and increased risk of arrhythmias), procainamide, disopyramide and ACE inhibitors, flecainide.
3. Others, e.g. chlorpropamide, insulin, H_2-antagonists.

Drugs which can be used in normal dose

1. Antimicrobials, e.g. cloxacillin, oxacillin, clindamycin, chloramphenicol, doxycycline, erythromycin, pyrimethamine, rifampicin and isoniazid (but increased risk of peripheral neuropathy)
2. Cardiovascular drugs, e.g. clonidine, calcium antagonists, hydralazine and prazosin, thiazide and loop diuretics.
3. Narcotic analgesics, e.g. codeine, morphine, naloxone, pentazocine and propoxyphene.
4. Psychotropic drugs, e.g. barbiturates, tricyclic antidepressants, haloperidol.
5. Oral anticoagulants, e.g. warfarin and phenindione.
6. Others, e.g. steroids, tolbutamide and theophylline.

ANTIDOTES USED IN OVERDOSE (Table 8.44)

Table 8.44 Antidotes used in overdose

Drug	Antidote
Digoxin	Fab antibody fragments to digoxin
Iron	Desferioxamine (chelating agent)
Lead	Penicillamine or calcium sodium edetate
Heavy metals (arsenic, mercury or gold)	Dimercaprol or D-penicillamine
Anticholinesterases	Pralidoxime (cholinesterase reactivator) and atropine (competitive antagonist at acetylcholine receptor)
Cyanide*	Sodium thiosulphate or cobalt edetate
Paracetamol (acetaminophen)	N-Acetyl cysteine[†] or methionine
Methanol	IV ethanol (competes with alcohol dehydrogenase)
Carbon monoxide	Oxygen
Opiates	Naloxone/naltrexone (competitive antagonist at opiate receptor)
Benzodiazepines	Flumazenil (a specific benzodiazepine antagonist, can precipitate seizures)
Warfarin	Vitamin K
Monoamine oxidase inhibitors	Hypertensive crisis: α-blocker, chlorpromazine and β-blocker
β-Blockers	Glucagon

*Mechanism: Inhibits cytochrome oxidase by complexing copper in the carrier. This prevents the reduction of molecular oxygen and causes the complete reduction of all electron transport carriers.

[†]Mechanism: After an overdose of paracetamol, the predominant pathways of elimination by conjugation to sulphate and glucuronic acid become saturated. An increasing amount of the drug is activated by the cytochrome P450 system and conjugated with the sulphahydryl group of glutathione. When the stores of glutathione are depleted, the reactive intermediates of paracetamol bind covalently to liver macromolecules, causing liver necrosis. Early administration of N-acetyl cysteine replenishes glutathione stores which protect against paracetamol toxicity.

Forced alkaline diuresis

Some drugs become un-ionized at urinary pH and may be reabsorbed in the distal tubule. Relatively small changes in urinary pH can produce large changes in the fraction of drug un-ionized. Sodium bicarbonate is used to increase the urinary pH. Used for overdoses with salicylates and phenobarbital.

Drugs for which dialysis or haemoperfusion in overdosage may be indicated

Drugs with small volume of distribution are largely restricted to plasma and can be removed by haemodialysis or perfusion

Salicylates
Aminophylline
Methanol
Barbiturates (haemoperfusion)
Lithium carbonate
Procainamide

Carbamazepine (haemoperfusion)
Disopyramide
Aminoglycosides
Cephalosporins
Sulphonamides.

Drugs not significantly removed by dialysis

Dextropropoxyphene
Benzodiazepines
Phenytoin
Phenothiazines
Tricyclic antidepressants
Oral hypoglycaemics
β-Blockers
Digoxin

Hydralazine
Rifampicin
Tetracycline
Benzylpenicillin
Flucloxacillin
Amphotericin
Erythromycin.

High concentrations of antimicrobial drugs in CSF, bile and urine

(Table 8.45)

Table 8.45 Antimicrobial drugs achieving high concentrations in CSF, bile and urine		
CSF	*Bile*	*Urine*
Chloramphenicol	Penicillins	Penicillins
Erythromycin	Cephalosporins	Cephalosporins
Isoniazid	Erythromycin	Aminoglycosides
Pyrazinamide		Sulphonamides
Rifampicin		Nitrofurantoin
Flucytosine		Nalidixic acid
		Ethambutol
		Flucytosine

SUMMARY OF DRUG-INDUCED DISEASE

CARDIOVASCULAR SYSTEM

HYPERTENSION

Corticosteroids, ACTH
Oral contraceptives
Non-steroidal anti-inflammatory drugs (NSAIDs)
MAOI with sympathomimetic agents
Clonidine and methyldopa withdrawal.

CONGESTIVE CARDIAC FAILURE/FLUID RETENTION

As above, plus:
Arterial vasodilators, e.g. minoxidil and hydralazine
β-Blockers
Verapamil.

EXACERBATION OF ANGINA

Vasopressin, oxytocin
β-Blocker withdrawal
Excessive thyroxine
α-Blockers
Hydralazine.

DIRECT MYOCARDIAL TOXICITY

Cytotoxic agents, e.g. doxorubicin, daunorubicin, vincristine
Anaesthetic agents, e.g. halothane
Alcohol.

SHORT QT INTERVAL

Digoxin
Other non-drug causes: hyperthermia, hypercalcaemia, hyperkalaemia.

PROLONGED QT INTERVAL

Class Ia and III anti-arrhythmic agents
Flecainide, terfenadine
Tricyclic antidepressants
Halofantrine
Other, non-drug causes: acute myocardial infarction, hypocalcaemia, hypokalaemia, hypertrophic cardiomyopathy, cerebral injury.

RESPIRATORY SYSTEM

BRONCHOSPASM

β-Blockers
Aspirin, NSAIDs
Cholinergic drugs, e.g. pilocarpine
Cholinesterase inhibitors, e.g. pyridostigmine
Prostaglandin $F_2\alpha$
Any drug causing anaphylaxis.

PULMONARY FIBROSIS

Cytotoxic agents, e.g. busulphan, bleomycin and methotrexate
Nitrofurantoin
Sulfasalazine
Prolonged high dose oxygen
Practolol
Amiodarone.

PLEURAL REACTION

Practolol
Drug-induced lupus syndrome, e.g. procainamide, hydralazine
Bromocriptine
Methotrexate.

ACUTE PULMONARY OEDEMA

Salicylates
β-Blockers
Narcotics, e.g. methadone and diamorphine
Contrast media.

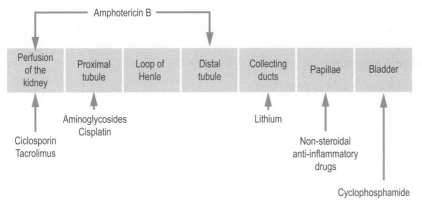

Fig. 8.16 Main sites of action of selected nephrotoxic drugs.

DIRECT NEPHROTOXICITY: ACUTE TUBULAR NECROSIS (Fig. 8.16)

Antibiotics, e.g. aminoglycosides, tetracyclines and amphotericin B
Cytotoxic agents (due to uric acid deposition)
Solvents, e.g. CCl_4, ethylene glycol
Paracetamol overdose
Heavy metals, e.g. mercury, bismuth
Radio-iodinated contrast media
Drug combinations:
1. Cephaloridine and furosemide
2. Gentamicin and furosemide.

ACUTE INTERSTITIAL NEPHRITIS

Antibiotics, e.g. penicillins, sulphonamides, tetracycline
Anti-TB drugs, e.g. rifampicin, streptomycin
Furosemide, thiazide diuretics
NSAIDs, analgesic abuse
Radiation nephritis
Phenytoin.

RENAL TUBULAR ACIDOSIS

Degraded tetracycline
Amphotericin B
Acetazolamide
Adefovir.

NEPHROTIC SYNDROME (ACCOUNTS FOR 2% CASES)

Penicillamine
Gold salts and other heavy metals
Mercurials
NSAIDs
Probenecid
Angiotensin-converting enzyme inhibitors, e.g. high dose captopril.

URINARY RETENTION

Diuretics with prostate enlargement
MAOI
Anticholinergic agents, e.g. tricyclic antidepressants, disopyramide.

GASTROINTESTINAL SYSTEM

OESOPHAGEAL ULCERATION

Tetracycline
Ferrous salts
Doxycycline
Disodium etidronate (bisphosphonate used in treatment of osteoporosis).

NAUSEA AND VOMITING

Digoxin
Opiates
Oestrogens
L-Dopa

Theophylline
Bromocriptine
Tetracycline
Quinidine.

PANCREATITIS

Azathioprine
Sulphonamides
Methyldopa
ddI ddc (antiretroviral drugs).

DIARRHOEA

Antibacterial drugs
Digoxin
Magnesium salts
Laxative abuse.

CONSTIPATION

Opiates
Anticholinergic drugs
Phenothiazines
Aluminium hydroxide
Ferrous salts.

HEPATITIS (2–3 WEEKS AFTER EXPOSURE)

Halothane (repeated administration)
MAOI
Anticonvulsants
Methyldopa
Anti-TB, e.g. rifampicin, isoniazid, pyrazinamide.

INTRAHEPATIC CHOLESTASIS ± HEPATITIS

(Hypersensitivity 3–6 weeks after exposure)
Phenothiazines
Tricyclic antidepressants
NSAIDs
Sulphonylureas
Anti-TB drugs, e.g. rifampicin, isoniazid
Antibiotics, e.g. erythromycin, carbenicillin, sulphonamides
Nevirapine (antiretroviral drug).

CHOLESTASIS ALONE

Anabolic steroids
Oral contraceptives.

HEPATOTOXINS

Tetracycline
CCl_4
Paracetamol
Methotrexate
Aflatoxin.

ENDOCRINE SYSTEM

GALACTORRHOEA

Methyldopa
Phenothiazines, haloperidol
L-Dopa
Metoclopramide

Cimetidine
Benzodiazepines
Oestrogens
Tricyclic antidepressants.

HYPERPROLACTINAEMIA

Antipsychotic drugs (dopamine antagonists)
Cimetidine
Verapamil
Opiates
Oestrogen therapy.

GYNAECOMASTIA

Anti-androgens:
Spironolactone
(without galactorrhoea)
Cimetidine (without galactorrhoea)
Methyldopa
Phenothiazines
Tricyclic antidepressants
Cytotoxic agents

Digoxin (without galactorrhoea)
Oestrogens.

HYPOTHYROIDISM

Iodides
Antithyroid drugs, e.g. carbimazole, thiouracil
Lithium
Amiodarone.

VAGINAL CARCINOMA

Diethylstilbestrol (administered to mother).

METABOLIC

HYPERGLYCAEMIA

Corticosteroids
Oral contraceptives
Diuretics (loop and thiazide).

HYPOGLYCAEMIA

Alcohol
Salicylates and NSAIDs
β-Blockers.

HYPERCALCAEMIA

Antacids (Ca^{2+} salts)
Vitamin D
Thiazide diuretics
Oestrogen therapy in cancer.

HYPERURICAEMIA

See page 277.

HYPERKALAEMIA

Potassium-sparing diuretics
Cytotoxic agents
Steroid withdrawal
ACE inhibitors, e.g. captopril, enalapril.

HYPOKALAEMIA

(See also p. 198.)
Diuretics
Laxative abuse
Corticosteroids
Amphotericin B
Insulin.

HYPONATRAEMIA/INAPPROPRIATE ADH

See pages 197–198.

NEPHROGENIC DIABETES INSIPIDUS

Lithium
Demethylchlortetracycline.

METABOLIC ACIDOSIS

See page 188.

OSTEOMALACIA

Anticonvulsants (long-term), e.g. phenytoin, barbiturates.

EXACERBATION OF PORPHYRIA

See page 273.

BLOOD DISEASES

APLASTIC ANAEMIA OR NEUTROPENIA

1. Cytotoxic agents
2. Antibiotics, e.g. chloramphenicol, sulphonamides, methicillin, ampicillin, co-trimoxazole
3. Anti-TB, e.g. rifampicin
4. Antimalarials, e.g. pyrimethamine, chloroquine
5. Antiretrovirals e.g. zidavodine
6. Antirheumatic agents, e.g. gold salts, penicillamine, NSAID (phenylbutazone)
7. Dapsone
8. Antithyroid, e.g. carbimazole
9. Oral hypoglycaemics, e.g. sulphonylureas
10. Anticonvulsants, e.g. carbamazepine, phenytoin
11. Tricyclic antidepressants
12. Anticoagulants, e.g. phenindione
13. Diuretics, e.g. thiazides, furosemide
14. Psychotropic drugs, e.g. phenothiazines, clozapine (agranulocytosis, 1:300)
15. Anti-arrhythmics, e.g. quinidine, procainamide.

THROMBOCYTOPENIA

As above, but especially:
Diuretics (thiazide and loop)
Antirheumatic agents, e.g. aspirin, NSAIDs
Antibiotics, e.g. rifampicin, carbenicillin, co-trimoxazole, quinine, quinidine
Methyldopa
Anticonvulsants, e.g. phenytoin, carbamazepine
Heparin.

MEGALOBLASTIC ANAEMIA (Fig. 8.17)

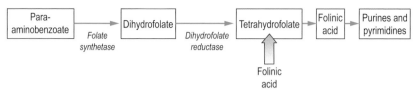

Fig. 8.17 Folate metabolism.

FOLATE DEFICIENCY

Dihydrofolate reductase inhibitors, e.g. methotrexate, pyrimethamine, trimethoprim
Sulphonamides
Impaired absorption, e.g. colestyramine, sulfasalazine
Uncertain mechanisms, e.g. anticonvulsants, ethanol and oral contraceptives.

HAEMOLYTIC ANAEMIA

- Mainly in G6PDH deficiency (see p. 344).
- Immune haemolysis
  - Type I: Antibodies directed against the drug, e.g. penicillin, quinidine, methyldopa, dapsone
  - Type II: Drug combines with an antibody and immune complex absorbed onto cells, e.g.
    Isoniazid
    Phenacetin
    Quinine, quinidine
    Sulphonamides
    Sulphonylureas
  - Type III: Autoimmune (autoimmune haemolytic anaemia)
    Methyldopa (+ve Coombs' test)
    L-Dopa
    Mefenamic acid
    Cephalosporins (+ve Coombs' test)
    Rifampicin.
- Drugs with direct toxicity, e.g. phenacetin abuse.

B$_{12}$ DEFICIENCY

Colchicine
Neomycin
Metformin.

METHAEMOGLOBINAEMIA

See page 275.

LYMPHADENOPATHY

Phenytoin
Phenylbutazone
Dapsone.

NEUROPSYCHIATRIC

ORGANIC PSYCHOSES

Amphetamines and amphetamine-derived designer drug 'ecstasy'
Anticholinergic drugs, e.g. atropine, trihexyphenidyl, L-dopa, and dopamine
agonists, e.g. bromocriptine
Steroids
Phencyclidine, e.g. PCP: 'angel dust'
Cannabis.

DRUG-WITHDRAWAL STATES

Benzodiazepines
Clonidine
Barbiturates
Opiates
Alcohol.

CONFUSIONAL STATES

Alcohol
Sedatives and hypnotics,
e.g. barbiturates,
benzodiazepines
Tricyclic antidepressants
Phenothiazines
Anticholinergic drugs

Antiparkinsonian drugs,
e.g. trihexyphenidyl, L-dopa
Opiates
Digoxin
Isoniazid
Efavirenz (antiretroviral drug).

DEPRESSION

Corticosteroids
Centrally acting
antihypertensives
e.g. methyldopa, clonidine
β-Blockers

Oral contraceptives
(4–6% of cases)
Phenothiazines
Opiates, benzodiazepines,
Alcohol
L-Dopa.

EXTRAPYRAMIDAL REACTIONS

Parkinsonism
Phenothiazines
e.g. chlorpromazine
Butyrophenones
e.g. haloperidol
Metoclopramide
Carbon monoxide

Dystonic reactions
Tricyclic antidepressants
L-Dopa, bromocriptine
Methyldopa
Oral contraceptives (chorea).

PERIPHERAL NEUROPATHY

Cytotoxic agents, e.g. vincristine, vinblastine
Antibiotics, e.g. nitrofurantoin, streptomycin, metronidazole nalidixic acid, chloramphenicol
Antiretroviral drugs e.g. ddI, ddc, d4T
Oral hypoglycaemics, e.g. sulphonylureas
Anti-TB, e.g. isoniazid, ethambutol
MAOI, e.g. phenelzine
Tricyclic antidepressants
Amiodarone.

PROXIMAL MYOPATHY

Corticosteroids
Chloroquine
Amiodarone

Oral contraceptives
Amphotericin B.

ACUTE RHABDOMYOLYSIS

Diamorphine
Barbiturates
Diazepam
Statins and fibrates

Isoniazid
Amphotericin B.

EXACERBATION OF MYASTHENIA

Aminoglycosides
Polymixins
Opiates.

BENIGN INTRACRANIAL HYPERTENSION

Corticosteroids
Oral contraceptives
Isotretinoin*

Tetracyclines
Hypervitaminosis A.

Other adverse effects: teratogenicity, dry skin and mucous membranes, epidermal fragility, allergic vasculitis, granulomatous lesions, increased triglyceride levels.

SEXUAL DYSFUNCTION

DECREASED LIBIDO AND ERECTILE DYSFUNCTION

Antihypertensives, e.g. clonidine, methyldopa, β-blockers and thiazide diuretics
Psychotropics, e.g. MAOIs, tricyclic antidepressants, phenothiazines, benzodiazepines
Sedatives, e.g. opiates, ethanol, anxiolytics
Cytotoxic drugs
Lithium
Antiandrogens, e.g. cimetidine, cyproterone acetate
Oestrogens.

FAILURE OF EJACULATION

Antihypertensives, e.g. methyldopa
Psychotropic agents
Tricyclic antidepressants.

OTOLOGICAL

DEAFNESS/TINNITUS/VERTIGO

Aminoglycosides
Quinine and quinidine ('cinchonism')
Salicylates
Furosemide.

EYE

CORNEAL OPACITIES

Phenothiazines,
esp. chlorpromazine
Chloroquine
Amiodarone
Indomethacin
Corticosteroids
Vitamin D.

CATARACT

Corticosteroids
Phenothiazines, esp. chlorpromazine
Cytotoxic agents, e.g. busulphan, chlorambucil.

RETINOPATHY

Chloroquine, quinine
Phenothiazines,
esp. high dose thioridazine
Penicillamine
Indomethacin.

OPTIC NEURITIS

Anti-TB, e.g. ethambutol,
streptomycin, isoniazid
Digoxin
Alcohol
Chloramphenicol.

DERMATOLOGICAL

FEVER (± other features of hypersensitivity)

Antihistamines
Hydralazine, methyldopa
Isoniazid, nitrofurantoin
Penicillin
Salicylates
Quinidine, procainamide
Phenytoin
Chlorambucil
6-Mercaptopurine
Abacavir (antiretroviral drug).

SERUM SICKNESS

Aspirin
Penicillins
Streptomycin
Sulphonamides.

SLE-LIKE SYNDROME

Antibiotics, e.g. griseofulvin, penicillin, streptomycin, tetracyclines, sulphonamides
Anti-TB drugs, e.g. isoniazid
Anticonvulsants, e.g. carbamazepine, phenytoin
Antihypertensives, e.g. hydralazine, methyldopa
Antiarrhythmics, e.g. practolol, procainamide
Antirheumatics, e.g. gold, phenylbutazone.

ERYTHEMA NODOSUM

Antibiotics, e.g. penicillin, sulphonamides
Dapsone
Salicylates, phenylbutazone
Sulphonylureas, e.g. chlorpropamide
Oral contraceptives
Gold salts.

FIXED DRUG ERUPTIONS

Antibiotics, e.g. penicillins, sulphonamides, tetracyclines
Phenytoin
Salicylates, phenylbutazone
Barbiturates
Antihistamines
Quinine
Captopril
Dapsone.

ERYTHEMA MULTIFORME OR STEVENS–JOHNSON SYNDROME

Barbiturates
Salicylates, phenylbutazone
Antibiotics, e.g. tetracycline, sulphonamide
Phenytoin, carbamazepine
Thiazide diuretics
Chlorpropamide.

TOXIC EPIDERMAL NECROLYSIS

Barbiturates
Phenytoin
Penicillin.

PIGMENTATION

ACTH
Phenothiazines
Amiodarone
Antimalarials, e.g. chloroquine, androgens
Cytotoxic agents, e.g. busulphan, cyclophosphamide
Phenytoin
Heavy metals, e.g. gold salts, mercury, arsenic
Corticosteroids,
Hypervitaminosis A
Oral contraceptives.

RAYNAUD'S SYNDROME

Ergotamine
β-Blockers
Clonidine.

PHOTOSENSITIVITY

Antibiotics, e.g. sulphonamides,
tetracyclines, griseofulvin,
nalidixic acid
Sulphonylureas

Thiazide diuretics
Phenothiazines
Oestrogens and progesterones.

LOSS OR ALTERATION OF TASTE

Penicillamine
Griseofulvin
Lithium

Metronidazole
Gold salts
ACE inhibitors.

HIRSUTISM/HYPERTRICHOSIS

Diazoxide
Minoxidil
Corticosteroids.

ALOPECIA

Cytotoxic agents
Anticoagulants, e.g. heparin
Withdrawal of oral contraceptives

Antithyroid agents
L-Dopa
Gold salts.

INDEX

Abacavir 390
Abdomen 175–178
  dermatomes 135
Abdominal reflexes 137
Abducent (VI) nerve 153, 159–60
Abetalipoproteinaemia 264
ABO blood group 123
Absolute risk 326
  reduction 327
Acanthamoeba spp. 75
Accessory (XI) nerve 154, 162
Accommodation reflex 152
Acetaminophen (paracetamol) overdose 400
Acetylation, genetic variants 345
Acetylcholine 141
  Alzheimer's disease therapeutic agents 374
  receptors 245, 346
Achondroplasia 22, 27
Aciclovir 73, 388
Acid phosphatase 295
Acid–base balance 183–6, 284, 287, 288
  disturbances 187–90
  mixed disorders 189
  prolonged vomiting 189
Acidosis
  hyperchloraemic 189
  hypochloraemic 189
  lactic 189–90, 250
  metabolic 187, 188
  mixed disorders 189
  respiratory 187–8
Acids 183
Acinetobacter spp. 53
Acquired hypogammaglobulinaemia 115
Acquired immune deficiency syndrome (AIDS) 68, 118
  see also Human immunodeficiency virus (HIV)
Actinomyces israelii 43
Action potential, cardiac cells 209
Acute intermittent porphyria 273, 344
Acute interstitial nephritis, drug-induced 403
Acute phase reactants 294
Acute tubular necrosis, drug-induced 403
Adaptive (acquired) immunity 92, 93
Adaptive immunotherapy 88
Adenine 7
Adenine arabinoside 6
Adenine phosphoribosyl transferase 276
Adenosine 354
Adenosine deaminase deficiency 18, 116
Adenosine diphosphate (ADP) 242
  agonists 356
Adenosine triphosphate (ATP) 242
Adenoviruses 69
Adenylate cyclase 246
Adhesion molecules 88, 89, 103, 244
Adipose tissue 258, 260
Adjuvant 88
Adrenal cortical steroids 230–2
  biosynthesis 231
  disorders of secretion 232
  urinary metabolites 231–2
Adrenal medulla 233
Adrenal sex steroids 232
Adrenaline 233, 278

Adrenergic receptors 143, 346
Adrenocorticotrophic hormone (ACTH) 194, 226
Adrenoleucodystrophy 25
Adult polycystic kidney disease 16, 22, 27
Adult respiratory distress syndrome (ARDS) 105
Adult T-cell leukaemia 68
Adverse drug reactions 346
Aeromonas hydrophilia 49
Affinity maturation 109
Afterload 216
Agammaglobulinaemia 23, 25
Ageing 36
  drug metabolism changes 398
  immune response 119
Agglutination assays 129
Aggregate (ecological) survey 331
AIDS 68, 118
  see also Human immunodeficiency virus (HIV)
Airway
  irritant receptors 208
  resistance (RAW) 205–6
Alanine amino transferase 295
Albendazole 78
Albinism 23, 269
Albumin 292
Alcohol consumption 375
Alcohol disinfectants 85
Aldehyde disinfectants 85
Aldosterone 193–195, 284
ALERT organisms 79
Alkaline phosphatase 295
Alkalosis
  metabolic 187, 188
  mixed disorders 189
  respiratory 187, 188
Alkaptonuria 269
Alkylating agents 11, 394
Alleles 2
Allergic contact dermatitis 114
Alloantibody 88
Allopurinol 381
Allotype 88, 109
Allylamines 75
Alopecia, drug-induced 413
α_1-antitrypsin 294
  deficiency 23, 28
α-fetoprotein 28, 297
α-glucosidase inhibitors 380
α-lipoprotein deficiency (Tangier disease) 264
α-thalassaemia 275
Alternative pathway 88
Alveolar ventilation 204
Alveolar–arterial oxygen difference ($P(\text{A-a})O_2$) 207
Alzheimer's disease 30, 105
  drug treatment 374
Amantadine 73, 388
Amine hormones 224
Amino acids 266
  inborn errors of metabolism 268, 270
  intestinal transport 267
  metabolic degradation 268
  renal reabsorption 199
  transport defects 270

Aminoaciduria 270
Aminoglycosides 59, 383
  induced deafness 26
Aminoquinolones 78, 387
Amiodarone 354
Amlyoidosis 120
Ammonium ion, renal secretion 186
Amniocentesis 29
Amoxicillin 59
Amphetamines 376
Amphotericin B 74, 75, 386
Ampicillin 59
Amplification, genetic 2
Amprenavir 392
Amyotrophic lateral sclerosis (motor neuron
    disease) 104
Anaemia
  drug-induced 407, 408
  stem cell transplantation 126
Anaerobes 53
Anaphylactic (type I) hypersensitivity reactions
    113, 114
Anaphylatoxins 88
Anatomy 133–77
Anchor residues 88
Ancylostoma duodenale 76
Andersen's disease 253
Androgen insensitivity (testicular feminization
    syndrome) 21
Androgens 232
Anencephaly 30
Aneuploidy 2
Angelman syndrome 20, 22
Angina, drug-induced 401
Angiotensin II 194
  antagonists 194, 350
Angiotensin-converting enzyme 195, 295
  inhibitors 349
Anion gap 183
Anomic aphasias 151
Anterior cerebral artery 148
Antiarrhythmic drugs 353–4
  classification 352
Antibiotics 58–62, 382–4
  antimalarials 387
  bactericidal/bacteriostatic 61
  bile levels 401
  cerebrospinal fluid levels 401
  combination therapy 61
  protein synthesis inhibitors 11
  resistance 61–2
  sites of action 60
  spectra of activity 58–60
  urine levels 401
Antibodies 109
  assay 129
  see also Immunoglobulins; Monoclonal
    antibodies
Antibody-dependent cellular cytotoxicity (ADCC)
    88, 99
Anticholinergic drugs 373
Anticholinesterase overdose 400
Anticoagulants 355–6
  elderly patients 398
  pregnant patients 397

Anticonvulsants 371–2
  pregnant patients 397
Antidepressants 364–6
Antidiuretic hormone (vasopressin) 192, 193,
    199–201, 229
  syndrome of inappropriate secretion 200–201
Antidotes 400
Antifibrinolytic agents 357, 358
Antifolates 60
  antimalarials 387
Antifungal drugs 74–5, 386
Antigen-presenting cells 88, 99
Antigenic determinants 109
Antigenic peptides 88
Antigens
  heterophile 90
  T-dependent 92
  T-independent 92
Antihypertensives 347–51
  elderly patients 398
Antilymphocyte globulin 395
Antimalarial drugs 360, 387
  pregnant patient 397
Antimanic drugs 368–9
Antimetabolites 394
Antimitochondrial antibodies 121
Antineutrophil cytoplasmic antibodies 123
Antinuclear antibodies 122
Antioxidants, dietary 104
Antiparkinsonian drugs 373
  elderly patients 398
Antiphospholipid antibody syndrome 120
Antipsychotic drugs 368–9
Antireticulin antibody 122
Antiretroviral drugs 389–92
Antisense technology 2, 16
Anti-smooth muscle antibody 121
Antitoxins 83
Antituberculous drugs 385
Antiviral agents 73, 388
Anxiolytic drugs 367
Aorta 163
Aortic arches 173
Aortic valve 173
Aplastic anaemia, drug-induced 407
Apolipoproteins 258, 259, 260
Apoptosis 35, 88, 105, 243
Aprotinin 358
Arenaviruses 63
Arterial blood gases 183
Arteries 163–5
Arylamino alcohol antimalarials 387
Ascaris lumbricoides 75
Ascorbic acid (vitamin C) 281
Aspartate aminotransferase 296
Aspergillus spp. 74
Aspirin 356, 357
Association 331
Asthma 30, 31
Astroviruses 63
Ataxic telangiectasia syndrome 117
Atazanavir 392
Atherosclerosis 104, 105
Atrial natriuretic peptide 196
Atrioventricular node 173

Atrophic gastritis 122
Attack rate 319
Attributable risk 327
Atypical mycobacteria 43
Atypical neuroleptics 369
Auerbach's plexus 176
Autoantibodies 120, 121–2
Autocrine signalling 246
Autoimmune disease 120
    autoantibodies 120, 121–2
    breakdown in self-tolerance 121
Autoimmune haemolytic anaemia 120
Autoimmune thrombocytopenia 120
Autoimmune thyroid disease 122
Autologous processes 88
Autonomic nervous system 141–5
Autosomal dominant disorders 22–3
    molecular basis 27
Autosomal recessive disorders 23–4
    ethnic associations 24
    molecular basis 28
Autosomes 2

B lymphocyte disorders, primary
        immunodeficiency 115
    combined T-cell disorders 116–17
B lymphocytes 93
    activation 109
    adhesion molecules 103
    development 109
    tumour immunology 128
Bacillus spp. 42
Bacteria 40–58
    ALERT organisms 79
    antibacterial chemotherapy 58–62
    classification 40
    conjugation 61
    enzyme-production 41
    exo/endotoxins 58
    lactose-fermentation 41
    neutrophil/macrophage phagocytosis 98
    opportunistic pathogens 79
    recurrent infection 112
    transduction 61
    transfection 61
    transformation 61
    zoonoses 79
Bactericidal/bacteriostatic antibiotics 61
Bacteriophages 13
Bacteroides spp. 53
Barbiturates 371
    elderly patients 398
Barr body 2
Bartonella spp. 55
Bartonellae 55–6
Basal ganglia 146, 147
Basal metabolic rate 291
Base excess 184
Bases 183
Basophils 98
bcl-2 35, 88, 105
bcr-abl 33, 127
Becker's muscular dystrophy 16, 25, 28
Bence Jones proteinuria 120
Benign intracranial hypertension, drug-induced
        410

Benign/essential fructosuria 254
Benzalkonium chloride 85
Benzodiazepines 367
    elderly patients 398
    overdose 400
Berry aneurysm 150
β-agonists 352
β-blockers 348
    overdose 400
11-β-hydroxylase deficiency 232
β-lactamase inhibitors 58
β-lipotrophin 226
β2-microglobulin 88
β-oxidation of fatty acids 260
β-thalassaemia 275
Bias 311
    lead time/length-time 334
    selection 311, 323
Bicarbonate
    carbon dioxide transport 273
    erythrocyte buffer system 185
    renal reabsorption 186, 198–199
Biguanides 85, 380
Bile 221
    antimicrobial drug levels 401
Bile acids 221
    sequestrant resins 361, 362
Bile pigments 222
Biliary system 221
Bilirubin 221, 222
Binomial distribution 310
Bioavailability 338
Biochemistry 239–78
Bioinformatics 14
Biotin 280
Bladder function 144–5
Blastomyces dermatidis 74
Bleomycin 11
Blood
    drug-induced disorders 407–8
    laboratory findings 300–1
    response to pregnancy 238
Blood groups 123–4
Blood pressure 216
    regulation 193–6
Blood transfusion 123
Blood vessels 217
Blood–gas barrier 206
Body fluids 180–1
    ion composition 181
Body mass index 291
Bohr effect 272
Bordetella pertussis 47
Borrelia spp. 54
Box and whisker plot 308
Brachial plexus 138
Bradykinin 193
Brain 146, 147, 148–51
    cerebral blood flow 217–218
Breast cancer, genetic aspects 30, 34
Breast feeding, drug safety 398
Breathing
    effect on heart murmurs 212
    regulation 208–9
    work of 204
Broca's dysphasia 151

Bronchi 169, 170
  surface markings 169
Bronchodilators 203
Bronchospasm, drug-induced 402
Brucella spp. 47
Brugia malayi 76, 78
Bruton's congenital agammaglobulinaemia 115
Buffer systems 184–5
Bullous skin disease 114
Bunyaviruses 63
Burkholderia spp. 52

c-myc 34
C-reactive protein 293
CA 19.9 297
CA 125 297
CA 153 297
Cadherins 103, 244
Calcitonin 233, 287
Calcium 286–8
  antagonists 350
  intracellular signalling 247
  urinary 303
Calciviruses 63
Calmodulin 286
Campylobacter fetus 49
Cancer
  cell cycle de-regulation 243
  familial syndromes 34
  somatic evolution 32–3
  therapy 394
  tumour immunology 127–8
  tumour products 297–8
Candida spp. 74, 116
Candins 75
Capillary hydrostatic pressure 181–2
Carbamazepine 372, 397
Carbamoyl phosphate synthetase 268
Carbapenems 59
Carbohydrates 247–8
  dietary requirements 291
  digestion 248
  inborn errors of metabolism 253–4, 255
  metabolism 240, 248–51
Carbon dioxide
  partial pressure 206
  regulation of breathing 208
  transport 273
Carbon monoxide
  diffusing capacity (T_{CO}) 207
  poisoning 400
Carboxyhaemoglobin 275
Carcinoembryonic antigen 127, 297
Carcinogenesis 33
Cardiac cycle 210, 211
  venous pressure changes 213
Cardiac failure, drug-induced 401
Cardiac glycosides 352
Cardiac output 214–16
Cardiac physiology 209–18
  response to pregnancy 238
Carotene 257
Carotid sheath 164
Carrier detection 16
Case fatality rate 319
Case-control study 322–3

Caspases 35, 105
Caspofungin 75, 386
Catalase 272
Cataract, drug-induced 411
Catecholamines 233
Catechol-*o*-methyltransferase (COMT) 233
Causation 331
Cause–effect studies 331
CC-type chemokines 103
CCR5 mutations 66
CD markers 88
  T lymphocytes 94, 95
CD2 (LFA-2) 91
CD3 94
CD4 T cells 94, 95
CD8 T cells 94, 95
CD10 127
CD11a/CD18 (LFA-1) 91
CD28 94, 95
CD45RA 95
CD45RO 95
CD50 (ICAM-3) 90
CD54 (ICAM-1) 90
CD58 (LFA-3) 91
CD62E (E-selectin) 91
CD62L (L-selectin) 91
CD62P (P-selectin) 91
CD95 (Fas) 35, 95
CD102 (ICAM-2) 90
cDNA 2
  library 3
Cell adhesion molecules (CAMs) 89, 103, 244
Cell compartments 240
Cell cycle 11, 242–3
  cytotoxic drug phase specificity 394
  regulation 243
Cell senescence 36
Cell signalling 244
  intracellular receptors 246
  mechanisms 245, 246
  membrane-bound receptors 245–6
Cell-bound (type II) hypersensitivity reactions
    113, 114
Cell–cell interactions 244
Cell-mediated/delayed (type IV) hypersensitivity
    reactions 114
Central limit theorem 311
Central nervous system 146, 147–163
Central tendency measures 307
Central venous pressure 213
Cephalosporins 59, 382
Cerebral blood flow 217–218
Cerebral cortex 148–52
  arterial supply 148–50
  location of function 150
Cerebrospinal fluid 151, 301–2
  antimicrobial drug levels 401
  low glucose 302
  raised protein 302
Cervical plexus 138
Cetrimide 85
Chagas' disease 103
Charcot–Marie–Tooth syndrome 22
Chediak–Higashi syndrome 117
Chemokines 102, 103
Chemoreceptors, respiratory 208

Chi-square test 317
Chimera 2
Chlamydia spp. 40, 57, 79
Chloral hydrate 367
Chlorambucil 11
Chloramphenicol 11, 59, 383
Chlorhexidine 85
Chloride 289
  renal transport 199
Chlorine disinfection 85
Chloroquine 78, 387
Chloroxylenols 85
Cholecystokinin-pancreatozymin 219, 220, 221, 222
Cholestasis, drug-induced 405
Cholesterol 257
  metabolism 260
  transport 258
Cholinesterase inhibitors 374
Chorionic villus sampling 29
Chromatids 2
Chromatin 7
Chromosomal abnormalities 18–22
  autosomes 19–20
  breakage syndromes 22
  microsatellite deletion syndromes 22
  prenatal diagnosis 29
  sex chromosomes 20–2
Chromosomes 7
  homologous 3
  mapping 2
Chronic active hepatitis 121, 122
Chronic external ophthalmoplegia 26
Chronic granulomatous disease 117
Chronic mucocutaneous candidiasis 116
Chronic myeloid leukaemia 20, 33
Chylomicrons 258, 259
Ciclosporin 395
Cidofovir 388
Circle of Willis 148
Circulation 217–18
  adaptations 218
  fetal 174–175
  pulmonary 207
Cis elements 9
Cisplatin 11
Citrobacter freundii 51
Class switching 89, 109
Claw hand 140
Clearance
  drug 338
  renal 190–1
Cleft lip/palate 30
Clinical chemistry 278–304
Clinitest reaction 303
Clonal selection 89
Clone 2
Clonidine 347
Cloning, genetic 2, 13–14
Clormethiazole 367
Clostridium spp. 42
Clotrimazole 75
Coagulation 298–300
  abnormalities 299–300
  cascade 299
  tests 300

Coccidia 76
Coccidioides immitis 74
Coefficient of variation 309
Coeliac disease 122
Coeliac plexus 162
Coenzymes 278
Cofactors 278
Cohort study 322, 323
Colchicine 381
Cold agglutinins 110
Collagen 276
Collecting duct function 193
Collectins 89
Colon 223
Colony-stimulating factors (CSFs) 89, 102
  immunotherapy 396
Colorectal cancer, inherited susceptibility 34
Colour blindness 25
Coma, eye signs 157
Common carotid artery 163
Common peroneal (lateral popliteal) nerve 141
Common variable immunodeficiency 115
Complement 111–12
  alternative pathway 111
  classical pathway 111
  deficiencies 112
  functions 112
  lectin pathway 111
Complement fixation tests 129–30
Compliance, respiratory 205
Concordant twins 2
Conduction aphasia 151
Confidence intervals 312–13, 314
Confounding bias 311
Confusional states, drug-induced 409
Congenital adrenal hyperplasia 23, 232
Congenital dislocation of hip 30
Congenital erythropoietic porphyria 23, 24
Congenital heart disease 30
Congenital malformations 30
Congenital thymic aplasia (DiGeorge's syndrome) 116
Conjugation 61
Connective tissue disorders 122
Conn's syndrome (primary hyperaldosteronism) 195
Conserved sequences
  amino acid motifs 9
  DNA 2
Constant regions 89
Constipation, drug-induced 404
Construction dyspraxia 151
Coombs' antiglobulin test 113, 129
Copper 290
Coreceptor activating molecules (immune response) 103
Cori cycle 250
Cori's limit dextrinosis 253
Cornea
  drug-induced opacities 411
  transplantation 125
Coronary arteries 171–172
Coronary blood flow 218
Coronavirus 63
Correlation 317

Correlation coefficient (*r*) 317
Corticosteroids 377
Corticosterone 232
Corticotrophin-like intermediate peptide (CLIP) 226
Corticotrophin-releasing hormone 225
Cortisol 231, 232, 278, 377
Corynebacterium diphtheriae 42
Cosmids 13
Cost–benefit analysis 335
Cost–effectiveness analysis 335
Cost–utility analysis 335
Co-stimulation 89
Countercurrent multiplier system 192
Coxiella burnetii 55
Cranial nerves 152–63
Creatine kinase 296
Creatine phosphate 242
Creatine phosphokinase 296
  isoenzymes 296
Creatinine clearance 191
CREST syndrome 122
Creutzfeldt–Jakob disease (CJD) 70
Cri du chat syndrome 20
Cricoid cartilage 167
Crohn's disease 122
Cross-over trial 325
Cross-sectional study 321
Cryoglobulins 110
Cryptococcus spp. 74
Cumulative frequency plot 306, 307
Cushing reflex 218
CXC-type chemokines 103
CXCR4 mutations 66
Cyanide poisoning 400
Cyanocobalamin *see* Vitamin B_{12}
Cyclic AMP 246, 247
  glycogen metabolism regulation 253
Cyclic GMP 247
Cyclin-dependent kinases (CDKs) 243
Cyclins 243
Cyclo-oxygenase 261–2
  COX-1 261
  COX-2 262
Cyclophosphamide 11
Cystic fibrosis 16, 18, 23, 28
Cystinosis 270
Cystinuria 270, 303
Cytarabine 73
Cytidine triphosphate (CTP) 242
Cytochrome P450 enzymes 345
  antiretroviral protease inhibitor drug interactions 393
Cytochromes 272
Cytokines 99–103
  dendritic cells 98
  disorders 103
  macrophages 98
  T_H1 cells 95, 96
  T_H2 cells 95, 96
Cytomegalovirus 73
Cytosine 7
Cytosine arabinoside 6
Cytotoxic drugs 360, 393–4
  cell cycle phase specificity 394
Cytotoxic T cells (T_C) 95

Dead space, airway 204
Deafness, drug-induced 26, 411
Defensins 89
Dehydration
  hyperosmotic (water depletion) 197
  hyposmotic (salt depletion) 196
Delayed hypersensitivity T cells (T_{DH}) 95
Delayed/cell-mediated (type IV) hypersensitivity reactions 114
Deleted in colorectal cancer (DCC) 34
Deletions 2, 20
β-aminolaevulinate synthetase 271
Dendritic cells 89, 98
Dengue fever 64
Depression, drug-induced 409
Dermatitis herpetiformis 122
Dermatomes 134–7
Dermatophyte infections 74
Descriptive studies 321
Diabetes with deafness 26
Diabetes insipidus
  cranial 201
  nephrogenic 25, 201
    drug-induced 407
Diabetes mellitus
  glycosylated haemoglobin 275
  insulin dependent 30
Diabetic ketoacidosis 255
Diagnostic tests 331
Dialysis, drug removal 400, 401
Diaminopyrimidines 78
Diaphragm 175–176
Diarrhoea, drug-induced 404
Didanosine 389
Dideoxycytidine 389
Dietary requirements 291
Diethylcarbamazine 78
Digestion
  carbohydrates 248
  fats 258
  proteins 267
Diglyceride system 247
Digoxin 353
  overdose 400
Dinucleotide repeats 13
2,3-Diphosphoglycerate 272, 273
Diphyllobothrium latum 76
Diploid 2, 7
Discordant twins 2
Disease modifying antirheumatic drugs (DMARDs) 359–60
Disinfection 84, 85
Disopyramide 353
Dispersion measures 307–9
Disseminated intravascular coagulation 299
Distal tubule function 193
Diuretics 351
  elderly patients 398
Dizygotic twins 2
DNA 6–7
  cis elements 9
  complementary (cDNA) 2
  conserved sequences 2
  fingerprinting 3
  hybridization 3, 12
  mitochondrial 7

DNA 6–7 (cont'd)
 recominant technology 11
 replication 8, 11
 satellite 7
 transcription 8–9
DNA polymerases 8
DNA viruses 69
Domains, immunoglobulins 89
Dopamine 225, 229
Dopamine D_2 receptor blockade 369, 370
Dopamine receptors 346
Dose–response curves 341
Double-blinding 325
Down's syndrome (trisomy 21) 19–20
 prenatal diagnosis 29
Doxazosin 349
Doxorubicin 11
Dracunculus medinensis 78
Dressing dyspraxia 151
Drug absorption 342
Drug concentration
 area under the curve 339
 first-order (linear) kinetics 340
 therapeutic monitoring 340
 zero-order (saturation) kinetics 340
Drug development, clinical trials 324
Drug elimination 340, 346
Drug interactions 342–6
Drug metabolism 342–5
 age-related changes 398
 genetic factors 344–5
Drug overdose 400
Drug-induced disorders 401–13
 acute porphyria 273
 blood disorders 407–8
 cardiovascular system 401–2
 dermatological 411–13
 endocrine system 405–6
 eye 411
 gastrointestinal system 404–5
 hyperuricaemia 278
 metabolic 406–7
 neuropsychiatric 409–10
 otological 26, 411
 renal system 403–4
 respiratory system 402
 sexual dysfunction 410–11
 systemic lupus erythematosus 120, 122, 345, 412
Drug-withdrawal states 409
Dubin–Johnson syndrome 273, 346
Duchenne muscular dystrophy 16, 18, 25, 28, 244
Duffy antigen 124
Duodenum 177
Dye dilution method 214
Dysgammaglobulinaemia 115
Dyslipoproteinaemias 263
Dysphasias 151
Dyspraxias 151
Dystonic drug reactions 409
Dystrophin 28, 244

E-selectin (CD62E) 91
Echinocandins 75, 386
Echinococcus granulosa 75

Ecological (aggregate) survey 331
Economic evaluation 335
Ecstasy (3,4-methylenedioxymethamphetamine; MDMA) 376
Edward's syndrome (trisomy 18) 20
Efavirenz 390
Effect measures 326–8
Effectiveness 324
Efficacy 324, 341, 342
Eflornithine 388
Ehlers–Danlos syndrome 22
 type VI 276
 type VIII 276
Ehrlichia spp. 56
Eicosanoid (prostanoid) metabolism 261–2
Eikonella corrodens 48
Ejaculation, drug-induced failure 410
Ejection fraction 214
Elderly people, drug safety 398
Electrocardiogram (ECG) intervals 213
Electron transport 242
Embden–Meyerhof (glycolytic) pathway 248–9
Endocrine signalling 246
Endocrine system 224–38
 drug-induced disorders 405–6
 response to pregnancy 238
Endoplasmic reticulum 240
Endorphins 226
Endothelin-1 196
Endothelins 196
Endotoxins 58
Energy
 metabolism 240–2
 requirements 291
Enkephalins 226
Entacapone 373
Entamoeba histolytica 75, 78
Enterobacter spp. 51
Enterobacteriae 50–2
Enterobius vermicularis 75
Enterohepatic circulation 221
Enteroviruses 62
Enzyme-linked immunoabsorbent assay (ELISA) 130
Eosinophils 98
Epidemiology 319–35
Epidermal growth factor receptor 245
Epidermophyton spp. 74
Epilepsy 30
Epitopes 89, 109
Epstein–Barr virus 127
Erb-Duchenne paralysis 138
Erectile dysfunction 374
 drug-induced 410
Error
 sampling 311
 type I/type II 315
Erythema multiforme, drug-induced 412
Erythema nodosum, drug-induced 412
Erythrocyte buffer systems 185
Erythromycin 11
Erythropoietic porphyria 22, 274
Erythropoietin 193, 209
Escherichia coli 50
Escherichia coli 0157:H7 50

Essential amino acids 266, 267
Essential fatty acids 256
Essential hypertension 30
Ethambutol 385
Ethnic groups, genetic disease associations 31
    autosomal recessive disorders 24
Etoposide 11
Evidence-based medicine 330
Exercise
    circulatory adaptations 218
    energy metabolism 250
Exons 3, 9, 10
Exotoxins 58
Experimental studies 321
Expiratory reserve volume 202
Expressed sequence tags (ESTs) 14
Expressivity, genetic 3
External carotid artery 164
Extracellular fluid 180
Extrapyramidal drug reactions 409
Eye
    drug-induced disorders 411
    movements 156
    muscles 158
    signs, comatose patient 157

Fab fragment 108
Fabry's disease 25
Facial (VII) nerve 153, 160–1
Faecal bile pigments 222
Famciclovir 73, 388
Familial adenomatous polyposis 22, 34
Familial breast cancer 27
Familial cancer syndromes 34
Familial hypercholesterolaemia 16, 22, 27
Fanconi syndrome 270
Fas (CD95) 35, 105
Fas ligand 89, 105
Fascioscapulohumeral muscular dystrophy 22
Fats
    dietary requirements 291
    metabolism 240
Fatty acid synthetase multienzyme complex
        260
Fatty acids 256
    β-oxidation 260
Fc fragment 108
Femoral artery 164
Ferritin 285, 286
Fetal circulation 174–175
Fetal haemoglobin 272
Fetoscopy 29
Fever, drug reactions 411
Fibrates 361, 362
Fibrinolysis 299
Fibroblast growth factor receptor 245
Fick principle 214
Filoviruses 63
First-order (linear) elimination 340
First-pass effect 338, 339
Fisher's exact probability test 317
Fixed drug eruptions 412
FK506 (tacrolimus) 395
Flaviviruses 63
Flow cytometry 130

Flow volume loops 204
Flucloxacillin 58
Fluconazole 75, 386
5-Flucytosine 75, 386
Fluid balance 180–3
5-Fluorouracil 6
Folate deficiency, drug-induced 408
Folic acid 281
Follicle-stimulating hormone 227–8
Fomiversen 73, 388
Food poisoning 80
Forced alkaline diuresis 400
Forced expiratory volume in one second
        (FEV$_1$) 203
Forced vital capacity 203
Formaldehyde 85
fos 243
Foscarnet 73, 388
Founder effect 31
Fragile X syndrome 21, 27
Francisella tularensis 48
Frank–Starling law 215
Free fatty acids (FFA) 256, 260
    transport 258
Free radicals 104
Frequency distributions 306
Friedreich's ataxia 23, 27
Fructose intolerance 254
Fructosuria, benign/essential 254
Functional residual capacity 202, 203
Fungal infections 74
    ALERT organisms 79
    opportunistic 79
Fusion inhibitors 391
Fusobacterium fusiforme 53
Fuzeon (T20) 391

G-proteins 245–6
GABA receptors 346
Gabapentin 372
Gait dyspraxia 151
Galactorrhoea, drug-induced 405
Galactosaemia 29, 254
Gall bladder, surface markings 175
Gametes 3
γ-glutamyltransferase 295
γ-lipotrophin 226
Ganciclovir 73, 388
Gardnerella vaginitis 48
Gardner's syndrome 22
Gastric acid secretion 219–20
Gastric emptying 220
Gastric inhibitory peptide 219, 220
Gastric juice 219
Gastric parietal cell antibody 122
Gastrin 219, 220, 221
    increased/decreased levels 222–3
Gastrinoma 222
Gastrointestinal polypeptide hormones 219
Gastrointestinal system 219–24
    drug-induced disorders 404–5
Gaucher's disease 265
Gaussian (normal) distribution 309
Gaze disturbance 156
Gene therapy 3, 18

Genes 3, 9
  analytic techniques 11–17
  cloning 13
  expression profiling 16
  libraries 13
  mapping 12–13
  Mendelian inheritance patterns 22
  microarray analysis 16
  regulation of expression 32
  reporter 5
  sequencing 14–15
  splicing 9
  targeting 14
Genetic anticipation 27
Genetic code 9–10
Genetic disorders
  chromosomal abnormalities 18–22
  ethnic associations 24, 31
  pre/postnatal diagnosis 28–9
  single-gene abnormalities 22–8
Genetic drift 31
Genetic factors, drug metabolism 344–5
Genetic restriction 89
Genetics 1–37
Genome 3
  library 3
Genotype 3
Giardia lamblia 76, 78
Gilbert's syndrome 273
Gilles de la Tourette syndrome 22
Glaucoma 30
Glitazones 380
Globin 271
  disorders of synthesis 275
Globulins 292, 293
Glomerular filtration rate 190
Glossopharyngeal (IX) nerve 154, 161
Glucagon 237–238, 278
  increased levels 223
Glucagonoma 223
Glucocorticoids 232
Gluconeogenesis 249–50
Glucose
  metabolism 248–50
  transport 237
Glucose-6-phosphate-dehydrogenase 251
Glucose-6-phosphate-dehydrogenase deficiency
      16, 25, 29, 32, 251
  haemolysis 344, 345
Gluteraldehyde 85
Glycogen 251
Glycogen storage disease type I 253, 278
Glycogen storage diseases 253, 255
Glycogen synthetase 252
Glycogenesis 251–2
Glycogenolysis 253
Glycolipids 247
Glycolytic (Embden–Meyerhof) pathway 248–9
Glycopeptide antibiotics 59, 384
Glycoprotein IIa/IIIb receptor antagonists 244, 356
Glycoproteins 247
Glycosaminoglycans 248
Glycosylated haemoglobin 275
Gold 360
Golgi apparatus 240

Gonadotrophin-releasing hormone 225
Gonococcus 46
Goodpasture's syndrome 120
Gout 278, 381
Gradenigo's syndrome 160
Graft rejection 125
Graft versus host disease 126
Gram-negative bacilli
  anaerobes 53
  enterobacteriae 50–2
  Parvobacteria 47–8
  Vibrios 49
Gram-negative bacteria 40
  bartonellae 55–6
  chlamydia 57
  rickettsiae 55–6
  spirochaetes 54
Gram-negative cocci 46
Gram-positive bacteria 40
Gram-positive cocci 44–5
Gram-positive rods 42–3
Granulocytes 98
Graves' disease 120, 122
Griseofulvin 75, 386
Growth factors 102
Growth hormone (somatotropin) 228–9, 278
Growth hormone-inhibiting hormone 225
Growth hormone-releasing hormone 225
Guanine 7
Guanine nucleotide-binding proteins 245–6
Guanosine triphosphate (GTP) 242
Gut-associated lymphoid tissue (GALT) 89
Guthrie test 29
Gynaecomastia, drug-induced 405

H_2-receptor antagonists 363
Haem 221, 271
  disorders of synthesis 273, 274
  pigments 272
  synthesis 271
Haemoglobin 271–5
  abnormal derivatives 275
  glycosylation 275
  oxygen dissociation curve 272
  oxygen transport 273
  structure 271
Haemoglobinopathies 23, 272, 275
Haemoglobinuria 303
Haemolytic anaemia, drug-induced 408
Haemolytic disease of newborn 124
Haemoperfusion, drug overdose 400
Haemophilia A 16, 18, 25
Haemophilia B 16, 25
Haemophilus spp. 47
Haemorrhage 218
Halogen disinfectants 85
Haploid 3
Haplotype 3, 90
Hapten 90
Hardy–Weinberg principle 31
Hartnup's disease 270
Hashimoto's thyroiditis 120, 122
Hazard ratio 330
Head and neck 167–168
  dermatomes 134

Heart 171–3
  cardiac cycle 210, 211
  conducting system 209–10
  exercise response 218
  innervation 172
  intracardiac pressures 211
  nodes 173
  performance 213–17
  sounds 212–13
  transplantation 126
  valves 173
Heart murmurs
  effect of drugs 212
  effect of respiration 212
Heat shock proteins 104
Heavy chain disease 120, 128
Heavy metal poisoning 400
Helicobacter pylori 49
Helper T cells *see* T helper (T_H) cells
Henderson–Hasselbach equation 184
Hepadnaviruses 69
Heparin 299, 357, 397
Hepatic plexus 162
Hepatic porphyrias 22
Hepatic portal vein 177–178
Hepatitis B 69, 73
  serology 71–2
  vaccination 82
Hepatitis C 63–4, 73
Hepatitis D 64
Hepatitis, drug-induced 404, 405
Hepatitis E 64
Hepatorenal syndrome 105
Hepatotoxic drugs 405
Hepatovirus 62
Hereditary angioneurotic oedema 112
Hereditary haemorrhagic telangiectasia 22
Hereditary non-polyposis coli (HNPCC) 35
Hereditary sensory and motor neuropathy 22
Hereditary spherocytosis 22
Hering–Bruer reflex 208
Heritability 30–31
Herpes simplex virus 73
Herpesviruses 69
Heterologous processes 90
Heterophile antigen 90
Heteroploidy 3
Heterozygotic advantage 32
Hexachlorophane 85
Hexokinase 248, 249
Hexose monophosphate shunt (pentose
    phosphate pathway) 250–1
High altitude acclimatization 209
High density lipoproteins (HDL) 258, 259, 263
High-energy phosphate compounds 242
Hirschsprung disease 30
Hirsutism, drug-induced 413
Histamine 220
  receptors 346
Histidinaemia 29
Histoplasma capsulatum 74
HLA antigens 36–7, 90
  disease associations 37
  tissue typing 125
Homocystinuria 269, 270, 276

Homologous chromosomes 3
Hookworm 76
Hormone replacement therapy 378
Hormone-sensitive lipase 258
Hormones 224
  endocrine signalling 246
  mode of action 224
Horner's syndrome 156
Human chorionic gonadotrophin 298
Human Genome Project 15
Human immunodeficiency virus (HIV) 35, 65–8
  AIDS indicator diagnoses 68
  chemokine receptor mutations 66
  clinical stages of infection 68, 118
  epidemiology 67
  life cycle 65–6
  opportunistic infections 118
  pathogenesis 67
  serology 72, 119
  site of drug actions 67
  structure 65
  T-cell depletion 118–19
Human papillomavirus 73, 127
Human slow virus infections 70
Human T-cell leukaemia virus (HTLV-1) 68
Hunter's syndrome 25, 265
Huntington's chorea 22, 27
Hurler's syndrome 265
Hybridization 3, 11–12
  in situ 3
Hydralazine 349
Hydrogen ions, renal secretion 198–199
5-Hydroxyindoleacetic acid 297
21-Hydroxylase deficiency 232
Hydroxymethyl-glutaryl-CoA reductase 260
  inhibitors (statins) 361, 362
5-Hydroxytryptamine IA agonists 367
Hydroxyurea 11
Hyper-IgM syndrome 116
Hyperaldosteronism, primary (Conn's syndrome)
    195
Hypercalcaemia 287–8
  drug-induced 406
Hyperchloraemia 289
Hyperchloraemic acidosis 189
Hypergammaglobulinaemia 119–20
Hyperglycaemia, drug-induced 406
Hyperhomocystinaemia 270
Hyperkalaemia 198–9, 285
  drug-induced 406
Hyperleucinaemia (maple syrup urine disease) 29,
    269, 270
Hyperlipidaemias 263
Hypermagnesaemia 289
Hypernatraemia 197
Hyperparathyroidism 287
Hyperphosphataemia 288
Hyperprolactinaemia, drug-induced 405
Hypersensitivity
  classification 113–14
  drug reactions 411
  skin disease 114
Hypertension, drug-induced 401
Hyperthyroidism 381
  treatment in pregnancy 397

Hypertrichosis, drug-induced 413
Hypertrophic cardiomyopathy with myopathy 26
Hyperuricaemia 278
Hypervariable regions 90
Hypnotics 367
Hypocalcaemia 288
Hypochloraemia 289
Hypochloraemic acidosis 189
Hypochlorhydria 289
Hypochlorite 85
Hypogammaglobulinaemia 118
Hypoglossal (XII) nerve 154, 162
Hypoglycaemia
  drug-induced 406
  spontaneous 255
Hypokalaemia 198, 284–5
  drug-induced 406
Hypolipoproteinaemias 264
Hypomagnesaemia 289
Hyponatraemia 197–198
Hypoparathyroidism 287
Hypophosphataemia 288
Hypothalamic regulatory hormones 224–5
Hypothermia 301
Hypothesis testing 313–15
Hypothyroidism 122
  drug-induced 405
Hypoxanthine guanine phosphoribosyl
    transferase 276
Hypoxia, acute/chronic adaptation 209
Hysteresis 205

ICAM-1 (CD54) 90
ICAM-2 (CD102) 90
ICAM-3 (CD50) 90
Ichthyosis 25
Idiopathic cirrhosis 121
Idiotype 90, 109
Idoxuridine 6, 73
Imidazoles 75, 386
Immune complex disease 112, 113
Immune complex (type III) hypersensitivity
    reactions 113, 114
Immune response 92–105
  adaptive (acquired) immunity 92, 93
  cells/molecules 93–105
  innate (non-specific) immunity 92, 93
  senescence 119
Immune system tumours 128
Immunization 81–4
  contraindications 83
  passive 83
  schedule (UK) 82
  travel vaccines 84
Immunodeficiency 112
  associated tumours 128
  B-cell disorders 115
  combined B- and T-cell disorders 116–17
  neutrophil disorders 117
  opportunistic infections 116, 117, 118
  primary 115
  secondary 118–20
  stem cell transplantation 126
  T-cell disorders 116
Immunodiffusion 131

Immunoenzyme assays 130–1
Immunofluorescence tests 130
Immunogenetics 36–7
Immunoglobulin A (IgA) 106, 108
  deficiency 115
Immunoglobulin D (IgD) 107
Immunoglobulin E (IgE) 107, 113
Immunoglobulin G (IgG) 106, 108
Immunoglobulin M (IgM) 106, 108
Immunoglobulins 105–11
  class switching 89, 109
  constant regions 89, 109
  domains 89
  heavy chains 108
  hypervariable regions 90
  light chains 108
  passive immunization 83
  replacement therapy 109
  structure 108–9
  subclasses 90
  superfamily 90, 244
  variable regions 109
  see also Antibodies
Immunology 87–131
Immunosuppression
  associated tumours 128
  drugs 393–5
Immunotherapy 396
In situ hybridization 3
Inborn errors of metabolism 23
  amino acids 268, 270
  carbohydrate 253–4, 255
  stem cell transplantation 126
Incidence rate 319
Incubation periods 80
  food poisoning 80
Index case (proband) 5
Indicator dilution method 180
Indinavir 392
Induction, protein synthesis 10
Infant mortality rate 321
Infantile polycystic disease 23
Inferior vena cava 166
Inflammation 105, 293
Influenza 73
Innate (non-specific) immunity 92, 93
Inotropes 352
Inspiration 206
Inspiratory capacity 202
Inspiratory reserve volume 202
Insulin 235–7, 278, 284
  glucose transport 237
  preparations 381
  resistance 237
Insulin growth factor receptor 245
Integrins 90, 103, 244
Intention to treat 325
Intercellular adhesion molecules 90
Interferons (IFNs) 73, 99, 100, 388
Interim analysis 325
Interleukin-1 (IL-1) 101
Interleukin-2 (IL-2) 101
Interleukins 101
Internal carotid artery 164
Internal jugular vein 166

Interquartile range 307, 308
Intestinal juice 222–3
Intestine
  amino acid transport 267
  blood supply 177
Intracardiac pressures 211
Intracellular fluid 181
  buffer systems 185
Intracellular receptors 246
Intradermal testing 114
Intrahepatic cholestasis, drug-induced 405
Intrapleural pressure 205
Introns 3, 9, 10
Iodine
  disinfection 85
  nutritional 290
Ion channels 245
Ions, body fluids 181
Iron 285–6
  deficiency anaemia 273
  overdose 400
Ischaemic heart disease 30
Isologous processes 90
Isoniazid 385
Isotype 90, 109
  class switching 109
Itraconazole 75, 386
Ivermectin 78

J (juxtacapillary) receptors 209
Job's syndrome 117
Joints
  motor root values 136–7
  muscle power tests 137

Kaplan–Meier life-tables 329
Karyotype 3
Kell antigen 124
Kendall's rank correlation coefficient 318
Kennedy syndrome (neuronopathy) 27
Ketoconazole 75, 386
Ketogenesis 252
Ketone bodies 252
Kidney
  amino acids reabsorption 199
  bicarbonate reabsorption 198–199
  buffer systems 185, 186
  chloride transport 199
  drug-induced disorders 403–4
  endocrine functions 193
  hydrogen secretion 198–199
  physiology 190–3
  potassium secretion 198–9
  response to pregnancy 238
  sodium transport 193
  sugars reabsorption 199
  surface markings 175
  transplantation 125
  tubule damage 270
  urea excretion 199
  water transport 199–201
Killer (K) cells 90
Klebsiella spp. 50
Kleinfelter's syndrome (seminiferous tubule
  dysgenesis) 21

Klumpke's paralysis 138
Koch–Weeks bacillus 47
Kruskal–Wallis test 317

L-dopa 373
L-selectin (CD62L) 91
Lactate dehydrogenase 296
Lactate production 250
Lactic acidosis 189–90, 250
Lamivudine 390
Lamotrigine 372
Langerhans cells 90, 98
Large intestine 223
  motility 224
Larynx 167–8
  innervation 167–168
  muscles 168
Lateral medullary circulation 150
Lateral popliteal (common peroneal) nerve 141
Latex agglutination test 121
Lazy leucocyte syndrome 117
Lead poisoning 273, 400
Lead time bias 334
Leber's hereditary optic neuropathy 26
Lecithin-cholesterolacyl transferase (LCAT) 258
  deficiency 258
Lectin pathway 91
Legionella pneumophila 48
Leishmania spp. 76, 78
  drug treatment 388
Length-time bias 334
Leptospira spp. 54
Lesch–Nyhan syndrome 25, 278
Leucocyte adhesion deficiency 117
Leucocyte alkaline phosphatase 295
Leucocyte functional antigens (LFAs) 91
Leucotrienes 261, 262
Leukaemia 128
  stem cell transplantation 126
LFA-1 (CD11a/CD18) 91
LFA-2 (CD2) 91
LFA-3 (CD58) 91
Li–Fraumeni syndrome 34
Libido, drug-induced impairment 410
Library, genetic 3, 13
Life-table (survival) analysis 329
Ligand-gated ion channels 245
Ligands, cell signalling 244
Light reflex 152
Lignocaine 354
Likelihood ratio 334
Limb-girdle muscular dystrophy 23
Limbic system 147
Lincosamides 60
Linear (first-order) elimination 340
Linezolid 59
Linkage disequilibrium 3
Linkage map 3
Lipid-lowering drugs 361–2
Lipids 256–7
  antihypertensive drug effects 351
  digestion 258
  metabolism 258–66
  peroxidation 104
  transport 258

Lipogenesis 260
Lipolysis 258, 260
Lipoprotein lipase 258
Lipoproteins 258
  antihypertensive drug effects 351
  disorders of metabolism 263
Listeria monocytogenes 42
Lithium carbonate 368
Live attenuated vaccines 81
Liver
  blood supply 177–178
  lipogenesis 260
  surface markings 175
  transplantation 126
Liver disease 273, 293, 299
  drug use 399
Loa loa 76, 78
Locus 4
Lod score 31
Log-normal distribution 310
Logistic regression 318
Loop of Henle function 192
Lopinavir 392
Losartan 194
Low density lipoproteins (LDL) 258, 259
Lower limb
  arteries 165
  dermatomes 135
  veins 166
Lumbosacral plexus 140–1
Lung
  blood–gas barrier 206
  capacities 202–3
  compliance 205
  diffusing capacity/transfer factor 206–207
  fissures 169
  respiratory segments 170
  root 171
  stretch receptors 208
  surface markings 169
  vascular resistance 207
  volumes 201–2
Luteinizing hormone 227–8
Lymphadenopathy, drug-induced 408
Lymphoma 128
Lysosome 240

Machado–Joseph disease 27
Macroglobulinaemia 120
Macroglobulins 110
Macrolides 60, 383
Macrophages 98, 99
Magnesium 289
Major histocompatibility complex (MHC) 36–7
  Class I/II restriction 89, 97
Malaria 32, 77–78
  prophylaxis 78
  treatment 78
Malassezia spp. 74
Malignant hyperpyrexia 344
Manic depression 31
Mann–Whitney U test 317
Mannose-binding lectin 111
Maple syrup urine disease (hyperleucinaemia) 29,
  269, 270

Marfan's syndrome 22, 27
Mast cells 98
Maternal screening tests 28–29
McArdle's disease 253
Mean, arithmetic/geometric 307
Mean arterial pressure 216
Measurement bias 311
Mebendazole 78
Medial popliteal (tibial) nerve 140–1
Median 307
Median nerve 139
Medulla 146, 147
Megaloblastic anaemia, drug-induced 408
Meiosis 4
Meissner's plexus 176
Melanocyte-stimulating hormone 228
Melarsoprol 78, 388
MELAS 26
Membrane-bound receptors 245–6
Memory cells 91
Mendelian inheritance 22
Meningitis 301
Meningococcus 46
Mercaptopurine 6
MERRF 26
Messenger RNA 7
  processing defects 10
  translation 9
Meta-analysis 326
Metabolic acidosis 187, 188
Metabolic alkalosis 187, 188
Metabolic bone disease 287
Metabolic disorders
  drug-induced 406–7
  see also Inborn errors of metabolism
Metabolic pathways 240–7
Metachromatic leucodystrophy 265
Methaemoglobin 275
Methaemoglobin-reductase deficiency 344
Methanol poisoning 400
Methicillin 58
Methisazone 73
Methotrexate 11
Methyldopa 347
3,4-Methylenedioxymethamphetamine (MDMA;
  ecstasy) 376
Metronidazole 78, 383
Miconazole 75, 386
Microbiology 39–85
Microsatellites 7, 13
  deletion syndromes 22
Microsporidia 76
Microsporum spp. 74
Midbrain 146, 147
Middle cerebral artery 148
Mineralocorticoids 232
Minerals 284–90
Minoxidil 349
Minute ventilation/minute volume 204
Miscarriage 18
Mismatch repair genes 35
Mitochondria 240
  DNA 7
  genetic disorders 26
Mitosis 4, 242

Mitral valve 173
Mixed connective tissue disorder 120
Mixed function oxidase system 345
Mixed lymphocyte reaction (MLR) 91
Mode 307
Molecular chaperones 104
Monoamine oxidase 233
Monoamine oxidase inhibitors (MAOIs) 364–5,
    366
  overdose 400
Monobactams 59
Monoclonal antibodies 110–11
Monoclonal hypergammaglobulinaemia 120
Monozygotic twins 4
Morganella morganii 51
Mortality rate 319
Motilin 219
Motor neuron disease (amyotrophic lateral
    sclerosis) 104
Motor root values 136–7
Moxonidine 347
Mucopolysaccharidoses 265
Mucor spp. 74
Mucosa-associated lymphoid tissue (MALT) 91
Multifactorial inheritance 29–31
Multiple endocrine neoplasia (MEN I) 298
Multiple endocrine neoplasia (MEN II) 298
Multiple linear regression 318
Multiple myeloma 120, 293
Multiple sclerosis 30
Muscles
  motor root values 136–7
  power screening tests 137
Muscular dystrophies 16
  inheritance 25
Mutation
  cancer-related 243
  single base (point) 10
  single-gene abnormalities 22–8
  see also Chromosomal abnormalities
Myasthenia gravis 120, 122
  drug-induced exacerbation 410
myc 33, 243
Mycobacterium spp. 43
Mycophenolate mofetil 395
Mycoplasma spp. 56
Myelofibrosis 20
Myeloma 128
Myeloperoxidase deficiency 118
Myocardial infarction 296
Myocardium
  arterial supply 171, 172
  conducting system 209–10
  contractility 215
  drug toxicity 402
  venous drainage 172
Myoglobin 272, 273
  oxygen dissociation curve 272
Myoglobinuria 303
Myopathy, drug-induced 410
Myotonic dystrophy 22, 27

Naegleria spp. 75
NARP 26
Natural killer (NK) cells 91, 99

Nausea, drug-induced 404
Neisseria spp. 46
Nelfinavir 392
Nephrotic syndrome 293
  drug-induced 403
Nephrotoxic drugs 403
Nerve root compression 137
Neural tube defects
  multifactorial inheritance 30
  prenatal diagnosis 28, 29
Neuraminidase inhibitors 388
Neurodegenerative disease 35
Neurofibromatosis I 22, 27
Neurofibromatosis II 22, 27
Neurofibromin 27
Neuroleptics 368–9
  atypical 369
Neuronopathy (Kennedy syndrome) 27
Neuropsychiatric disorders, drug-induced 409–10
Neutropenia, drug-induced 407
Neutrophils 98
  disorders 117
Nevirapine 390
NfKB 91
Niacin (vitamin B$_3$) 279
Niclosamide 78
Nicorandil 349
Nicotinic acid 279, 361, 362
Niemann–Pick disease 265
Nitrates/nitrites 349
Nitric oxide 104, 105, 196
Nitric oxide synthase 104
Nitrofurantoin 383
Nitrogen balance 268
Nocardia asteroides 43
Non-dysjunction 4
Non-esterified free fatty acids (NEFA) 256, 260
Non-nucleoside reverse transcriptase inhibitors
    (NNRTIs) 390
Non-parametric tests 316–18
Non-steroidal anti-inflammatory drugs (NSAIDs)
    359
Noonan's syndrome 21
Noradrenaline 233
Normal (Gaussian) distribution 309
Northern blot technique 13
Nucleic acids 6–11
  structure 6–8
Nucleoside reverse transcriptase inhibitors
    (NRTIs) 389–90
Nucleotides 6
Nucleus 240
Null hypothesis 313
Number needed to treat 328
Nutrition
  deficiencies 291
  pregnancy 238
Nystatin 74

Observational studies 321
Octreotide 238
Oculomotor (III) nerve 153, 157, 158
Odds ratio 328, 329
Oedema 182
Oesophageal plexus 162

Oesophagus
  blood supply 176
  drug-induced ulceration 404
  surface markings 176
Oestradiol 227
Oestrogens 232
  hormone replacement therapy 378
  oral contraceptives 378
Olfactory (I) nerve 152, 153
Oligonucleotide primer 5
Onchocerca volvulus 76, 78
Oncogenes 4, 33, 243
Oncogenic viruses 71
One-tailed tests 314
Opiate overdose 400
Opioid receptors 346
Opportunistic infections 79, 115, 116, 117
  HIV/AIDS 118
  immunodeficiency 116, 118
Optic (II) nerve 152, 153, 155
Optic neuritis, drug-induced 411
Optic tract 155
Oral contraceptives 301, 378
Oral hypoglycaemics 379–80
Organelles 240
Ornithine transcarbamoylase 268
Orthomyxoviruses 62
Oseltamivir 73, 388
Osmolality 182–3
Osmolar gap 183
Osmolarity 183
Osteogenesis imperfecta 22, 23
Osteomalacia, drug-induced 407
Osteoporosis 360
Ototoxic drugs 411
Ovarian dysgenesis (Turner's syndrome) 20–1
Oxidative phosphorylation 242
Oxygen
  dissociation curve 272
  intracardiac saturation 211
  partial pressure 206
  regulation of breathing 208
  transport 273
Oxytocin 229, 230

p values 314
p53 34, 35, 243
  mutations 34, 35
P-selectin (CD62P) 91
Pacemaker 210
Paclitaxel (taxol) 394
Pancreas 220
  endocrine functions 235–8
  transplantation 125
Pancreatic islet cells 235
Pancreatic juice 220
Pancreatic polypeptide 219
Pancreatitis, drug-induced 404
Pantothenic acid 279
Papovaviruses 69
Paracetamol (acetaminophen) overdose 400
Paracoccidioides brasiliensis 74
Paracrine signalling 246
Parametric tests 315–16
Paramyxoviruses 62

Paraprotein 109
Paraproteinaemia 120
Parasitic infections 75–9
  chemotherapy 78
  opportunistic 79
  zoonoses 79
Parasympathetic nervous system 144–5
  outflow 144
Parathyroid hormone 287
Parkinsonism
  drug treatment 373, 398
  drug-induced 409
Paroxysmal nocturnal haemoglobinuria 112
Partial pressure 184
Partial thromboplastin time 300
Parvobacteria 47–8
Parvoviruses 69
Passive immunization 83
  antitoxins 83
  immunoglobulin preparations 83
Pasteurella multocida 48
Pasteurization 84
Patau's syndrome (trisomy 13) 20
Patch test 114
Peak flow 203
  flow volume loops 204
Pearson syndrome 26
Pearson's correlation 315
Pearson's product moment correlation coefficient 317
Pemphigoid 120
Pemphigus 120
Penetrance 4
Penicillamine 360
Penicillins 58, 382
Penicillium marneffei 74
Pentamidine 78, 388
Pentavalent antimony 388
Pentose phosphate pathway (hexose monophosphate shunt) 250–1
Peptic ulcer disease 30, 31, 363
Percentiles 307, 308
Perforin 91
Perinatal mortality rate 320
Period prevalence 319
Peripheral nervous system 134–41
Peripheral neuropathy, drug-induced 410
Peripheral resistance 216–17
Pernicious anaemia 120, 122
Peroxidase 272
Peroxisome 240
Person-time at risk 320
pH 184
Phage 4
Phagocytosis 98
Pharmacodynamics 338
Pharmacogenetics 344, 345
Pharmacokinetics 338
  pregnant patient 397
Pharmacology 337–413
Phase I/phase II enzymes 343
Phenacetin-induced methaemoglobinaemia 345
Phenol 85
Phenolic disinfectants 85

Phenothiazines 368–9
  elderly patients 398
Phenotype 4
Phenylketonuria 16, 18, 269, 270
  postnatal screening 29
Phenytoin 371
Philadelphia chromosome 20, 33
Phosphate 288
  renal excretion 186
Phosphodiesterase inhibitors 352
Phosphofructokinase 248, 249
6-Phosphogluconate dehydrogenase 251
Phosphoglycerides 256
Phospholipids 256–7
  transport 258
Phosphorylase 253
Photosensitivity, drug-induced 413
Phrenic nerve 138
Physical mapping, genes 4
Physiology 179–238
Picornaviruses 62
Pigmentation, drug-induced changes 412
Piperazine 78
Pituitary, anterior 224, 225
  hormones 225–9
Pituitary, posterior 224, 225
  hormones 229–30
pKa 184
Placebo 325
Plasma
  buffer systems 185
  enzymes 295
  oncotic pressure 181–2
  osmolality 182–3
  tissue compartment fluid flow 181–2
  urea:creatinine ratio 199
  volume 180
Plasma cell tumours 128
Plasma half-life 338
Plasma proteins 292–4
  drug binding 342
Plasmids 4, 13
  antibiotic resistance 61
  DNA cloning technique 14
Plasmodium spp. 76–8
  life cycle 77–8
  prophylaxis/treatment 78
Platelet activating factor 298
Platelet count 300
Pleiotropy 4
Pleura, surface marking 169
Pleural reaction, drug-induced 402
Pneumocystis carinii 76, 78, 116
Point prevalence 319
Point (single base) mutation 10
Poisson distribution 310
Polycystin 27
Polycythaemia 209
Polycythaemia rubra vera 20
Polyene macrolides 74
Polymerase chain reaction (PCR) 16–17
  applications 17
Polymorphic genetic markers 13
Polymorphisms 4
Polypeptide hormones 224

Polyploidy 5
Pompe's disease 253
Pons 146, 147
Population attributable fraction 327
Population attributable risk 327
Population genetics 31
Porphyria
  acute attack precipitants 273
  acute intermittent 344
  cutanea tarda 274
  erythropoietic 274
  hepatic 274
Porphyrins
  excessive excretion 273
  synthesis 271
Post-translational processing 9
  defects 10
Posterior cerebral artery 148
Posture, circulatory adaptations 218
Potassium 284
  renal secretion 198–9
Potency, drug 341, 342
Power, statistical test 315
Poxviruses 69
Prader–Willi syndrome 20, 22
Praziquantel 78
Prazosin 349
Predictive value of test 331, 332–333
Pregnancy 301
  adverse drug effects 396–7
  maternal screening tests 29
  pharmacokinetics 397
  physiological response 238
Preload 215
Premature ovarian failure 120
Prenatal diagnosis 16, 28–9
Prevalence rate 319
Primary biliary cirrhosis 120, 121
Primer DNA 5
Prion diseases (transmissible spongiform
    encephalopathies) 70
Probability distributions 309
Proband 5
Probe, genetic hybridization 5, 12
  preparation technique 12
Probenecid 381
Probucol 361
Procainamide 353
Progesterone 232
Progestogen-only pill 378
Prolactin 229
Prolactin-inhibiting factor 225
Prolactin-releasing hormone 225
Promoter 32
Pro-opiocortin 228
Proportionate mortality rate 319–20
Propositus 5
Prostacyclin 261, 262
Prostaglandins 193, 261
Prostanoid (eicosanoid) metabolism 261–2
Prostate specific antigen 298
Protease inhibitors 391–2
  cytochrome P450-metabolized drug
      interactions 393
Protein metabolism 240, 269

Protein synthesis 8–9
  defects 10
  inhibitors 11
  regulation 10
Proteins 266–267
  biological value 267
  dietary requirements 291
  digestion 267
Proteinuria 303
Proteoglycans 248
Proteus spp. 51
Prothrombin time 300
Prothrombin-gene mutation G20210A 299
Proton pump inhibitors 363
Protooncogenes 33
Providencia spp. 51
Proximal tubule function 192
Pseudocholinesterase 295, 345
Pseudomonas aeruginosa 52
Psychosis, drug-induced 409
Pulmonary arterial pressure 207
Pulmonary circulation 207
Pulmonary dynamics 204–6
Pulmonary fibrosis, drug-induced 402
Pulmonary hypertension 105, 209
Pulmonary oedema, drug-induced 402
Pulmonary plexus 162
Pulmonary surfactant 205
Pulmonary valve 173
Pulse pressure 216
Pupillary reflexes 152, 155
Purine analogues 11
Purines 6, 276
  metabolic disorders 278
  metabolism 276–7
Pyloric stenosis 30
Pyrazinamide 385
Pyridoxine (vitamin B_6) 279
Pyrimethamine 78
Pyrimidine analogues 11
Pyrimidines 6, 276
  metabolic disorders 278
  metabolism 276–7
Pyruvate 249
Pyruvate kinase 248, 249
  deficiency 249

QT interval, drug effects 402
Qualitative variables 306
Quantitative variables 306
Quartiles 307
Quaternary ammonium compounds 85
Quinghaosu 387
Quinidine 353
Quinolones 59, 383, 385

Radial nerve 138–9
Radioimmunoassay 131
Raloxifene 395
Random error 311
Randomization 324
Randomized clinical trial 324–6
  measures of effect 326–8
Rapamycin 395
ras 33, 243
Raynaud's syndrome, drug-induced 413

Reactive oxygen/nitrogen intermediates 91
Receiver operator curve (ROC) 333
Recombinant DNA technology 11
  applications 16
Recurrent laryngeal nerve 168
Regression 318
Relative risk 326, 329
  reduction 328
Renal blood flow 191–2
Renal clearance 190–1
Renal disease 399
Renal hypertension 105
Renal plasma flow 192
Renal plexus 162
Renal transport maximum 192
Renal tubular acidosis, drug-induced 403
Renin 193, 194, 195
Renin–angiotensin system 194
Reoviruses 62
Reperfusion injury 104
Reporter gene 5
Repression, protein synthesis 10
Reproducibility of test 334
Residual volume 203
Resistance (R) factors 61
Respiratory acidosis 187–8
Respiratory alkalosis 187, 188
Respiratory centres 208
Respiratory cycle 206
  see also Breathing
Respiratory gases
  blood–gas barrier 206
  diffusing capacity/transfer factor 206–207
  partial pressures 206
Respiratory physiology 201–9
  drug-induced disorders 402
  response to pregnancy 238
Resting energy expenditure 291
Resting potential, cardiac cells 209
Restriction enzymes 5, 12
Restriction fragment length polymorphisms
  (RFLPs) 13
Retinitis pigmentosa 22
Retinoblastoma 22, 34
Retinopathy, drug-induced 411
Retroviruses 63
Reverse transcriptase 9, 71
Reverse transcriptase polymerase chain reaction
  (RT-PCR) 17
Reverse transcription 5
Rhabdomyolysis, drug-induced 410
Rhabdoviruses 63
Rhesus blood group 124
Rheumatoid arthritis 30, 120, 121, 122
Rheumatoid factor 122
Rhinoviruses 62
Rhizopus spp. 74
Ribavarin 73, 388
Riboflavin (vitamin B_2) 279
Ribonuclear proteins 9
Ribosomal RNA 8
Ribosomes 9
Rickettsia spp. 55
Rickettsiae 40, 55–6
  zoonoses 79
Rifampicin 11, 60, 385

Rimantadine 73, 388
Ritonavir 392
RNA 6, 7
  synthesis (transcription) 8–9
RNA polymerase 9
RNA viruses 62–9
Rose–Waaler test 121
Roundworms 75, 78

Salmonella spp. 51
Sample range 307
Sample size 312, 315
Sampling 311–13
Sampling error 311
Saquinavir 391
Satellite DNA 7
Saturated fatty acids 256
Saturation kinetics 340
Scattergrams 318
Schilling test 284
Schistosoma spp. 76
Schizophrenia 30
Sciatic nerve 140–1
Scleroderma (CREST variant) 120, 122
Screening tests 331, 332
  criteria 334
  evaluation biases 334
Scurvy 276
Second messengers 224, 244, 246–7
Secretin 219, 220, 221, 222
Selectins 91, 103, 244
Selection bias 311, 323
Selective serotonin reuptake inhibitors (SSRIs)
    365, 366
Selegiline 373
Seminiferous tubule dysgenesis (Kleinfelter's
    syndrome) 21
Sensitivity 332, 333, 334
Septic shock 103, 105
Sequence-tagged sites (STSs) 14
Serological tests 71–2
Serotonin-noradrenaline reuptake inhibitors
    (SNRIs) 365
Serratia marcescens 51
Serum amylase 295
Serum sickness, drug-induced 411
Severe combined immunodeficiency (SCID) 25,
    116
Sex-linked disorders
  carrier detection 26
  dominant 25
  recessive 25–6, 28
Sexual dysfunction, drug-induced 410–11
Sheep red cell agglutination test 121
Shigella spp. 52
Short bowel syndrome 222
Sickle cell disease 16, 18, 23, 32, 275
Sideroblastic anaemia 273
Signal transduction 244
Significance
  clinical 314
  statistical 313–14
  tests 315–18
Significance level (α) 313, 315
Sildenafil 374
Single base (point) mutation 10

Single nucleotide polymorphism 13
Single-gene abnormalities 22–8
  autosomal dominant 22–3, 27
  autosomal recessive 23–4, 28
  mitochondrial genome 26
  molecular basis 27–8
  sex-linked dominant 25
  sex-linked recessive 25–6, 28
  triplet/trinucleotide repeat diseases 27
Sinoatrial node 173, 210
Sjögren's syndrome 122
Skewed distribution 310
Skin disease
  drug reactions 411–13
  hypersensitivity reactions 114
Skin prick test 113, 114
Skull
  foramina 152
  fossae 152
Small intestine 222–3
  digestion/absorption 223
  digestive enzymes 222
  intestinal juice 222–3
  motility 223
Small round viruses (SRVs) 63
Sodium 284
  balance abnormalities 197–8
  balance regulation 193–6
  depletion 196, 198
  excess 197
  renal transport 193–8
Sodium stibogluconate 78
Sodium valproate 372
Somatomedins 228
Somatostatin 225, 238
Somatostatinoma 223
Somatotropin (growth hormone) 228–9
Southern blot technique 13
Spearman's correlation coefficient 318
Specificity 332, 333, 334
Sphingolipidoses 265
Sphingolipids 256–7
Spina bifida 30
Spinal cord 148
Spinal nerves 138–41
Spinocerebellar ataxia 27
Spirochaetes 54
Spirometric measures 202–3
Spleen, surface markings 175
Splicesome 9
Splicing
  genes 9
  messenger RNA 5
Sporothrix schenckii 74
Standard deviation 308, 312
Standard error of the mean 312
Standardized mortality ratio 320
Staphylococcus aureus 45
  toxins 45
Staphylococcus spp. 45
Starling equation 181
Starvation 250, 252
Statins 361, 362
Statistical inference 311
Statistical significance 313–14
Statistics 305–18

Stavudine 390
Steady state concentration 338
Stem cell transplantation 126
Stenotrophomonas maltophilia 52
Stercobilinogen 222
Sterilization 84, 85
Sternal angle 169
Steroid hormones 224, 230
    structure 230
Stevens-Johnson syndrome, drug-induced
        412
Still birth rate 320
Stomach 219–20
    blood supply 176
    innervation 176
Streptobacillus moniliformis 48
Streptococcal haemolysis 44
Streptococcus spp. 44
Streptogramins 60
Streptokinase 357
Streptomycin 11
Stroke 105
Stroke volume 214
Student's *t*-test 315
Study design 321–6
Subclavian artery 164
Subclavian steal syndrome 164
Subclavian vein 166
Sugars, renal reabsorption 199
Sulfasalazine 360
Sulphadiazine 78
Sulphamethoxazole 78
Sulphonamides 384
Sulphonylureas 379
Superantigens 91
Superior laryngeal nerve 168
Superior vena cava 165
Suppressor (TS) cell 91
Suramin 78, 388
Survival curve 329–330
Survival (life-table) analysis 329
Suxamethonium sensitivity 345
Sympathectomy 144
Sympathetic nervous system 142–144
    effects 143
    outflow 142
    trunk anatomy 144
Syndrome of inappropriate anti-diuretic hormone
        secretion 200–201
Syngenic individuals 91
Synovial fluid 304
Syphilis, serology 72
Systematic error (bias) 311
Systemic lupus erythematosus 120, 122
drug-induced 120, 122, 345, 412

T cytotoxic (T$_C$) cells 95
T delayed hypersensitivity (T$_{DH}$) cells 95
T helper (T$_H$) cells 90, 95
    B cell interactions 109
    T$_H$1 subset 94, 95, 96
    T$_H$2 subset 94, 95, 96
T lymphocyte disorders, primary
        immunodeficiency 116
    combined B-cell disorders 116–17

T lymphocytes 93–4
    adhesion molecules 103
    antigen recognition 97
    coreceptor activating molecules 103
    deficiency 118–19
    $\gamma\delta$ subset 97–98
    regulatory/effector populations 95
    subsets 94, 95
    surface antigens/CD markers 94, 95
    tumour immunology 128
T supressor (T$_S$) cells 95
T-cell receptor (TCR) 92, 95, 96, 97
T-dependent antigens 92
T-independent antigens 92
Tacrolimus (FK506) 395
Taenia spp. 75, 76
Tamoxifen 395
Tandem repeat sequences 5
Tangier disease (α-lipoprotein deficiency) 264
TAP transporters 92
Tapeworms 75, 76, 78
Taste alteration, drug-induced 413
Taxol (paclitaxel) 394
Tay–Sachs disease 265
Telomerase 36
Telomeres 36
Tendon jerks 137
Tenofovir 390
Teratogenic drugs 396
Terbinafine 75
Termination signals 9
Testicular feminization syndrome (androgen
        insensitivity) 21, 25
Tetracyclines 11, 59, 382
Tetraploid *see* Polyploidy
Thalassaemia 16, 18, 23, 32, 275
Therapeutic index 340
Therapeutic monitoring 340
Thermic effect of muscle/food 291
Thermodilution principle 215
Thiabendazole 78
Thiamine (vitamin B$_1$) 279
Thioguanine 6
Thiouracils 381
Thoracic cage compliance 205
Thoracic duct 176
Thorax 169–175
    dermatomes 135
Threadworms 75
Thrombin time 300
Thrombocytopenia, drug-induced 407
Thrombolytic agents 357
Thromboxanes 261, 262
Thymidine 7
Thyroglobulin 233
Thyroid autoantibodies 122
Thyroid function tests 301
    postnatal screening 29
Thyroid gland 167, 233
    hormones 234
Thyroid-stimulating hormone 226–7
Thyrotrophin-releasing hormone 225
Thyroxine (T$_4$) 234
Thyroxine-binding globulin 234, 235
Tibial (medial popliteal) nerve 140–1

Tidal volume 202
Tinidazole 78
Tinnitus, drug-induced 411
Tissue typing 125
Tissue-type plasminogen activators (t-PAs) 357
Titre 92
Togaviruses 63
Toll receptors 92
Tongue, sensory innervation 161
TORCH screen 28
Torulopsis spp. 74
Total body water 180
Total lung capacity 202, 203
Toxic epidermal necrolysis 412
Toxic shock syndrome 103
Toxins
  endo/exotoxins 58
  Staphylococcus aureus 45
Toxocara canis 75
Toxoplasma gondii 76, 78
Trace elements 289, 290
Trachea, surface markings 169
Tranexamic acid 358
Transactivating factors 9
Transcortical dysphasias 151
Transcription 8–9
  defects 10
Transcription factors 9, 32, 246
Transduction 61
Transfection 5, 61
Transfer factor 206–207
Transfer RNA 7, 9
Transferrin 285, 286
Transformation
  bacterial 61
  of data 310
Transforming growth factor-beta (TGF-β) 102
Transforming growth factors 92
Transgenic analysis 15
Transient hypogammaglobulinaemia of infancy
    115
Translation 9
  defects 10
Translocation 5
Transmissible spongiform encephalopathies
    (prion diseases) 70
Transplantation 9, 124–7
  graft rejection 125
  graft survival 125–6
  stem cells 126
  terminology 124
  tissue typing 125
Transposition 5
Transposon 5
Travel vaccines 84
Trematodes 78
Treponema spp. 54
Triazoles 75
Tricarboxylic acid–citric acid cycle 240–2
Trichinella spiralis 76
Trichomonas vaginalis 76, 78
Trichophyton spp. 74
Tricuspid valve 173
Tricyclic antidepressants 364
Trigeminal (V) nerve 153, 159

Triglycerides 256
  digestion 258
  synthesis 260
Tri-iodothyronine (T_3) 234
Trimethoprim 78
Triple X syndrome 22
Triplet/trinucleotide repeat diseases 16, 27
Triploid *see* Polyploidy
Trisomies 5, 19–20
Trisomy 13 (Patau's syndrome) 20
Trisomy 18 (Edward's syndrome) 20
Trisomy 21 (Down's syndrome) 19–20, 29
Trochlear (IV) nerve 153, 158–9
Trypanosoma spp. 76, 78, 103
  drug treatment 388
Tuberculosis 385
Tuberous sclerosis 22
Tumour immunology 127–8
Tumour products 297–8
Tumour suppressor genes 34, 243
Tumour-associated antigens 127–8
Tunour necrosis factor (TNF) 92, 101, 102
Turner's syndrome (ovarian dysgenesis) 20–1
Twins 2, 4
Two-tailed tests 314
Tyrosine kinase receptors 245

Ulnar nerve 139–40
Unsaturated fatty acids 256
Upper limb dermatomes 135
Urea:creatinine ratio 199
Urea
  cycle 268
  renal excretion 199
Ureaplasma urealyticum 56
Uric acid metabolism 277
Uridine triphosphate (UTP) 242
Urinary retention, drug-induced 404
Urine
  antimicrobial drug levels 401
  bile pigments 222
  biochemistry 302–3
  casts 302
Urobilinogen 222
Urticaria 114

Vaccines 81
  travel 84
Vaginal carcinoma 405
Vagus (X) nerve 154, 162
Valaciclovir 73, 388
Validity of test 332
Valsalva manoevre 218
Vanillyl mandelic acid 297
Variable number tandem repeats (VNTRs) 13
Variables 306
Variance 308
Varicella zoster virus 73
Vascular tone 216, 217
Vasculitis 114, 120
Vasoactive intestinal peptide 219
  increased levels 223
Vasoconstriction 217
Vasodilatation 217
Vasodilators 348–9

Vasopressin (antidiuretic hormone) 192, 193, 199–201, 229
Vectors 6
  gene therapy 18
Veins 165–6
Ventilation/perfusion ratio (V/Q) 208
Ventricles of brain 151
Ventricular end-diastolic volume 213
Ventricular end-systolic volume 213
Verapamil 353
Vertebrobasilar circulation 149
Vertigo, drug-induced 411
Very low density lipoproteins (VLDL) 258, 259
Vestibulocochlear (VIII) nerve 154, 161
Vibrio spp. 49
Vibrios 49
Vigabatrin 372
Vinca alkaloids 394
Vincristine 11
VIPoma 223
Viral haemorrhagic fever 64
Viruses 40, 62–73
  ALERT organisms 79
  DNA-containing 69
  oncogenic 71
  opportunistic pathogens 79
  RNA-containing 62–9
  structure 62
  zoonoses 79
Vital capacity 202
Vitamin A 257, 282
Vitamin B_1 (thiamine) 279
Vitamin B_2 (riboflavin) 279
Vitamin B_3 (niacin/nicotinamide) 279
Vitamin B_6 (pyridoxine) 279
Vitamin B_{12} (cyanocobalamin) 280
  drug-induced deficiency 408
  Schilling test 284
Vitamin C (ascorbic acid) 281
Vitamin D 193, 257, 282, 287
Vitamin D-resistant rickets 24
Vitamin E 257, 283
Vitamin K 257, 283, 299
Vitamins 278–84
  fat-soluble 282–3
  mode of action 278
  water-soluble 279–81
Voltage-gated ion channels 245
Volume of distribution 339

Vomiting
  drug-induced 404
  prolonged 189
von Gierke's disease 253
Von Hipple–Lindau disease 22
Von Willebrand's disease 22
Voriconazole 75, 386

Waldenström's macroglobulinaemia 110, 120, 128
Warfarin 299, 355
  overdose 400
Water
  depletion (hyperosmotic dehydration) 197
  excess 197
  excretion regulation 199
  renal transport 199–201
WDHA syndrome 223
Weber's syndrome 158
Werdnig–Hoffman disease 23
Werner–Morrison syndrome 223
Wernicke's dysphasia 151
Wilcoxon rank sum test 317
Wilcoxon signed rank test 317
Wilson's disease 23, 28
Wiscott–Aldrich syndrome 25, 117
Work of breathing 204
Wuchereria bancrofti 76, 78

X-linked spinobulbal muscular atrophy (SMBA) 27
Xanthine oxidase 277
Xenotransplantation 127
Xeroderma pigmentosa 23
47 XYY 21

Yates' correction factor 317
Yeast infections 74
Yersinia spp. 53

Z score 313
Zanamivir 73, 388
Zero-order elimination 340
Zidovudine (AZT) 389
Zinc 290
Zollinger–Ellison syndrome 222
Zoonoses 79
Zopliclone 367
Zygotes 6